THE
ULTIMATE
COLLECTION
OF
BARBARA
O'NEILL

7 BOOKS IN 1

550+ Revolutionary Herbal and Natural
Remedies for Everyday Ailments, Life-
Changing Holistic Health and Wellness

By
Serena Moss

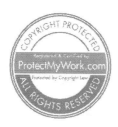

TABLE OF CONTENT

A Transformation Anecdote

Dear reader,

Welcome to *"The Ultimate Collection of Barbara O'Neill: 550+ Revolutionary Herbal and Natural Remedies for Everyday Ailments, Life-Changing Holistic Health and Wellness"*.

Before you dive in, I want to share a little anecdote.

One day, while Barbara was conducting a workshop, a participant shared how a simple change in her diet, suggested by Barbara, had drastically improved her health. This story inspired many others present to try Barbara's advice.

If you also find something surprising in these pages, I invite you to share it with a review on Amazon. Your experiences can inspire other readers to take charge of their health.

Leaving feedback is simple, and I treasure each piece of insight. Just go to the ORDERS section of your Amazon account and click on the "Write a product review" button, or SCAN THIS QR CODE to go directly to the review section.

Remember, every review counts and plays a crucial role in guiding and inspiring fellow readers.

Should you feel any aspect of the book might be enhanced, your constructive feedback is warmly welcomed at **info [at] herbulharmony [dot] com.**

For ongoing updates, additional resources, and to join a community of like-minded individuals, please visit ***www.herbfulharmony.com***.

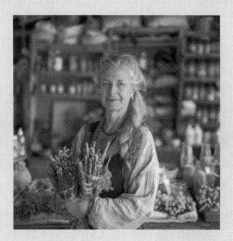

Happy reading and thank you for your contribution!

Serena Moss

BOOK 1: THE COMPLETE HERBAL ENCYCLOPEDIA

Chapter 1: Introduction to Herbal Remedies

1.1 Who is Barbara O'Neill?

Barbara O'Neill's journey as a prominent naturopath and health educator began in her early years. Growing up in a family that valued natural living, she developed a keen interest in wellness and herbal remedies. This early exposure laid the foundation for her lifelong passion for natural health.

Barbara pursued formal education in naturopathy, earning her qualifications from esteemed institutions. Her academic journey was marked by a deep commitment to understanding the intricate connections between the human body and natural therapies. This dedication was further fueled by pivotal moments in her life, where she witnessed the transformative power of natural remedies in addressing health challenges.

Over the years, Barbara has made significant contributions to the field of naturopathy. She has authored numerous books and articles, sharing her extensive knowledge and practical insights with a global audience. Her seminars and workshops have empowered countless individuals to take charge of their health through natural means.

Barbara's achievements have not gone unnoticed. She has received various recognitions for her work, including awards from prestigious naturopathic associations. Her commitment to promoting natural wellness has also led her to collaborate with other experts in the field, further advancing the understanding and application of herbal remedies.

Through her dedication and expertise, Barbara O'Neill has become a respected figure in the world of naturopathy, inspiring many to explore the benefits of natural health practices.

1.2 Barbara O'Neill's Health Philosophy

Natural Wellness Principles

Barbara O'Neill's health philosophy is deeply rooted in the principles of natural wellness. She advocates for a holistic approach to health that encompasses a clean diet, adequate rest, and regular exercise. According to Barbara, these elements are crucial for achieving and maintaining optimal health.

Barbara emphasizes the importance of a clean diet, rich in whole foods and devoid of processed ingredients. She believes that the food we consume directly impacts our physical and mental well-being. Her teachings often include practical advice on how to incorporate more fruits, vegetables, and natural herbs into daily meals, promoting a balanced and nutritious diet.

Rest and relaxation are also fundamental aspects of Barbara's wellness philosophy. She stresses the need for sufficient sleep and downtime to allow the body to repair and rejuvenate. In her view, rest is not merely the absence of activity but an essential component of a healthy lifestyle that supports both mental clarity and physical vitality.

Exercise is another pillar of Barbara's approach to natural health. She advocates for regular physical activity as a means to strengthen the body, improve cardiovascular health, and enhance overall well-being. Whether through walking, yoga, or more vigorous forms of exercise, Barbara encourages incorporating movement into daily routines.

Barbara O'Neill integrates these principles into her own life and teachings, serving as a living example of the benefits of natural wellness. Her holistic approach not only addresses the symptoms of illness but also aims to prevent health issues by fostering a balanced and healthy lifestyle.

Clean Diet

Barbara O'Neill advocates for a clean diet as a cornerstone of natural wellness. According to Barbara, a clean diet primarily consists of whole, organic, and minimally processed foods. This approach emphasizes the consumption of fresh fruits and vegetables, whole grains, nuts, seeds, and lean proteins. Barbara believes that these food choices not only give essential nutrients but also aid the body's natural detoxification processes.

Barbara advises avoiding foods that are heavily processed, laden with artificial additives, or high in refined sugars and unhealthy fats. She is particularly critical of fast food, sugary snacks, and beverages, as well as foods containing preservatives and artificial colors. In her view, these substances can provide to a variety of health issues, from digestive issue to chronic diseases.

The benefits of consuming organic and minimally processed foods are numerous. Barbara highlights that organic foods are matured without the use of synthetic pesticides and fertilizers, which can have harmful effects on health. Moreover, minimally processed foods retain more of their natural nutrients which are essential for an optimal health.

In her teachings, Barbara integrates these principles by encouraging her followers to make gradual, sustainable changes to their diets. She often shares practical tips on meal planning, shopping for organic produce, and preparing nutritious meals at home. By adopting a clean diet, Barbara believes individuals can achieve better mental clarity, augmented energy levels, and increased overall well-being.

Rest and Exercise

In Barbara O'Neill's health philosophy, rest and exercise are pivotal components for achieving optimal well-being. She emphasizes that a balanced approach to physical activity and adequate sleep are essential for maintaining mental and physical health.

Barbara advocates for a variety of exercises that cater to different fitness levels and preferences. She recommends incorporating activities such as:

- Walking and hiking for cardiovascular health
- Yoga and stretching for flexibility and stress relief
- Strength training to build muscle and support bone health
- Swimming for a full-body workout with low impact on joints

Barbara believes that regular exercise not only enhances physical fitness but also plays a crucial role in mental wellness. Physical activity aids to diminish stress, augment mood, and increase energy levels.

Equally important in her philosophy is the need for adequate rest. Barbara stresses that sleep is a fundamental aspect of health, as it allows the body to repair and rejuvenate. She encourages practices that promote good sleep hygiene.

By integrating rest and exercise into daily routines, Barbara O'Neill teaches that individuals can achieve a harmonious balance that supports overall well-being. Her holistic approach underscores the interconnectedness of physical activity, rest, and mental health, advocating for lifestyle changes that foster long-term health and vitality.

1.3 Barbara's Detox Principles

Barbara O'Neill emphasizes the importance of natural detoxification as a cornerstone of her health philosophy. She advocates for methods that cleanse the body gently and effectively, promoting long-term health and well-being. One of her primary recommendations is the use of herbal teas. These teas, often made from dandelion, milk thistle, and burdock root, are known for their detoxifying properties and can help to cleanse the liver and kidneys.

Fasting is another method Barbara champions for detoxification. She suggests periodic fasting, which can range from intermittent fasting to longer, more structured fasts. This practice allows the body to rest and repair, reducing the burden on the digestive system and promoting cellular regeneration. Barbara believes that fasting, when done correctly, can lead to increased energy levels and improved mental clarity.

In addition to herbal teas and fasting, Barbara also recommends other natural remedies such as dry brushing and Epsom salt baths. Dry brushing helps to stimulate the lymphatic system, aiding in the removal of toxins through the skin. Epsom salt baths, rich in magnesium, can aid to relax the muscles and draw out impurities from the body.

Integrating these detoxification methods into a daily routine can be simple and highly beneficial. Barbara encourages individuals to start with small, manageable changes, such as incorporating a daily herbal tea or practicing intermittent fasting a few times a week. Over time, these practices can become a natural part of one's lifestyle, contributing to a healthier, more vibrant life.

1.4 Holistic Approach to Health

Barbara O'Neill's holistic approach to health emphasizes the integration of mental, physical, and spiritual wellness. Her philosophy diverges from conventional medicine by focusing on the interconnectedness of these aspects to achieve overall well-being. Barbara believes that true health cannot be achieved by addressing only one part of the body; instead, it requires a balanced approach that nurtures the mind, body, and spirit.

Mental Wellness

Barbara advocates for practices such as mindfulness, meditation, and stress management techniques to maintain mental clarity and emotional stability. She emphasizes the importance of mental health in preventing and managing stress, which can have detrimental effects on physical health.

Physical Wellness

Physical wellness, according to Barbara, involves regular exercise, a clean diet, and adequate rest. She recommends a variety of exercises, including yoga, walking, and strength training, to keep the body fit and functioning optimally. Additionally, she underscores the importance of consuming organic and minimally processed foods to fuel the body with the necessary nutrients.

Spiritual Wellness

Spiritual wellness is another cornerstone of Barbara's approach. She encourages practices such as prayer, meditation, and spending time in nature to foster a deeper connection with oneself and the universe. This spiritual grounding helps individuals find purpose and meaning in their lives, contributing to overall happiness and contentment.

By advocating for a holistic approach, Barbara O'Neill provides a comprehensive framework for achieving balance and harmony in all areas of life, promoting long-term health and well-being.

Chapter 2: Introduction to Herbal Remedies

2.1 Importance of Nutrition

Barbara O'Neill places a significant emphasis on the role of nutrition in both preventing and treating illnesses. She believes that a diet rich in whole foods is fundamental to maintaining good health and warding off disease. According to Barbara, the body thrives on natural, unprocessed foods that give essential nutrients and aid the body's natural healing processes.

Her philosophy underscores the importance of consuming a variety of vegetables, fruits, nuts, whole grains, and seeds. These foods are dense in vitamins, minerals, and antioxidants, which are crucial for bolstering the immune system and reducing inflammation. Barbara advocates for the elimination of processed foods, refined sugars, and artificial additives, which she believes contribute to the development of chronic diseases and overall poor health.

In her teachings, Barbara often highlights the benefits of organic produce, which is free from harmful pesticides and chemicals. She argues that organic foods are not only better for individual health but also for the environment. By choosing organic, individuals can reduce their exposure to toxins and support sustainable farming practices.

Barbara's approach to nutrition is holistic, viewing food as medicine. She encourages her followers to be mindful of their dietary choices and to prioritize nutrient-dense foods that nourish the body. By doing so, she believes that individuals can achieve optimal health, prevent illness, and enhance their overall well-being.

2.2 Whole Foods and Preparation

Barbara O'Neill emphasizes the importance of whole foods in her nutritional philosophy. Whole foods are those that are unprocessed or minimally processed, retaining their natural nutrients and fiber. Barbara advocates for a diet rich in vegetables, fruits, whole grains, nuts, and seeds. These foods provide essential vitamins, minerals, and antioxidants that support overall health and prevent chronic diseases.

One of the key principles in Barbara's approach is the preparation of these foods to preserve their nutritional value. She recommends consuming raw foods whenever possible, as cooking can sometimes degrade certain nutrients. For instance, raw vegetables and fruits are excellent sources of enzymes and vitamins that can be lost during cooking. However, when cooking is necessary, methods such as steaming or blanching are preferred because they minimize nutrient loss compared to boiling or frying.

Fermentation is another technique Barbara encourages. Fermented foods which are beneficial for gut health. These foods not only enhance digestion but also boost the immune system and improve mental health by promoting a healthy gut microbiome.

By integrating these whole foods and preparation methods into daily routines, individuals can maximize their nutritional intake and support long-term health and well-being. Barbara's approach underscores the belief that proper nutrition is a cornerstone of preventive healthcare, offering a natural and effective way to maintain balance and vitality.

2.3 Barbara's Detox Principles

Barbara O'Neill emphasizes the importance of natural detoxification as a cornerstone of her health philosophy. She advocates for methods that cleanse the body gently and effectively, promoting long-term health and well-being. One of her primary recommendations is the use of herbal teas. These teas, often made from dandelion, milk thistle, and burdock root, are known for their detoxifying properties and can help to cleanse the liver and kidneys.

Fasting is another method Barbara champions for detoxification. She suggests periodic fasting, which can range from intermittent fasting to longer, more structured fasts. This practice allows the body to rest and repair, reducing the burden on the digestive system and promoting cellular regeneration. Barbara believes that fasting, when done correctly, can lead to increased energy levels and improved mental clarity.

In addition to herbal teas and fasting, Barbara also recommends other natural remedies such as dry brushing and Epsom salt baths. Dry brushing helps to stimulate the lymphatic system, aiding in the removal of toxins through the skin. Epsom salt baths, rich in magnesium, can aid to relax the muscles and draw out impurities from the body.

Integrating these detoxification methods into a daily routine can be simple and highly beneficial. Barbara encourages individuals to start with small, manageable changes, such as incorporating a daily herbal tea or practicing intermittent fasting a few times a week. Over time, these practices can become a natural part of one's lifestyle, contributing to a healthier, more vibrant life.

Chapter 3: Herbal Highlights - Key Plants

3.1 Introduction to Key Plants

Herbs have been used for centuries across cultures for their healing and therapeutic properties. Understanding these diverse plants, their origins, and uses is crucial for anyone interested in herbal medicine.

In this chapter, we explore the rich profiles of various herbs, categorized by their therapeutic properties and traditional uses. We delve into the calming effects of herbs like lavender and chamomile, and the skin benefits of aloe vera and calendula.

From promoting relaxation to enhancing skin health, these herb profiles provide essential knowledge. This foundation allows for the integration of ancient wisdom into modern wellness practices, enriching our daily lives.

Categories of Herbs and Their Uses

Herbs can be thoughtfully organized based on their therapeutic properties, which allows for a more targeted approach to herbal remedies. Among these classifications are:

- **Anti-inflammatory herbs**, such as turmeric and ginger, are celebrated for their ability to reduce inflammation within the body, offering relief from various ailments, including joint pain and digestive issues.
- **Antioxidant-rich herbs** like green tea and milk thistle play a crucial role in combating oxidative stress and supporting the body's natural detoxification processes, contributing to overall health and wellness.
- **Calming herbs**, including lavender and chamomile, are prized for their soothing effects on the mind and body, assisting in stress relief and promoting relaxation and better sleep.

Understanding these categories and their corresponding herbs facilitates a comprehensive approach to selecting herbal remedies, tailored to the specific health needs and wellness goals of individuals.

Regions of Origin and Traditional Uses

The geographical origins of herbs are as diverse as their uses, spanning continents and cultures. For instance, Lavender, known for its soothing aroma, hails from the Mediterranean region but has been enthusiastically adopted worldwide for its calming effects. Similarly, Chamomile, with its gentle stress-relieving properties, has European origins, while Holy Basil, revered in Ayurvedic medicine for its balancing effects, originates from India. The traditional uses of these herbs in their native cultures have laid the groundwork for modern applications in wellness and medicine. For example, the use of Neem from India in promoting skin health mirrors its long-standing Ayurvedic applications for cleansing and detoxification. The cross-cultural adoption and blending of herbal practices underscore the universal recognition of their significant health benefits, illustrating a rich tapestry of herbal wisdom that continues to evolve and influence contemporary herbalism.

Overview of Herbal Benefits

Herbal remedies offer a multitude of benefits, encompassing the support of physical, mental, and emotional health. By harnessing the therapeutic properties of herbs, individuals can adopt a more holistic approach to wellness, addressing ailments at their root and nurturing the body in a gentle, natural manner. The use of herbs encourages a balanced lifestyle, promoting relaxation, skin and hair health, and safe, gentle remedies for children. Embracing herbalism not only connects us to ancient traditions but also offers sustainable options for enhancing well-being in our modern world, encouraging a harmonious relationship between nature and ourselves.

3.2 Herbs for Relaxation and Meditation

Herbs for Relaxation and Meditation

In today's fast-paced world, the ancient wisdom of using herbs for relaxation and meditation is more relevant than ever. This section delves into the serene world of calming herbs, each with its unique history and properties. These botanicals offer a gentle, natural approach to alleviating stress, enhancing relaxation, and supporting meditation practices without the need for specific recipes, allowing for versatile application in daily life.

Calming Properties of Lavender

Lavender, with its soothing purple blooms, is renowned for its calming effects. Historically used in Roman baths to relax the body and spirit, it has traversed centuries to become a cornerstone in modern aromatherapy and herbal teas. Lavender's gentle sedative properties make it a popular choice for reducing stress, easing anxiety, and promoting a restful sleep. Its aromatic essence is believed to directly impact the limbic system, the part of the brain responsible for emotions, making it a valuable ally in creating a tranquil environment for relaxation and meditation.

Chamomile for Stress Relief

Chamomile, another gem in the herbal kingdom, is revered for its stress-relieving qualities. Widely used across various cultures, this daisy-like herb has been a go-to remedy for calming the mind and soothing the digestive system. Its popularity as a herbal tea spans globally, offering a gentle way to unwind after a stressful day. The active compound in chamomile, bisabolol, is thought to have anti-inflammatory and anti-anxiety effects, contributing to its effectiveness in promoting relaxation and peaceful sleep.

Holy Basil in Meditation Practices

Holy basil, or Tulsi, holds a sacred place in Ayurvedic medicine as an adaptogen, helping the body adapt to stress and fostering mental balance. Its use in meditation practices stems from its reputed ability to clear the mind, calm the nerves, and bring the body into a state of harmony and balance. By reducing stress-related hormones and promoting a sense of well-being, holy basil serves not only as a tool for deep meditation but also as a daily supplement for maintaining mental clarity and emotional stability.

Valerian Root for Sleep and Relaxation

Valerian root has a long history of use as a remedy for insomnia and nervous anxiety. Known for its potent sedative properties, it works by increasing levels of gamma-aminobutyric acid (GABA) in the brain, which helps regulate nerve impulses and calm anxiety. While its strong, earthy odor may be off-putting to some, its effectiveness in promoting deep, restorative sleep and relaxation is well-documented, making it a valuable herb for those seeking natural solutions to sleep disorders and stress management.

Lemon Balm for Reducing Anxiety

Lemon balm, with its delicate lemon-scented leaves, is considered a mood-lifting herb. Historically, it was used by the Greeks to dress wounds and by medieval Europeans to reduce stress and anxiety, improve sleep, and enhance digestion. Modern studies support its traditional use, highlighting its ability to ease symptoms of anxiety and promote a sense of calmness. Its mild sedative effect makes lemon balm an excellent herb for reducing agitation, elevating mood, and supporting cognitive function, thereby aiding in relaxation and contemplative practices.

These herbs embody the essence of nature's pharmacy, offering gentle, effective ways to enhance relaxation, support mental health, and deepen meditation practices. By tapping into the ancient wisdom of herbal remedies, we can find solace in nature's serenity, fostering a holistic well-being of body, mind, and spirit.

3.3 Herbs for Radiant Skin

Herbal remedies have been a cornerstone of natural beauty and skin health across various cultures for centuries. These natural treasures offer an array of benefits for the skin, thanks to their soothing, anti-inflammatory, and antioxidant properties. Understanding the specific attributes and applications of these herbs can empower individuals to address a wide range of skin concerns, from acne and inflammation to premature aging and skin regeneration.

Calendula, known for its vibrant orange blossoms, is celebrated for its exceptional soothing properties. It has been traditionally used to calm skin irritations and inflammations, making it a staple in natural skincare formulations. The herb's gentle nature makes it suitable for even the most sensitive skin, providing a comforting remedy for conditions such as eczema and diaper rash.

Aloe Vera is synonymous with skin healing. Its gel, extracted from the leaves of the plant, is renowned for its ability to soothe burns, cuts, and other skin abrasions. The healing properties of Aloe Vera stem from its rich composition of vitamins, amino acids, and minerals, which collectively promote skin regeneration and hydration. This herb's widespread use in topical applications underscores its significance in natural skincare.

Neem has long been revered in Ayurvedic medicine for its detoxifying effects. It plays a crucial role in promoting overall skin health by combatting bacterial infections that can lead to acne and other skin conditions. Neem's leaves and oil contain compounds that offer anti-inflammatory and antimicrobial benefits, making it an effective ingredient in cleansers and creams aimed at purifying the skin and maintaining its clarity.

Rosehip is highly acclaimed for its regenerative properties, particularly in diminishing scars and fine lines. Rich in vitamins A and C, along with essential fatty acids, rosehip oil is a powerful ally in enhancing skin's texture and elasticity. Its high antioxidant content aids in combating oxidative stress, making it an excellent choice for anti-aging remedies.

Green Tea is another potent antioxidant that has gained popularity for its anti-aging benefits. The catechins found in green tea are effective in neutralizing harmful free radicals and reducing inflammation, thereby slowing the aging process. Its inclusion in skincare products and oral consumption contributes to a radiant, youthful complexion.

These herbs highlight the holistic approach to skin health, emphasizing the use of natural ingredients to nurture and protect the skin. By incorporating these herbal remedies into skincare routines, individuals can leverage the healing power of nature to achieve a radiant, healthy complexion. It's a testament to the timeless wisdom of herbalism and its relevance in modern-day beauty practices.

Calendula for Soothing Skin

Calendula, known for its vibrant golden petals, holds a prestigious place in the realm of natural remedies due to its soothing properties. Historically, it has been a go-to herb for alleviating skin irritations and inflammations, thanks to its anti-inflammatory and healing compounds. Modern skincare products frequently harness calendula's gentle yet potent effectiveness in treating cuts, scrapes, and a variety of skin conditions, making it a cherished ingredient in the formulation of creams, oils, and balms designed for sensitive or damaged skin. Its application extends beyond mere topical use, embodying the holistic approach to skin health and wellness.

Aloe Vera's Healing Properties

Aloe vera, renowned for its remarkable healing properties, stands out as a cornerstone in the realm of natural remedies, especially for skin care. This succulent plant is highly valued for its ability to soothe burns, cuts, and other skin irritations, thanks to its cooling, moisturizing, and healing benefits. The clear gel found inside the fleshy leaves contains bioactive compounds, including vitamins, minerals, and amino acids, which contribute to its skin-regeneration qualities. Aloe vera's widespread use in topical applications spans from everyday skincare products to after-sun lotions, underscoring its indispensable role in promoting skin health and recovery.

Neem for Skin Health and Detoxification

Neem, known scientifically as Azadirachta indica, is celebrated for its potent detoxifying properties that contribute significantly to skin health. Rooted deeply in Ayurvedic medicine, neem has been used for centuries in India to clear up toxins from the body, support the immune system, and treat a wide array of skin issues like acne, psoriasis, and eczema. Its antibacterial, antifungal, and anti-inflammatory qualities make it an invaluable herbal ally in promoting clear, healthy skin. Neem oil and extracts are commonly found in skincare products, demonstrating its modern applications while honoring traditional uses.

Rosehip for Skin Regeneration

Rosehip is celebrated for its potent regenerative properties, offering a natural solution for diminishing scars and fine lines. This herb is rich in vitamins, especially Vitamin C, and antioxidants, which are crucial for skin repair and rejuvenation. Rosehip's oil, extracted from the seeds, is a valuable ingredient in many skincare products due to its ability to improve skin elasticity, promote collagen production, and enhance skin's overall radiance. Its use in traditional medicine spans centuries, with applications that leverage its healing benefits not just for the skin, but for overall health, underscoring its versatility and importance in herbal skincare regimens.

Green Tea for Anti-Aging

Green tea, revered for its high antioxidant content, particularly epigallocatechin gallate (EGCG), plays a crucial role in skin health and anti-aging. These antioxidants combat free radicals, reducing damage that can lead to wrinkles and fine lines, thus preserving the skin's youthful appearance. Beyond its topical applications in skincare products, green tea's benefits are maximized when incorporated into a daily diet, promoting overall health from the inside out. Its widespread use in both beauty products and health supplements underscores green tea's versatility and effectiveness in supporting skin vitality and combating the signs of aging.

3.4 Herbs for Hair Health

Herbs have been used for centuries to enhance hair health, with practices that extend far back into various traditional medicines around the world. Today, the wisdom gleaned from these ancient practices can still be applied, offering natural ways to nourish, strengthen, and protect our hair. This section delves into some of the most effective herbs known for their beneficial properties in hair care.

Rosemary is renowned for its role in promoting hair growth. This herb's ability to improve circulation to the scalp, coupled with its antioxidant properties, makes it a powerful tool in preventing hair loss. Historically utilized in Mediterranean cultures as a rinse to darken and strengthen hair, modern applications have seen rosemary oil used in shampoos and conditioners to stimulate hair follicles and encourage growth.

Hibiscus, often referred to as the "flower of hair care," serves multiple functions for hair health. Rich in vitamins and amino acids that nourish the hair, hibiscus flowers and leaves have been used in Ayurvedic remedies to create hair masks and oils. These treatments are believed to prevent premature graying, encourage hair growth, and even combat dandruff, making hibiscus a versatile choice for a variety of hair concerns.

Nettle is another herb with a long history of use, traditionally employed to stimulate the scalp and improve the strength of hair. Packed with minerals like iron and magnesium, nettle leaves can be brewed into a tea and used as a hair rinse, or extracted into oil for direct scalp application. Its natural properties are said to reduce scalp inflammation and block excess DHT, a hormone linked to hair loss.

Fenugreek, with its high content of proteins and nicotinic acid, is celebrated for its ability to combat hair fall and dandruff while promoting healthy hair growth. Fenugreek seeds, when ground into a paste and applied to the scalp, can condition the hair, leaving it smooth and shiny. Its use in traditional medicine spans across various cultures, from the Middle East to South Asia, underscoring its global appeal as a remedy for hair loss prevention.

Sage is praised for its ability to improve scalp circulation and treat fungal infections. Its antiseptic and anti-inflammatory qualities make it an excellent option for soothing itchy scalps and reducing dandruff. Sage tea has been used as a rinse to darken hair and prevent thinning, showcasing this herb's multifaceted benefits for hair care.

In incorporating these herbal remedies into our daily routines, it's important to acknowledge the holistic approach of herbalism in hair care. While these herbs offer specific benefits for hair health, their effectiveness can be enhanced by a balanced diet and healthy lifestyle. Moreover, as with any remedy, it's crucial to understand that results may vary based on individual factors such as genetics and underlying health conditions. By embracing the natural properties of these herbs, we can explore gentle, sustainable methods to maintain and improve the health of our hair.

Rosemary for Hair Growth

Rosemary is revered not only for its aromatic qualities but also for its robust ability to stimulate hair growth. Historically, it has been utilized in various cultures as a natural remedy to enhance blood circulation to the scalp, thus encouraging hair growth. Its application in modern hair care products continues to thrive, as rosemary oil is commonly found in shampoos and conditioners designed to strengthen hair, reduce hair loss, and improve scalp health. This versatile herb, backed by both traditional use and emerging scientific research, stands as a testament to nature's capacity to foster beauty and wellness.

Hibiscus for Hair Nourishment

Hibiscus, often celebrated for its vibrant blooms, extends its beauty beyond ornamental purposes to nurturing hair health. Historically, it has been a cornerstone in traditional hair care regimens, particularly in cultures where the importance of natural, botanical remedies prevails. The petals and leaves of hibiscus are rich in vitamins and amino acids that nourish the scalp and strands, combating dryness and promoting a lustrous sheen. Regular use of hibiscus can stimulate hair follicles, supporting growth and preventing premature graying. Its conditioning properties leave hair soft and manageable, making hibiscus a valued ingredient in natural hair care products today.

Nettle for Strengthening Hair

Nettle, scientifically known as Urtica dioica, has been a staple in traditional medicine for centuries, primarily for its ability to strengthen hair and stimulate growth. Its rich composition includes vitamins A, C, and K, along with minerals like iron and magnesium, which are vital for hair health. Nettle works by improving circulation and reducing inflammation in the scalp, thereby creating an ideal environment for hair growth. Modern hair care routines have embraced nettle, incorporating it into shampoos, conditioners, and scalp treatments, leveraging its natural potency to combat hair loss and thinning, proving itself as a valuable ally in the quest for healthy, strong hair.

Fenugreek for Preventing Hair Loss

Fenugreek, renowned for its multifaceted herbal benefits, plays a significant role in preventing hair loss, a concern for many across the globe. Its seeds are rich in hormones that promote hair growth and proteins that strengthen hair follicles, making it an invaluable ingredient in hair care treatments. Traditional applications have seen fenugreek used in various cultures as a paste applied directly to the scalp, encouraging healthy hair growth and combating root weakness. Scientific studies support its efficacy, attributing its benefits to the high concentration of folic acid, vitamins A, K, and C, as well as minerals such as potassium and calcium found within the seeds. This makes fenugreek not just a traditional remedy but a scientifically backed solution for maintaining lush, healthy hair.

Sage for Scalp Health

Sage, renowned for its potent herbal properties, is not only a culinary staple but also a valuable resource for scalp health. Its natural antiseptic and anti-inflammatory qualities make it an effective remedy for reducing dandruff and soothing scalp irritations. Traditionally used in herbal medicine to promote hair growth and prevent thinning, sage's benefits have been scientifically recognized in modern hair care formulations. Incorporating sage into shampoos, conditioners, or as a herbal rinse can invigorate the scalp, enhance hair vitality, and maintain a healthy, dandruff-free head of hair, proving its enduring value in natural hair care practices.

3.5 Safe Herbs for Children

In the realm of herbal remedies, special consideration must be given to the youngest members of our families. Children, with their developing bodies and immune systems, require gentle, safe herbal treatments for various ailments and wellness support. This segment of our herbal guide focuses on mild herbs that have been traditionally used to soothe, nourish, and protect children's health while emphasizing their safety and gentle effects.

Chamomile for Calming Children

Chamomile is renowned for its calming properties, making it an excellent choice for children. Its mild sedative effects can help soothe anxiety, induce sleep, and relieve irritability, thereby being a staple in bedtime teas. Historically, chamomile tea has been used to alleviate colic symptoms and soothe teething babies, attesting to its safety profile and effectiveness in promoting relaxation and comfort in young ones.

Fennel for Digestive Health

Fennel is another herb that is particularly beneficial for children, especially in aiding digestion. Its mild carminative properties help relieve gas, bloating, and stomach cramps, often seen in colicky infants. Fennel tea can also stimulate appetite in children who may be finicky eaters. The gentle nature of fennel, combined with its pleasant licorice-like taste, makes it highly acceptable to young palates.

Lemon Balm for Gentle Relaxation

Lemon balm, with its mild sedative properties, serves as a wonderful herb for children needing gentle relaxation support. It can help alleviate symptoms of stress and anxiety, promote restful sleep, and soothe hyperactivity. Its antiviral properties also make it beneficial for treating colds and flu in children, thereby supporting both mental and physical aspects of child health.

Elderflower for Boosting Immunity

Elderflower is a potent herb for boosting immunity in children. Its antiviral and antibacterial properties make it particularly effective in preventing and treating colds, flu, and other respiratory infections. Elderflower can be administered as a tea or syrup, offering a delightful flavor that appeals to children. Furthermore, its immune-boosting effects are complemented by its fever-reducing properties, making it a holistic remedy for common childhood ailments.

Marshmallow Root for Soothing Irritations

Marshmallow root is a soothing herb ideal for children experiencing digestive or respiratory irritations. Its mucilaginous properties provide a protective layer over irritated mucous membranes, offering relief from coughs, sore throats, and gastrointestinal upset. Marshmallow root can be prepared as a mild tea, making it a soothing remedy for children dealing with discomfort or inflammation in the digestive tract or respiratory system.

Incorporating these gentle herbs into a child's wellness routine offers a natural, safe, and effective way to support their health and well-being. However, it is always advisable to consult with a healthcare professional before introducing any new herb to ensure it is appropriate for the child's specific health situation. By choosing mild, safe herbs such as chamomile, fennel, lemon balm, elderflower, and marshmallow root, parents and caregivers can confidently provide their children with the healing benefits of nature's bounty, fostering a foundation for lifelong wellness.

Chapter 4: The Ultimate Guide to Over 150 Herbs

Acerola (Malpighia emarginata)

Botanical Description: Acerola is a small, bushy tree native to tropical regions of the Western Hemisphere. It has bright green leaves and small pink or white flowers, producing cherry-like fruits that are red or purple when ripe. The fruit is highly perishable and rich in vitamin C.

Health Benefits:

- **Rich in Vitamin C**: Boosts the immune system and helps skin health.
- **Antioxidant Properties**: Helps combat oxidative stress and inflammation.
- **Supports Digestive Health**: High in fiber, aiding digestion and preventing constipation.
- **Improves Metabolic Function**: May help regulate blood sugar levels and improve metabolic function.

Recommended Dosage: 1/8-1/4 tsp of acerola extract per day, divided into two doses. Fresh fruit can be consumed in moderation, typically 1-2 fruits per day.

Preparation Methods:

- **Juice**: Fresh acerola can be juiced and consumed directly.
- **Powder**: Dried acerola can be ground into a powder and added to smoothies or drinks.
- **Capsules**: Acerola extract is available in capsule form for convenient supplementation.
- **Infusions**: Acerola powder can be added to teas or other beverages for added vitamin C.

Agrimony (Agrimonia eupatoria)

Botanical Description: Agrimony is a perennial herb with slender stems and bright yellow flowers arranged in long spikes. It grows in temperate regions and prefers sunny, well-drained habitats. The entire plant, including leaves, stems, and flowers, is used for medicinal purposes.

Health Benefits:

- **Anti-inflammatory**: Helps reduce inflammation and soothe digestive issues.
- **Astringent**: Effective in treating skin conditions and minor wounds.
- **Diuretic**: Promotes urine production, helping to detoxify the body.
- **Digestive Aid**: Supports liver and gallbladder function, aiding in digestion.

Recommended Dosage: 1-2 tsp of dried agrimony per day, typically consumed as a tea. Tincture dosage is usually 1/2-1 tsp, three times daily.

Preparation Methods:

- **Tea**: Steep 1-2 tsp of dried agrimony in hot water for 12-14 min.
- **Tincture**: Agrimony tinctures can be added to water or juice for easy consumption.
- **Poultice**: Crushed fresh agrimony can be applied directly to the skin to treat wounds.
- **Infusions**: Dried agrimony can be infused in oil for topical use in skincare products.

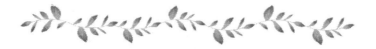

Alfalfa (Medicago sativa)

Botanical Description: Alfalfa is a perennial flowering plant in the pea family. It has deep roots, small clusters of purple flowers, and compound leaves with three leaflets. It thrives in temperate climates and is often grown as forage for livestock.

Health Benefits:

- **Nutrient-Rich**: High in vitamins A, C, E, and K, as well as minerals like calcium and potassium.
- **Digestive Health**: Helps alleviate digestive disorders and promotes healthy gut flora.
- **Cholesterol Reduction**: May help reduce cholesterol levels and improve heart health.
- **Detoxification**: Acts as a natural detoxifier, supporting liver function.

Recommended Dosage: 1-2 tsp of alfalfa powder or 1/8-1/4 tsp of alfalfa extract daily. Fresh alfalfa sprouts can be consumed in salads or smoothies.

Preparation Methods:

- **Sprouts**: Fresh alfalfa sprouts can be added to salads, sandwiches, or smoothies.
- **Tea**: Steep 1-2 tsp of dried alfalfa leaves in hot water for 12-14 min.

- **Capsules**: Alfalfa extract is available in capsule form for convenient supplementation.
- **Powder**: Alfalfa powder can be added to juices, smoothies, or other beverages.

Allspice (Pimenta dioica)

Botanical Description: Allspice is derived from the dried unripe berries of the Pimenta dioica tree, that comes from the Caribbean and Central America. The tree has aromatic leaves and produces small, dark brown berries resembling large peppercorns.

Health Benefits:

- **Digestive Aid**: Helps relieve indigestion, bloating, and gas.
- **Anti-inflammatory**: Reduces inflammation and may alleviate pain from arthritis.
- **Antioxidant**: Rich in antioxidants, helping to protect cells from damage.
- **Antimicrobial**: Possesses antimicrobial properties, which can help fight infections.

Recommended Dosage: Typically used as a spice, with 1-2 tsp added to recipes. For medicinal purposes, a tea made from 1-2 tsp of crushed allspice berries can be consumed up to three times daily.

Preparation Methods:

- **Spice**: Ground allspice is commonly used in cooking and baking.
- **Tea**: Crush allspice berries and steep in hot water for 12-14 min.
- **Essential Oil**: Allspice essential oil can be used in aromatherapy or diluted for topical application.
- **Infusions**: Infuse allspice in alcohol or oil for use in cooking or as a topical rub.

Amalaki (Phyllanthus emblica)

Traditional Applications: Amalaki, also known as Indian gooseberry or Amla, is widely used in Ayurvedic medicine. It is employed to promote longevity, improve digestion, and strengthen the immune system. It is known for its high vitamin C content.

Health Benefits:

- **Immunomodulatory**: Enhances immune function and fights infections.
- **Antioxidant**: Protects cells from oxidative stress.
- **Digestive Aid**: Improves digestion and alleviates constipation.
- **Anti-inflammatory**: Reduces inflammation and supports overall health.
- **Anti-aging**: Promotes healthy skin and delays aging signs.

Recommended Dosage: 1/8-1/4 tsp of amla extract per day, typically divided into two doses. Fresh amla fruit can be consumed in moderation, usually 1-2 fruits per day.

Preparation Methods:

- **Juice**: Fresh amla can be juiced and consumed directly.
- **Powder**: Dried amla can be ground into a powder and added to smoothies or drinks.
- **Capsules**: Amla extract is available in capsule form for convenient supplementation.
- **Infusions**: Amla powder can be added to teas or other beverages for added benefits.

Andrographis (Andrographis paniculata)

Traditional Applications: Andrographis, also known as the "King of Bitters," is used in traditional Asian medicine to treat infections, fever, and digestive disorders. It is known for its bitter properties and powerful immune-boosting effects.

Health Benefits:

- **Immune Support**: Boosts the immune system and helps fight infections.
- **Anti-inflammatory**: Reduces inflammation and alleviates symptoms of arthritis and other inflammatory conditions.
- **Antimicrobial**: Fights bacteria, viruses, and parasites.
- **Liver Health**: Supports liver function and detoxification.
- **Digestive Health**: Aids in digestion and alleviates gastrointestinal issues.

Recommended Dosage: 1/8-1/4 tsp of andrographis extract per day, divided into two doses. For acute conditions, higher doses may be used under medical supervision.

Preparation Methods:

- **Capsules**: Andrographis extract is commonly available in capsule form for easy consumption.
- **Tea**: Steep 1-2 tsp of dried andrographis leaves in hot water for 12-14 min.
- **Tincture**: Andrographis tinctures can be added to water or juice for easy consumption.
- **Powder**: Andrographis powder can be mixed into smoothies or other beverages.

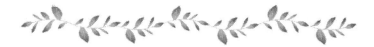

Angelica (Angelica archangelica)

Traditional Applications: Angelica has been used in European medicine for centuries, particularly for digestive and respiratory issues. Angelica root is often used to make infusions and tonics.

Health Benefits:

- **Digestive Aid**: Improves digestion and alleviates gastrointestinal issues.
- **Respiratory Health**: Helps treat respiratory infections and coughs.
- **Anti-inflammatory**: Reduces inflammation and pain.
- **Menstrual Health**: Helps regulate menstrual cycles and alleviate menstrual pain.
- **Detoxification**: Supports liver health and detoxification processes.

Recommended Dosage: 1/4-1/2 tsp of dried angelica root per day, typically consumed as a tea. Tincture dosage is usually 1-2 ml, three times daily.

Preparation Methods:

- **Tea**: Steep 1-2 tsp of dried angelica root in hot water for 12-14 min.
- **Tincture**: Angelica tinctures can be added to water or juice for easy consumption.
- **Capsules**: Angelica root powder is available in capsule form for convenient supplementation.
- **Infusions**: Dried angelica root can be infused in oil for topical use in skincare products.

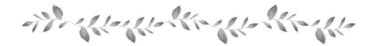

Amla (Phyllanthus emblica)

Traditional Applications: Amla, also known as Amalaki, is used in Ayurvedic medicine to promote overall health and longevity. It is known for its high vitamin C content and antioxidant properties.

Health Benefits:

- **Immune Support**: Enhances immune function and fights infections.
- **Antioxidant**: Protects cells from oxidative stress.
- **Digestive Health**: Improves digestion and alleviates constipation.
- **Anti-inflammatory**: Reduces inflammation and supports overall health.
- **Anti-aging**: Promotes healthy skin and delays aging signs.

Recommended Dosage: 1/8-1/4 tsp of amla extract per day, typically divided into two doses. Fresh amla fruit can be consumed in moderation, usually 1-2 fruits per day.

Preparation Methods:

- **Juice**: Fresh amla can be juiced and consumed directly.
- **Powder**: Dried amla can be ground into a powder and added to smoothies or drinks.
- **Capsules**: Amla extract is available in capsule form for convenient supplementation.
- **Infusions**: Amla powder can be added to teas or other beverages for added benefits.

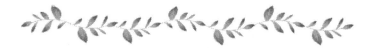

Anise (Pimpinella anisum)

Traditional Applications: Anise has been used for centuries in traditional medicine to treat digestive issues such as bloating and flatulence. It is also used to enhance the flavor of many herbal preparations.

Health Benefits:

- **Digestive Health**: Helps relieve bloating, indigestion, and gas.
- **Respiratory Support**: Alleviates coughs and asthma symptoms.
- **Antimicrobial**: Fights bacterial and fungal infections.
- **Hormonal Balance**: Can help regulate menstrual cycles.
- **Antioxidant Properties**: Protects cells from oxidative damage.

Recommended Dosage: 1/4-1 tsp of dried anise seeds per day, or 1/4-1/2 tsp of anise tincture three times daily.

Preparation Methods:

- **Tea**: Steep 1-2 tsp of crushed anise seeds in hot water for 12-14 min.

- **Tincture**: Anise tinctures can be added to water or juice for easy consumption.
- **Powder**: Ground anise seeds can be added to baked goods or culinary dishes.
- **Essential Oil**: Anise oil can be used in aromatherapy or diluted for topical use.

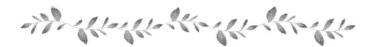

Arnica (Arnica montana)

Traditional Applications: Arnica is traditionally used to treat bruises, sprains, and muscle pain. It is valued for its anti-inflammatory and analgesic properties.

Health Benefits:

- **Anti-inflammatory**: Reduces swelling and inflammation.
- **Pain Relief**: Alleviates muscle pain, bruises, and sprains.
- **Wound Healing**: Speeds up the healing process of minor wounds and insect bites.
- **Circulation Boost**: Improves blood flow to affected areas.

Recommended Dosage: Typically used topically. Arnica gel or cream can be applied to the affected area 2-3 times per day. Not recommended for internal use without medical supervision.

Preparation Methods:

- **Topical Gel/Cream**: Apply arnica gel or cream directly to the skin.
- **Infused Oil**: Arnica flowers can be infused in oil and used for massage.
- **Compress**: Soak a cloth in a diluted arnica tincture solution and apply to the skin.

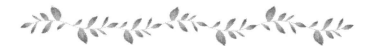

Arjuna (Terminalia arjuna)

Traditional Applications: Arjuna is a plant used in Ayurvedic medicine for cardiovascular health. It is known for strengthening the heart and improving blood circulation.

Health Benefits:

- **Cardiovascular Health**: Strengthens heart muscles and improves cardiac function.
- **Blood Pressure Regulation**: Helps maintain healthy blood pressure levels.

- **Antioxidant**: Protects the heart from oxidative stress.
- **Anti-inflammatory**: Reduces inflammation in the cardiovascular system.
- **Liver Health**: Supports liver function and detoxification.

Recommended Dosage: 1/8-1/4 tsp of arjuna bark extract per day, typically divided into two doses.

Preparation Methods:

- **Tea**: Boil 1-2 tsp of dried arjuna bark in water for 12-14 min.
- **Capsules**: Arjuna extract is available in capsule form for easy consumption.
- **Tincture**: Arjuna tinctures can be added to water or juice.
- **Powder**: Dried arjuna bark can be ground into a powder and added to smoothies or drinks.

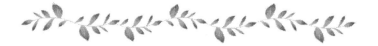

Artichoke (Cynara scolymus)

Traditional Applications: Artichoke is used in traditional European medicine to support liver health and improve digestion. It is known for its detoxifying properties.

Health Benefits:

- **Liver Health**: Promotes liver function and detoxification.
- **Digestive Aid**: Improves digestion and alleviates symptoms of indigestion.
- **Cholesterol Regulation**: Helps lower cholesterol levels.
- **Antioxidant**: Protects cells from oxidative stress.
- **Anti-inflammatory**: Reduces inflammation in the body.

Recommended Dosage: 1/8-1/4 tsp of artichoke extract per day, divided into two doses. Fresh artichoke can be consumed as part of the diet.

Preparation Methods:

- **Tea**: Boil 1-2 tsp of dried artichoke leaves in water for 12-14 min.
- **Capsules**: Artichoke extract is available in capsule form for convenient supplementation.
- **Tincture**: Artichoke tinctures can be added to water or juice.
- **Culinary Use**: Fresh artichokes can be steamed, boiled, or grilled and added to salads or main dishes.

Ashitaba (Angelica keiskei)

Traditional Applications: Ashitaba is traditionally used in Japan to promote longevity and overall health. It is known as the "longevity herb" due to its numerous health benefits.

Health Benefits:

- **Antioxidant**: Protects cells from oxidative damage.
- **Anti-inflammatory**: Reduces inflammation and supports immune function.
- **Digestive Health**: Promotes healthy digestion and relieves gastrointestinal issues.
- **Blood Sugar Regulation**: Helps maintain stable blood sugar levels.
- **Longevity**: Supports overall health and longevity.

Recommended Dosage: 1/4-1/2 tsp of dried ashitaba powder per day, or 1-2 cups of ashitaba tea.

Preparation Methods:

- **Tea**: Steep 1 tsp of dried ashitaba leaves in hot water for 10 min.
- **Powder**: Add ashitaba powder to smoothies, juices, or soups.
- **Capsules**: Ashitaba is available in capsule form for easy supplementation.
- **Fresh Leaves**: Can be added to salads or used in cooking.

Ashwagandha (Withania somnifera)

Traditional Applications: Ashwagandha is one of the primary herbs in Ayurvedic medicine, used to reduce stress, enhance vitality, and support the immune system.

Health Benefits:

- **Stress Relief**: Reduces stress and anxiety levels.
- **Energy Boost**: Enhances physical performance and energy levels.
- **Immune Support**: Strengthens the immune system.
- **Cognitive Function**: Improves memory and cognitive abilities.
- **Anti-inflammatory**: Reduces inflammation and supports joint health.

Recommended Dosage: 1/8 tsp of ashwagandha extract per day, divided into two doses.

Preparation Methods:

- **Tea**: Boil 1 tsp of ashwagandha root powder in water for 10 min.
- **Capsules**: Ashwagandha is available in capsule form for easy supplementation.
- **Tincture**: Ashwagandha tinctures can be added to water or juice.
- **Powder**: Mix ashwagandha powder into smoothies, warm milk, or soups.

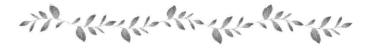

Astragalus (Astragalus membranaceus)

Traditional Applications: Astragalus is used in traditional Chinese medicine to strengthen the immune system and increase physical endurance.

Health Benefits:

- **Immune Support**: Boosts immune system function.
- **Anti-inflammatory**: Reduces inflammation in the body.
- **Antioxidant**: Protects cells from oxidative stress.
- **Cardiovascular Health**: Supports heart health and improves circulation.
- **Energy Boost**: Enhances physical endurance and reduces fatigue.

Recommended Dosage: 1/8-1/4 tsp of astragalus extract per day, divided into two doses.

Preparation Methods:

- **Tea**: Simmer 1-2 tsp of dried astragalus root in water for 20-30 min.
- **Capsules**: Astragalus extract is available in capsule form for convenient use.
- **Tincture**: Astragalus tinctures can be added to water or juice.
- **Powder**: Add astragalus powder to smoothies, soups, or teas.

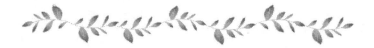

Baikal Skullcap (Scutellaria baicalensis)

Traditional Applications: Baikal Skullcap is used in traditional Chinese medicine for its anti-inflammatory and antioxidant properties. It is known to support the immune system and liver health.

Health Benefits:

- **Anti-inflammatory**: Reduces inflammation and supports joint health.
- **Antioxidant**: Protects cells from oxidative damage.
- **Immune Support**: Enhances immune system function.
- **Liver Health**: Supports liver detoxification and health.
- **Respiratory Health**: Helps alleviate respiratory conditions and allergies.

Recommended Dosage: 1/8-1/4 tsp of Baikal skullcap extract per day, divided into two doses.

Preparation Methods:

- **Tea**: Steep 1-2 tsp of dried Baikal skullcap root in hot water for 12-14 min.
- **Capsules**: Baikal skullcap is available in capsule form for easy supplementation.
- **Tincture**: Baikal skullcap tinctures can be added to water or juice.
- **Powder**: Mix Baikal skullcap powder into smoothies, teas, or soups.

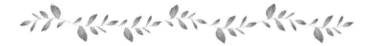

Baobab (Adansonia)

Traditional Applications: Baobab is traditionally used in Africa for its nutritional and medicinal properties. Known as the "tree of life," its parts are used to promote overall health and wellness.

Health Benefits:

- **Antioxidant**: High in antioxidants, which protect cells from damage.
- **Digestive Health**: Rich in fiber, aiding digestion and promoting gut health.
- **Vitamin C**: Extremely high in vitamin C, boosting the immune system.
- **Hydration**: Contains electrolytes that help maintain hydration.
- **Anti-inflammatory**: Reduces inflammation and supports joint health.

Recommended Dosage: 1-2 tablespoons of baobab powder per day.

Preparation Methods:

- **Powder**: Add baobab powder to smoothies, juices, or yogurt.
- **Tea**: Mix baobab powder with hot water and honey.
- **Capsules**: Baobab is available in capsule form for easy supplementation.
- **Baking**: Incorporate baobab powder into baking recipes for an added nutritional boost.

Barberry (Berberis vulgaris)

Traditional Applications: Barberry has been used in traditional European and Asian medicine to treat a variety of ailments, including digestive issues and infections.

Health Benefits:

- **Digestive Health**: Stimulates appetite and improves digestion.
- **Antimicrobial**: Fights bacteria and other pathogens.
- **Anti-inflammatory**: Reduces inflammation in the body.
- **Liver Health**: Supports liver function and detoxification.
- **Cardiovascular Health**: Helps regulate blood sugar and cholesterol levels.

Recommended Dosage: 1/8-1/4 tsp of barberry extract per day, divided into two doses.

Preparation Methods:

- **Tea**: Steep 1 tsp of dried barberry root or berries in hot water for 12-14 min.
- **Tincture**: Barberry tinctures can be added to water or juice.
- **Capsules**: Barberry extract is available in capsule form for easy supplementation.
- **Powder**: Add barberry powder to smoothies or teas.

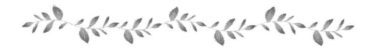

Basil (Ocimum basilicum)

Traditional Applications: Basil is widely used in Mediterranean and Asian cuisine and is also valued for its medicinal properties, such as treating digestive and respiratory disorders.

Health Benefits:

- **Antioxidant**: Protects cells from oxidative stress.
- **Anti-inflammatory**: Reduces inflammation and supports joint health.
- **Digestive Health**: Aids digestion and relieves gastrointestinal discomfort.
- **Antimicrobial**: Fights bacterial and fungal infections.
- **Mental Health**: Supports mental clarity and reduces stress.

Recommended Dosage: 1-2 tsp of dried basil leaves per day, or 1-2 fresh basil leaves per meal.

Preparation Methods:

- **Tea**: Steep fresh or dried basil leaves in hot water for 5-10 min.
- **Culinary Use**: Add fresh basil leaves to salads, sauces, and soups.
- **Pesto**: Blend fresh basil leaves with olive oil, garlic, and nuts to make pesto.
- **Essential Oil**: Use diluted basil essential oil for aromatherapy or topical application.

Bayberry (Myrica cerifera)

Traditional Applications: Bayberry is used in traditional North American medicine to treat infections and digestive issues. Its roots and bark are particularly valued for their astringent properties.

Health Benefits:

- **Digestive Health**: Aids in treating diarrhea and other gastrointestinal issues.
- **Anti-inflammatory**: Reduces inflammation and soothes mucous membranes.
- **Antimicrobial**: Fights bacterial and fungal infections.
- **Circulatory Health**: Supports blood circulation and reduces varicose veins.
- **Respiratory Health**: Eases congestion and respiratory infections.

Recommended Dosage: 1/8-1/4 tsp of bayberry extract per day, divided into two doses.

Preparation Methods:

- **Tea**: Boil 1 tsp of dried bayberry root or bark in water for 12-14 min.
- **Tincture**: Bayberry tinctures can be added to water or juice.
- **Capsules**: Bayberry extract is available in capsule form for easy supplementation.

- **Poultice**: Make a poultice with bayberry powder and water for topical use.

Bee Balm (Monarda didyma)

Traditional Applications: Bee Balm, also known as Oswego Tea, has been traditionally used by Native Americans to treat colds, flu, and respiratory issues. It is also used as a digestive aid and for its antimicrobial properties.

Health Benefits:

- Anti-inflammatory properties
- Antimicrobial and antifungal effects
- Digestive aid
- Relieves respiratory congestion

Recommended Dosage:

- Tea: 1-2 tsp of dried Bee Balm leaves per cup of boiling water, steep for 10 min, up to 3 times daily
- Tincture: 1-2 dropperfuls up to 3 times daily

Preparation Methods:

- Tea: Steep dried Bee Balm leaves in boiling water for 10 min.
- Tincture: Take directly under the tongue or diluted in water.
- Infused Oil: Steep dried Bee Balm in a carrier oil for topical applications.

Betony (Stachys officinalis)

Traditional Applications: Betony has been traditionally used in European herbal medicine for its calming and nerve-soothing properties. It is often used to treat headaches, anxiety, and digestive disorders.

Health Benefits:

- Calms the nervous system
- Eases headaches and migraines

- Supports digestive health
- Alleviates anxiety and stress

Recommended Dosage:

- Tea: 1-2 tsp of dried Betony leaves per cup of boiling water, steep for 12-14 min, up to 3 times daily
- Tincture: 1-2 dropperfuls up to 3 times daily

Preparation Methods:

- Tea: Steep dried Betony leaves in boiling water for 12-14 min.
- Tincture: Take directly under the tongue or diluted in water.
- Compress: Soak a cloth in Betony tea and apply to the affected area for headaches.

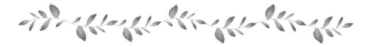

Bilberry (Vaccinium myrtillus)

Traditional Applications: Bilberry has been used traditionally in Europe for improving vision and treating various eye conditions. It is also known for its benefits to cardiovascular health and blood sugar regulation.

Health Benefits:

- Supports eye health and improves vision
- Antioxidant properties
- Enhances cardiovascular health
- Regulates blood sugar levels

Recommended Dosage:

- Tea: 1-2 tsp of dried Bilberry leaves or berries per cup of boiling water, steep for 10 min, up to 3 times daily
- Extract: 1/4 to 1/2 tsp of Bilberry extract, standardized to contain 25% anthocyanosides, taken up to 3 times daily

Preparation Methods:

- Tea: Steep dried Bilberry leaves or berries in boiling water for 10 min.

- Extract: Take as directed on the product label.
- Capsules: Take as directed on the product label.

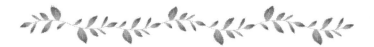

Bitter Melon (Momordica charantia)

Traditional Applications: Bitter Melon is widely used in traditional Asian and African medicine for its ability to regulate blood sugar levels. It is also used to treat digestive issues and support liver health.

Health Benefits:

- Regulates blood sugar levels
- Supports liver health
- Aids in digestion
- Antimicrobial properties

Recommended Dosage:

- Juice: 1-2 tbsp of fresh Bitter Melon juice, taken 1-2 times daily
- Tea: 1-2 tsp of dried Bitter Melon slices per cup of boiling water, steep for 10 min, up to 3 times daily
- Capsules: 1/4 to 1/2 tsp of Bitter Melon extract, taken up to 3 times daily

Preparation Methods:

- Juice: Extract juice from fresh Bitter Melon using a juicer.
- Tea: Steep dried Bitter Melon slices in boiling water for 10 min.
- Capsules: Take as directed on the product label.

Black Cohosh (Actaea racemosa)

Traditional Applications: Black Cohosh has been traditionally used by Native Americans and later by European settlers to treat menstrual cramps, menopause symptoms, and as a remedy for rheumatism and muscle pain.

Health Benefits:

- Alleviates menopause symptoms such as hot flashes and night sweats
- Eases menstrual cramps and PMS
- Anti-inflammatory properties
- Supports overall women's health

Recommended Dosage:

- Tea: 1 tsp of dried Black Cohosh root per cup of boiling water, steep for 12-14 min, up to 2 times daily
- Tincture: 1-2 dropperfuls up to 3 times daily

Preparation Methods:

- Tea: Steep dried Black Cohosh root in boiling water for 12-14 min.
- Tincture: Take directly under the tongue or diluted in water.
- Capsules: Take as directed on the product label.

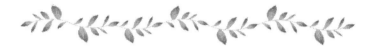

Black Currant (Ribes nigrum)

Traditional Applications: Black Currant has been traditionally used in European medicine for its immune-boosting properties and to treat sore throats and respiratory infections. It is also known for its anti-inflammatory benefits.

Health Benefits:

- Boosts the immune system
- Rich in antioxidants and vitamins
- Reduces inflammation
- Supports cardiovascular health

Recommended Dosage:

- Tea: 1-2 tsp of dried Black Currant leaves or berries per cup of boiling water, steep for 10 min, up to 3 times daily
- Extract: 1/4 to 1/2 tsp of Black Currant extract, taken up to 3 times daily

Preparation Methods:

- Tea: Steep dried Black Currant leaves or berries in boiling water for 10 min.
- Extract: Take as directed on the product label.
- Capsules: Take as directed on the product label.

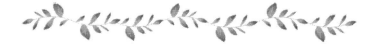

Black Horehound (Ballota nigra)

Traditional Applications: Black Horehound has been traditionally used in European herbal medicine for its antiemetic and antispasmodic properties. It is commonly employed to treat nausea, vomiting, and digestive disturbances, as well as respiratory conditions like coughs and bronchitis.

Health Benefits:

- Relieves nausea and vomiting
- Eases digestive discomfort
- Acts as an antispasmodic to reduce muscle spasms
- Supports respiratory health

Recommended Dosage:

- Tea: 1-2 tsp of dried Black Horehound leaves per cup of boiling water, steep for 10-15 min, up to 3 times daily
- Extract: 1/4 to 1/2 tsp of Black Horehound extract, taken up to 3 times daily

Preparation Methods:

- Tea: Steep dried Black Horehound leaves in boiling water for 10-15 min.
- Extract: Take as directed on the product label.
- Capsules: Take as directed on the product label.

Black Walnut (Juglans nigra)

Traditional Applications: Black Walnut has been used traditionally by Native Americans and herbalists for its antifungal, antiparasitic, and antiviral properties. It is often employed to treat skin conditions and intestinal parasites.

Health Benefits:

- Antifungal and antiparasitic properties
- Supports digestive health
- Promotes healthy skin
- Antiviral effects

Recommended Dosage:

- Tincture: 1-2 dropperfuls up to 3 times daily
- Infusion: 1-2 tsp of dried Black Walnut hulls per cup of boiling water, steep for 12-14 min, up to 3 times daily

Preparation Methods:

- Tincture: Take directly under the tongue or diluted in water.
- Infusion: Steep dried Black Walnut hulls in boiling water for 12-14 min.
- Capsules: Take as directed on the product label.

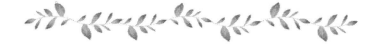

Blessed Thistle (Cnicus benedictus)

Traditional Applications: Blessed Thistle has been traditionally used in European and Native American medicine to stimulate appetite, aid digestion, and treat respiratory infections. It is also known for its use in supporting lactation.

Health Benefits:

- Stimulates appetite and aids digestion
- Supports lactation in nursing mothers

- Antimicrobial properties
- Alleviates respiratory infections

Recommended Dosage:

- Tea: 1-2 tsp of dried Blessed Thistle leaves per cup of boiling water, steep for 12-14 min, up to 3 times daily
- Tincture: 1-2 dropperfuls up to 3 times daily

Preparation Methods:

- Tea: Steep dried Blessed Thistle leaves in boiling water for 12-14 min.
- Tincture: Take directly under the tongue or diluted in water.
- Capsules: Take as directed on the product label.

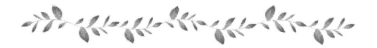

Blueberry (Vaccinium corymbosum)

Traditional Applications: Blueberry has been traditionally used by Native Americans for its medicinal properties, including improving vision and treating diarrhea. It is also known for its high antioxidant content.

Health Benefits:

- Rich in antioxidants, supports overall health
- Improves vision and eye health
- Supports cardiovascular health
- Enhances cognitive function

Recommended Dosage:

- Fresh Berries: 1/2 to 1 cup daily
- Tea: 1-2 tsp of dried Blueberry leaves per cup of boiling water, steep for 10 min, up to 3 times daily
- Extract: 1/4 to 1/2 tsp of Blueberry extract, taken up to 3 times daily

Preparation Methods:

- Fresh Berries: Consume as a snack or in smoothies and salads.

- Tea: Steep dried Blueberry leaves in boiling water for 10 min.
- Extract: Take as directed on the product label.
- Capsules: Take as directed on the product label.

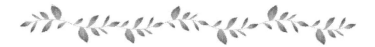

Boneset (Eupatorium perfoliatum)

Traditional Applications: Boneset has been traditionally used by Native Americans and early settlers to treat fevers, colds, and flu. It is known for its bitter properties and is often used as a herbal tonic.

Health Benefits:

- Reduces fever and alleviates cold and flu symptoms
- Supports immune system health
- Anti-inflammatory properties
- Aids digestion

Recommended Dosage:

- Tea: 1-2 tsp of dried Boneset leaves per cup of boiling water, steep for 12-14 min, up to 3 times daily
- Tincture: 1-2 dropperfuls up to 3 times daily

Preparation Methods:

- Tea: Steep dried Boneset leaves in boiling water for 12-14 min.
- Tincture: Take directly under the tongue or diluted in water.
- Capsules: Take as directed on the product label.

Broom (Cytisus scoparius)

Traditional Applications: Broom has been traditionally used in European folk medicine to treat urinary tract infections and as a diuretic. It is also used to support cardiovascular health.

Health Benefits:

- Diuretic properties, supports urinary tract health
- Supports cardiovascular health
- Anti-inflammatory properties
- Aids in detoxification

Recommended Dosage:

- Tea: 1 tsp of dried Broom tops per cup of boiling water, steep for 10 min, up to 3 times daily
- Tincture: 1-2 dropperfuls up to 3 times daily

Preparation Methods:

- Tea: Steep dried Broom tops in boiling water for 10 min.
- Tincture: Take directly under the tongue or diluted in water.
- Capsules: Take as directed on the product label.

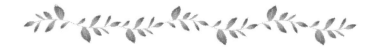

Buckthorn (Rhamnus cathartica)

Traditional Applications: Buckthorn has been traditionally used in European herbal medicine as a laxative and to treat constipation. It is also known for its detoxifying properties.

Health Benefits:

- Natural laxative, alleviates constipation
- Supports digestive health
- Detoxifying properties
- Anti-inflammatory effects

Recommended Dosage:

- Tea: 1 tsp of dried Buckthorn bark per cup of boiling water, steep for 12-14 min, up to 2 times daily
- Tincture: 1-2 dropperfuls up to 2 times daily

Preparation Methods:

- Tea: Steep dried Buckthorn bark in boiling water for 12-14 min.
- Tincture: Take directly under the tongue or diluted in water.

- Capsules: Take as directed on the product label.

Bugbane (Cimicifuga racemosa)

Traditional Applications: Bugbane, also known as Black Cohosh, has been traditionally used by Native Americans and in European herbal medicine to treat menopausal symptoms, menstrual cramps, and inflammation.

Health Benefits:

- Alleviates menopausal symptoms
- Reduces menstrual cramps
- Anti-inflammatory properties
- Supports hormonal balance

Recommended Dosage:

- Tea: 1-2 tsp of dried Bugbane root per cup of boiling water, steep for 12-14 min, up to 3 times daily
- Tincture: 1-2 dropperfuls up to 3 times daily

Preparation Methods:

- Tea: Steep dried Bugbane root in boiling water for 12-14 min.
- Tincture: Take directly under the tongue or diluted in water.
- Capsules: Take as directed on the product label.
-

Bur Marigold (Bidens tripartita)

Traditional Applications: Bur Marigold has been traditionally used in European and Asian herbal medicine to treat wounds, skin conditions, and as a diuretic. It is also known for its anti-inflammatory properties.

Health Benefits:

- Treats wounds and skin conditions
- Diuretic properties
- Anti-inflammatory effects
- Supports urinary tract health

Recommended Dosage:

- Tea: 1-2 tsp of dried Bur Marigold leaves per cup of boiling water, steep for 12-14 min, up to 3 times daily
- Tincture: 1-2 dropperfuls up to 3 times daily

Preparation Methods:

- Tea: Steep dried Bur Marigold leaves in boiling water for 12-14 min.
- Tincture: Take directly under the tongue or diluted in water.
- Capsules: Take as directed on the product label.

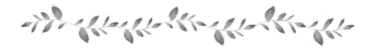

Burdock (Arctium lappa)

Traditional Applications: Burdock has been traditionally used in both European and Asian herbal medicine to detoxify the body, treat skin conditions, and support liver health. It is also known for its blood-purifying properties.

Health Benefits:

- Detoxifies the body
- Supports liver health
- Treats skin conditions like eczema and acne
- Acts as a diuretic
- Has anti-inflammatory properties

Recommended Dosage:

- Tea: 1-2 tsp of dried Burdock root per cup of boiling water, steep for 12-14 min, up to 3 times daily
- Tincture: 1-2 dropperfuls up to 3 times daily

Preparation Methods:

- Tea: Steep dried Burdock root in boiling water for 12-14 min.
- Tincture: Take directly under the tongue or diluted in water.
- Capsules: Take as directed on the product label.
- Food: Young Burdock roots can be eaten as a vegetable.

Butcher's Broom (Ruscus aculeatus)

Traditional Applications: Butcher's Broom has been traditionally used in European herbal medicine to improve circulation, treat varicose veins, and reduce swelling. It is also known for its diuretic properties.

Health Benefits:

- Improves circulation
- Treats varicose veins and hemorrhoids
- Reduces swelling and inflammation
- Acts as a diuretic

Recommended Dosage:

- Tea: 1-2 tsp of dried Butcher's Broom root per cup of boiling water, steep for 12-14 min, up to 3 times daily
- Tincture: 1-2 dropperfuls up to 3 times daily

Preparation Methods:

- Tea: Steep dried Butcher's Broom root in boiling water for 12-14 min.
- Tincture: Take directly under the tongue or diluted in water.
- Capsules: Take as directed on the product label.

Butternut (Juglans cinerea)

Traditional Applications: Butternut has been traditionally used in Native American and early American herbal medicine as a gentle laxative and to support liver health. It is also used for its anti-inflammatory properties.

Health Benefits:

- Acts as a gentle laxative
- Supports liver health
- Has anti-inflammatory properties
- Aids in detoxification

Recommended Dosage:

- Tea: 1-2 tsp of dried Butternut bark per cup of boiling water, steep for 12-14 min, up to 2 times daily
- Tincture: 1-2 dropperfuls up to 2 times daily

Preparation Methods:

- Tea: Steep dried Butternut bark in boiling water for 12-14 min.
- Tincture: Take directly under the tongue or diluted in water.
- Capsules: Take as directed on the product label.

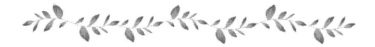

Calendula (Calendula officinalis)

Traditional Applications: Calendula has been traditionally used in European herbal medicine to heal wounds, treat skin conditions, and as an anti-inflammatory agent. It is often used topically in creams and salves.

Health Benefits:

- Heals wounds and skin conditions like eczema and dermatitis
- Reduces inflammation
- Acts as an antimicrobial
- Supports digestive health when taken internally

Recommended Dosage:

- Tea: 1-2 tsp of dried Calendula flowers per cup of boiling water, steep for 12-14 min, up to 3 times daily
- Tincture: 1-2 dropperfuls up to 3 times daily

- Topical: Apply Calendula cream or salve to affected areas as needed

Preparation Methods:

- Tea: Steep dried Calendula flowers in boiling water for 12-14 min.
- Tincture: Take directly under the tongue or diluted in water.
- Topical: Use Calendula-infused oils, creams, or salves for skin conditions.
- Infused Oil: Infuse dried Calendula flowers in a carrier oil for topical use.

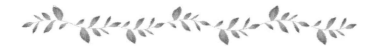

California Poppy (Eschscholzia californica)

Traditional Applications: California Poppy has been traditionally used by Native Americans as a mild sedative and to alleviate pain. It is also used to promote relaxation and improve sleep quality.

Health Benefits:

- Promotes relaxation and reduces anxiety
- Improves sleep quality
- Acts as a mild sedative
- Alleviates pain and muscle tension

Recommended Dosage:

- Tea: 1-2 tsp of dried California Poppy per cup of boiling water, steep for 12-14 min, up to 3 times daily
- Tincture: 1-2 dropperfuls up to 3 times daily

Preparation Methods:

- Tea: Steep dried California Poppy in boiling water for 12-14 min.
- Tincture: Take directly under the tongue or diluted in water.
- Capsules: Take as directed on the product label.

Cardamom (Elettaria cardamomum)

Traditional Applications: Cardamom has been traditionally used in Ayurvedic and Chinese medicine to treat digestive issues, improve oral health, and enhance respiratory function. It is also used as a flavoring spice in many culinary dishes.

Health Benefits:

- Aids digestion and relieves bloating
- Freshens breath and improves oral health
- Enhances respiratory function
- Acts as an antioxidant

Recommended Dosage:

- Tea: 1-2 tsp of crushed Cardamom seeds per cup of boiling water, steep for 12-14 min, up to 3 times daily
- Tincture: 1-2 dropperfuls up to 3 times daily
- Powder: 1/2-1 tsp added to food or beverages daily

Preparation Methods:

- Tea: Steep crushed Cardamom seeds in boiling water for 12-14 min.
- Tincture: Take directly under the tongue or diluted in water.
- Powder: Add to food or beverages as a spice.

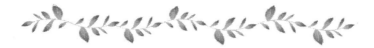

Caraway (Carum carvi)

Traditional Applications: Caraway has been traditionally used in European and Middle Eastern herbal medicine to aid digestion, relieve colic, and treat respiratory issues. It is also a common culinary spice.

Health Benefits:

- Aids digestion and relieves bloating
- Eases colic and intestinal cramps
- Treats respiratory issues like coughs and bronchitis
- Acts as an antimicrobial

Recommended Dosage:

- Tea: 1-2 tsp of crushed Caraway seeds per cup of boiling water, steep for 12-14 min, up to 3 times daily
- Tincture: 1-2 dropperfuls up to 3 times daily
- Powder: 1/2-1 tsp added to food or beverages daily

Preparation Methods:

- Tea: Steep crushed Caraway seeds in boiling water for 12-14 min.
- Tincture: Take directly under the tongue or diluted in water.
- Powder: Add to food or beverages as a spice.

Carob (Ceratonia siliqua)

Traditional Applications: Carob has been traditionally used in Mediterranean and Middle Eastern cultures as a natural sweetener and a remedy for digestive issues. It is also used to support heart health and as a chocolate substitute.

Health Benefits:

- Aids digestion and relieves diarrhea
- Supports heart health
- Acts as a natural sweetener and chocolate substitute
- Provides antioxidants

Recommended Dosage:

- Powder: 1-2 tbsp added to food or beverages daily
- Syrup: 1-2 tbsp taken directly or diluted in water up to 3 times daily

Preparation Methods:

- Powder: Add to smoothies, baked goods, or as a chocolate substitute in recipes.
- Syrup: Take directly or dilute in water for a sweet drink.
- Capsules: Take as directed on the product label.

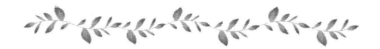

Cascara Sagrada (Rhamnus purshiana)

Traditional Applications: Cascara Sagrada has been traditionally used by Native Americans and later by European settlers as a natural laxative. It is known for its effectiveness in relieving constipation.

Health Benefits:

- Acts as a natural laxative
- Supports bowel regularity
- Aids in detoxification

Recommended Dosage:

- Capsules: 1-2 capsules taken with water at bedtime
- Tea: 1-2 tsp of dried bark per cup of boiling water, steep for 12-14 min, taken once daily
- Tincture: 1-2 dropperfuls taken in water at bedtime

Preparation Methods:

- Capsules: Take with water as directed.
- Tea: Steep dried bark in boiling water for 12-14 min.
- Tincture: Take directly under the tongue or diluted in water.

Cat's Claw (Uncaria tomentosa)

Traditional Applications: Cat's Claw has been traditionally used in South American medicine to boost the immune system, reduce inflammation, and treat digestive disorders. It is also known for its antioxidant properties.

Health Benefits:

- Boosts immune function
- Reduces inflammation
- Supports digestive health

- Provides antioxidants

Recommended Dosage:

- Capsules: 1-2 capsules taken 1-2 times daily
- Tea: 1-2 tsp of dried Cat's Claw per cup of boiling water, steep for 12-14 min, up to 3 times daily
- Tincture: 1-2 dropperfuls taken in water 1-2 times daily

Preparation Methods:

- Capsules: Take with water as directed.
- Tea: Steep dried Cat's Claw in boiling water for 12-14 min.
- Tincture: Take directly under the tongue or diluted in water.

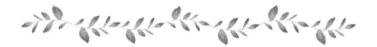

Catnip (Nepeta cataria)

Traditional Applications: Catnip has been traditionally used in European and Native American medicine to promote relaxation, reduce anxiety, and treat digestive issues. It is also used to alleviate cold symptoms.

Health Benefits:

- Promotes relaxation and reduces anxiety
- Supports digestive health
- Relieves cold and flu symptoms
- Acts as a mild sedative

Recommended Dosage:

- Tea: 1-2 tsp of dried Catnip per cup of boiling water, steep for 12-14 min, up to 3 times daily
- Tincture: 1-2 dropperfuls taken in water 1-2 times daily
- Capsules: 1-2 capsules taken 1-2 times daily

Preparation Methods:

- Tea: Steep dried Catnip in boiling water for 12-14 min.
- Tincture: Take directly under the tongue or diluted in water.

- Capsules: Take with water as directed.

Carrot (Daucus carota)

Traditional Applications: Carrots have been traditionally used in various cultures for their nutritional benefits and to improve vision. They are also used to support digestive health and enhance the immune system.

Health Benefits:

- Rich in beta-carotene, which supports eye health
- Enhances immune function
- Promotes healthy digestion
- Provides antioxidants

Recommended Dosage:

- Juice: 1 cup of fresh carrot juice daily
- Raw: 1-2 raw carrots daily
- Supplement: Follow the product label instructions

Preparation Methods:

- Raw: Eat fresh carrots as a snack or in salads.
- Juice: Blend fresh carrots to make juice.
- Cooked: Add to soups, stews, and casseroles.
- Supplement: Take as directed on the product label.

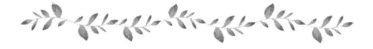

Chicory (Cichorium intybus)

Traditional Applications: Chicory has been used traditionally in European herbal medicine as a liver tonic, digestive aid, and for its anti-inflammatory properties. The roots are often roasted and used as a coffee substitute.

Health Benefits:

- Supports liver health
- Aids digestion
- Reduces inflammation
- Promotes healthy gut flora

Recommended Dosage:

- Tea: 1-2 tsp of dried chicory root per cup of boiling water, steep for 12-14 min, up to 3 times daily
- Roasted Root: 1-2 tsp of roasted chicory root per cup of boiling water, used as a coffee substitute
- Tincture: 1-2 dropperfuls taken in water 1-2 times daily

Preparation Methods:

- Tea: Steep dried chicory root in boiling water for 12-14 min.
- Roasted Root: Roast chicory root until dark brown and use as a coffee substitute.
- Tincture: Take directly under the tongue or diluted in water.

Cinnamon (Cinnamomum verum)

Traditional Applications: Cinnamon has been used in traditional medicine worldwide for its warming properties, to improve circulation, and as a digestive aid. It is also known for its antimicrobial and antioxidant properties.

Health Benefits:

- Enhances circulation
- Supports digestive health
- Provides antimicrobial and antioxidant benefits
- Helps regulate blood sugar levels

Recommended Dosage:

- Powder: 1/2 to 1 tsp of ground cinnamon daily
- Tea: 1-2 cinnamon sticks or 1 tsp of ground cinnamon per cup of boiling water, steep for 12-14 min, up to 3 times daily

- Tincture: 1-2 dropperfuls taken in water 1-2 times daily

Preparation Methods:

- Powder: Add to food or beverages.
- Tea: Steep cinnamon sticks or ground cinnamon in boiling water for 12-14 min.
- Tincture: Take directly under the tongue or diluted in water.

Clove (Syzygium aromaticum)

Traditional Applications: Clove has been used traditionally for its analgesic properties, particularly for toothaches and dental pain. It is also employed as a digestive aid and for its antimicrobial effects.

Health Benefits:

- Provides pain relief
- Supports digestive health
- Offers antimicrobial benefits
- Acts as an anti-inflammatory

Recommended Dosage:

- Oil: 1-2 drops of clove oil diluted in a carrier oil, applied topically
- Tea: 1/2 to 1 tsp of ground cloves per cup of boiling water, steep for 12-14 min, up to 3 times daily
- Powder: 1/4 to 1/2 tsp of ground cloves daily

Preparation Methods:

- Oil: Dilute in a carrier oil and apply topically.
- Tea: Steep ground cloves in boiling water for 12-14 min.
- Powder: Add to food or beverages.

Club Moss (Lycopodium clavatum)

Traditional Applications: Club Moss has been used in traditional European herbal medicine for its diuretic properties and to support urinary health. It is also known for its use in treating digestive disorders and respiratory issues.

Health Benefits:

- Acts as a diuretic
- Supports urinary health
- Aids digestion
- Relieves respiratory issues

Recommended Dosage:

- Tea: 1 tsp of dried club moss per cup of boiling water, steep for 12-14 min, up to 3 times daily
- Powder: 1/4 to 1/2 tsp of dried club moss powder daily
- Tincture: 1-2 dropperfuls taken in water 1-2 times daily

Preparation Methods:

- Tea: Steep dried club moss in boiling water for 12-14 min.
- Powder: Add to food or beverages.
- Tincture: Take directly under the tongue or diluted in water.

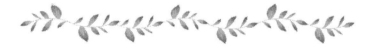

Cocoa (Theobroma cacao)

Traditional Applications: Cocoa has been used for centuries in Central and South American cultures as a sacred and medicinal plant. It is commonly consumed as a beverage and used for its energizing, mood-enhancing, and cardiovascular benefits.

Health Benefits:

- Boosts mood and cognitive function
- Supports cardiovascular health
- Provides antioxidant properties
- Enhances energy levels

Recommended Dosage:

- Powder: 1-2 tbsp of raw cocoa powder daily
- Nibs: 1-2 tbsp of cocoa nibs daily
- Drink: 1-2 tbsp of cocoa powder mixed with hot water or milk, up to 2 times daily

Preparation Methods:

- Powder: Add to smoothies, baked goods, or hot beverages.
- Nibs: Use as a topping for yogurt, oatmeal, or salads.
- Drink: Mix cocoa powder with hot water or milk for a rich beverage.

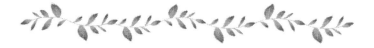

Coconut (Cocos nucifera)

Traditional Applications: Coconut has been a staple in tropical diets and traditional medicine, valued for its nutritional and hydrating properties. It is used for its meat, water, oil, and milk.

Health Benefits:

- Supports hydration and electrolyte balance
- Promotes skin and hair health
- Provides healthy fats for energy
- Aids digestion and nutrient absorption

Recommended Dosage:

- Water: 1-2 cups of coconut water daily
- Oil: 1-2 tbsp of coconut oil daily
- Meat: 1/4 to 1/2 cup of fresh coconut meat daily

Preparation Methods:

- Water: Drink fresh or bottled coconut water.
- Oil: Use in cooking, baking, or as a topical treatment.
- Meat: Consume fresh, dried, or added to recipes.

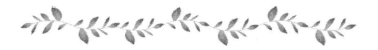

Coffee (Coffea arabica)

Traditional Applications: Coffee has been used for centuries as a stimulant beverage. It is known for its energizing properties and is commonly consumed to enhance alertness and mental focus.

Health Benefits:

- Increases energy and alertness
- Enhances mental focus and cognitive function
- Provides antioxidants
- May support metabolic health

Recommended Dosage:

- Brewed: 1-3 cups of brewed coffee daily
- Ground: 1-2 tbsp of ground coffee per cup of water
- Instant: 1-2 tsp of instant coffee per cup of water

Preparation Methods:

- Brewed: Use a coffee maker, French press, or pour-over method.
- Ground: Brew in a coffee maker or espresso machine.
- Instant: Mix with hot water for a quick beverage.

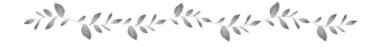

Coleus (Coleus forskohlii)

Traditional Applications: Coleus has been used in traditional Indian medicine (Ayurveda) for its ability to support heart health and respiratory function. It is known for its active compound forskolin.

Health Benefits:

- Supports cardiovascular health
- Enhances respiratory function
- Promotes weight management

- Aids in lowering blood pressure

Recommended Dosage:

- Powder: 1/4 to 1/2 tsp of Coleus forskohlii powder daily
- Capsules: 1-2 capsules (250-500 mg) of standardized extract daily
- Tincture: 1-2 dropperfuls taken in water 1-2 times daily

Preparation Methods:

- Powder: Add to smoothies or water.
- Capsules: Take with water as directed on the label.
- Tincture: Take directly under the tongue or diluted in water.

Cola Nut (Cola acuminata)

Traditional Applications: Cola nut has been used traditionally in West African cultures as a stimulant and for its medicinal properties. It is commonly chewed to reduce hunger and fatigue and used in various ceremonial contexts.

Health Benefits:

- Enhances energy and alertness
- Supports digestive health
- Provides antioxidants
- May aid in weight management

Recommended Dosage:

- Powder: 1/4 to 1/2 tsp of cola nut powder daily
- Tincture: 1-2 dropperfuls taken in water up to 3 times daily
- Chewed: 1-2 nuts daily

Preparation Methods:

- Powder: Add to smoothies or beverages.
- Tincture: Take directly under the tongue or diluted in water.

- Chewed: Consume the raw nuts as is.

Coltsfoot (Tussilago farfara)

Traditional Applications: Coltsfoot has been used traditionally in European and Native American medicine for its ability to soothe respiratory issues. It is commonly used in teas, syrups, and poultices.

Health Benefits:

- Supports respiratory health
- Soothes coughs and colds
- Provides anti-inflammatory properties
- Aids in relieving sore throats

Recommended Dosage:

- Tea: 1-2 tsp of dried coltsfoot leaves per cup of boiling water, up to 3 times daily
- Syrup: 1-2 tbsp up to 3 times daily
- Tincture: 1-2 dropperfuls in water up to 3 times daily

Preparation Methods:

- Tea: Steep dried leaves in boiling water for 12-14 min.
- Syrup: Make by boiling leaves in water and adding honey.
- Tincture: Take directly under the tongue or diluted in water.

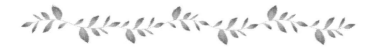

Comfrey (Symphytum officinale)

Traditional Applications: Comfrey has been used traditionally in European herbal medicine for its wound-healing and anti-inflammatory properties. It is often used in poultices, ointments, and teas.

Health Benefits:

- Supports wound healing

- Provides anti-inflammatory properties
- Aids in reducing pain and swelling
- Promotes skin health

Recommended Dosage:

- Poultice: Apply as needed to affected areas
- Ointment: Apply to skin 2-3 times daily
- Tea: 1-2 tsp of dried leaves per cup of boiling water, up to 3 times daily

Preparation Methods:

- Poultice: Crush fresh leaves and apply directly to the skin.
- Ointment: Use comfrey-infused oil or ointment on the skin.
- Tea: Steep dried leaves in boiling water for 12-14 min.

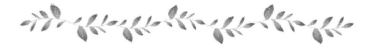

Coriander (Coriandrum sativum)

Traditional Applications: Coriander has been used in traditional medicine and cuisine in many cultures for its digestive and anti-inflammatory properties. Both the seeds and leaves (cilantro) are used in culinary and medicinal preparations.

Health Benefits:

- Supports digestive health
- Provides anti-inflammatory properties
- Helps lower blood sugar levels
- Offers antioxidant benefits

Recommended Dosage:

- Seeds: 1-2 tsp of crushed seeds daily
- Leaves: 1/4 to 1/2 cup of fresh leaves daily
- Tincture: 1-2 dropperfuls in water up to 3 times daily

Preparation Methods:

- Seeds: Use crushed seeds in cooking or as a tea.
- Leaves: Add fresh leaves to salads, salsas, and dishes.
- Tincture: Take directly under the tongue or diluted in water.

Corn Poppy (Papaver rhoeas)

Traditional Applications: Corn poppy, also known as field poppy, has been used traditionally in European folk medicine for its calming and mild sedative properties. It is often used in teas and infusions to promote relaxation and sleep.

Health Benefits:

- Promotes relaxation and sleep
- Provides mild sedative effects
- May help alleviate mild pain
- Supports respiratory health

Recommended Dosage:

- Tea: 1-2 tsp of dried petals per cup of boiling water, up to 3 times daily
- Tincture: 1-2 dropperfuls taken in water up to 3 times daily

Preparation Methods:

- Tea: Steep dried petals in boiling water for 12-14 min.
- Tincture: Take directly under the tongue or diluted in water.

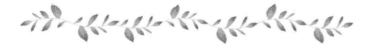

Cranberry (Vaccinium macrocarpon)

Traditional Applications: Cranberry has been traditionally used by Native Americans for its medicinal properties, particularly for urinary tract health. It is commonly used in juices, sauces, and as dried fruit.

Health Benefits:

- Supports urinary tract health
- Provides antioxidant benefits
- May help prevent urinary tract infections (UTIs)
- Supports overall immune health

Recommended Dosage:

- Juice: 8-16 oz of unsweetened cranberry juice daily
- Capsules: 1-2 capsules (equivalent to 400-800 mg) up to 3 times daily
- Dried Fruit: 1/4 to 1/2 cup daily

Preparation Methods:

- Juice: Drink pure, unsweetened cranberry juice.
- Capsules: Take as a dietary supplement with water.
- Dried Fruit: Add to cereals, salads, or eat as a snack.

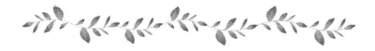

Cubeb (Piper cubeba)

Traditional Applications: Cubeb, also known as tailed pepper, has been used in traditional Chinese and Ayurvedic medicine for its digestive and respiratory benefits. It is often used as a spice and in herbal remedies.

Health Benefits:

- Supports digestive health
- Provides anti-inflammatory properties
- May help relieve respiratory issues
- Offers antimicrobial benefits

Recommended Dosage:

- Powder: 1/4 to 1/2 tsp daily
- Tincture: 1-2 dropperfuls taken in water up to 3 times daily

Preparation Methods:

- Powder: Add to food or beverages.
- Tincture: Take directly under the tongue or diluted in water.

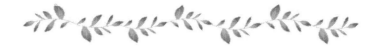

Cumin (Cuminum cyminum)

Traditional Applications: Cumin has been used in traditional medicine and cooking across various cultures for its digestive and anti-inflammatory properties. It is commonly used as a spice in culinary dishes and herbal preparations.

Health Benefits:

- Supports digestive health
- Provides anti-inflammatory properties
- May help boost immune function
- Offers antioxidant benefits

Recommended Dosage:

- Seeds: 1-2 tsp of ground cumin seeds daily
- Tea: 1-2 tsp of whole seeds per cup of boiling water, up to 3 times daily

Preparation Methods:

- Seeds: Use ground seeds as a spice in cooking.
- Tea: Steep whole seeds in boiling water for 12-14 min.

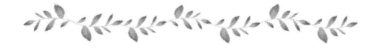

Curry Leaf (Murraya koenigii)

Traditional Applications: Curry leaf has been traditionally used in Indian and Ayurvedic medicine for its digestive and anti-inflammatory properties. It is commonly used in cooking to enhance the flavor of dishes.

Health Benefits:

- Supports digestive health
- Provides anti-inflammatory properties
- May help regulate blood sugar levels
- Offers antioxidant benefits

Recommended Dosage:

- Fresh Leaves: 1-2 tbsp daily
- Powder: 1-2 tsp daily
- Juice: 1/4 cup fresh leaf juice daily

Preparation Methods:

- Fresh Leaves: Use in cooking, soups, and stews.
- Powder: Add to food or beverages.
- Juice: Extract fresh juice from leaves and drink directly.

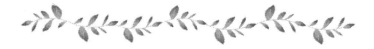

Damiana (Turnera diffusa)

Traditional Applications: Damiana has been used traditionally in Central and South American medicine as an aphrodisiac and for treating various conditions like depression and anxiety. It is often consumed as a tea or tincture.

Health Benefits:

- May help reduce anxiety and depression
- Supports sexual health and libido
- Provides mild stimulant effects
- Supports digestive health

Recommended Dosage:

- Tea: 1-2 tsp of dried leaves per cup of boiling water, up to 3 times daily
- Tincture: 1-2 dropperfuls up to 3 times daily

Preparation Methods:

- Tea: Steep dried leaves in boiling water for 12-14 min.
- Tincture: Take directly under the tongue or diluted in water.

Dandelion (Taraxacum officinale)

Traditional Applications: Dandelion has been used in traditional herbal medicine for its diuretic and detoxifying properties. It is commonly used to support liver and kidney health.

Health Benefits:

- Supports liver health and detoxification
- Acts as a natural diuretic
- Provides antioxidant benefits
- Supports digestive health

Recommended Dosage:

- Tea: 1-2 tsp of dried root or leaves per cup of boiling water, up to 3 times daily
- Tincture: 1-2 dropperfuls up to 3 times daily
- Capsules: 1-2 capsules (equivalent to 400-800 mg) up to 3 times daily

Preparation Methods:

- Tea: Steep dried root or leaves in boiling water for 12-14 min.
- Tincture: Take directly under the tongue or diluted in water.
- Capsules: Take as a dietary supplement with water.

Devil's Claw (Harpagophytum procumbens)

Traditional Applications: Devil's Claw has been traditionally used in African medicine for its anti-inflammatory and analgesic properties. It is often used to treat arthritis, back pain, and other inflammatory conditions.

Health Benefits:

- Provides anti-inflammatory and analgesic effects
- May help reduce pain and swelling
- Supports joint health
- May aid in digestive issues

Recommended Dosage:

- Tea: 1-2 tsp of dried root per cup of boiling water, up to 3 times daily
- Tincture: 1-2 dropperfuls up to 3 times daily
- Capsules: 1-2 capsules (equivalent to 400-800 mg) up to 3 times daily

Preparation Methods:

- Tea: Steep dried root in boiling water for 12-14 min.
- Tincture: Take directly under the tongue or diluted in water.
- Capsules: Take as a dietary supplement with water.

Dittany (Origanum dictamnus)

Traditional Applications: Dittany, also known as Cretan Dittany, has been traditionally used in Greek and Mediterranean medicine for its healing and antiseptic properties. It is often used for wound healing and as a digestive aid.

Health Benefits:

- Supports wound healing and skin health
- Provides antiseptic and antibacterial properties
- Aids in digestive health
- Offers anti-inflammatory benefits

Recommended Dosage:

- Tea: 1-2 tsp of dried leaves per cup of boiling water, up to 3 times daily
- Infusion: 1-2 tsp of dried leaves steeped in hot water for 12-14 min

Preparation Methods:

- Tea: Steep dried leaves in boiling water for 12-14 min.
- Infusion: Prepare by steeping dried leaves in hot water and consuming as a tea.

Dong Quai (Angelica sinensis)

Traditional Applications: Dong Quai, often referred to as "female ginseng," is widely used in Traditional Chinese Medicine (TCM) for supporting women's health, particularly in regulating menstruation and relieving menopausal symptoms.

Health Benefits:

- Supports women's reproductive health
- Helps regulate menstrual cycles
- Relieves menopausal symptoms
- Provides anti-inflammatory properties

Recommended Dosage:

- Decoction: 1-2 tsp of dried root per cup of boiling water, up to 3 times daily
- Tincture: 1-2 dropperfuls up to 3 times daily
- Capsules: 1-2 capsules (equivalent to 500-1000 mg) up to 3 times daily

Preparation Methods:

- Decoction: Simmer dried root in water for 20-30 min.
- Tincture: Take directly under the tongue or diluted in water.
- Capsules: Take as a dietary supplement with water.

Echinacea (Echinacea purpurea)

Traditional Applications: Echinacea has been used traditionally by Native Americans and in Western herbal medicine to boost the immune system and fight off infections, particularly colds and flu.

Health Benefits:

- Boosts immune system function
- Helps fight off colds and flu
- Provides anti-inflammatory effects
- Supports wound healing

Recommended Dosage:

- Tea: 1-2 tsp of dried root or leaves per cup of boiling water, up to 3 times daily
- Tincture: 1-2 dropperfuls up to 3 times daily
- Capsules: 1-2 capsules (equivalent to 400-800 mg) up to 3 times daily

Preparation Methods:

- Tea: Steep dried root or leaves in boiling water for 12-14 min.
- Tincture: Take directly under the tongue or diluted in water.
- Capsules: Take as a dietary supplement with water.

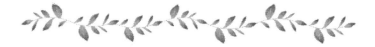

Elder (Sambucus nigra)

Traditional Applications: Elder, particularly the berries and flowers, has been used in traditional European medicine for its immune-boosting and antiviral properties. It is commonly used to treat colds, flu, and respiratory infections.

Health Benefits:

- Boosts immune system function
- Provides antiviral and antibacterial effects
- Helps alleviate cold and flu symptoms
- Supports respiratory health

Recommended Dosage:

- Tea: 1-2 tsp of dried flowers or berries per cup of boiling water, up to 3 times daily
- Tincture: 1-2 dropperfuls up to 3 times daily
- Syrup: 1-2 tbsp up to 3 times daily

Preparation Methods:

- Tea: Steep dried flowers or berries in boiling water for 12-14 min.
- Tincture: Take directly under the tongue or diluted in water.
- Syrup: Take as a dietary supplement, often prepared by simmering berries with honey.

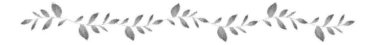

Elderberry (Sambucus nigra)

Traditional Applications: Elderberry has a long history in European folk medicine for treating respiratory issues and boosting the immune system. It is particularly known for its use in combating colds and flu.

Health Benefits:

- Strengthens the immune system
- Provides antiviral properties
- Reduces the severity and duration of cold and flu symptoms
- Offers antioxidant benefits

Recommended Dosage:

- Tea: 1-2 tsp of dried berries per cup of boiling water, up to 3 times daily
- Tincture: 1-2 dropperfuls up to 3 times daily
- Syrup: 1-2 tbsp up to 3 times daily

Preparation Methods:

- Tea: Steep dried berries in boiling water for 12-14 min.
- Tincture: Take directly under the tongue or diluted in water.
- Syrup: Often made by simmering elderberries with honey or sugar.

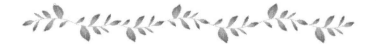

Elecampane (Inula helenium)

Traditional Applications: Elecampane has been used traditionally in European and Chinese medicine to treat respiratory conditions, such as bronchitis and asthma. It is also known for its digestive benefits.

Health Benefits:

- Supports respiratory health
- Provides expectorant properties to clear mucus
- Aids in digestion
- Offers antibacterial and antifungal effects

Recommended Dosage:

- Decoction: 1-2 tsp of dried root per cup of water, simmered for 20 min, up to 3 times daily
- Tincture: 1-2 dropperfuls up to 3 times daily

Preparation Methods:

- Decoction: Simmer dried root in water for 20 min.
- Tincture: Take directly under the tongue or diluted in water.

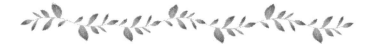

Eleuthero (Eleutherococcus senticosus)

Traditional Applications: Eleuthero, also known as Siberian ginseng, has been used in traditional Chinese and Russian medicine to enhance physical performance, reduce stress, and improve overall vitality.

Health Benefits:

- Increases energy and stamina
- Reduces stress and fatigue
- Enhances mental clarity
- Supports immune function

Recommended Dosage:

- Tea: 1-2 tsp of dried root per cup of boiling water, up to 3 times daily
- Tincture: 1-2 dropperfuls up to 3 times daily
- Capsules: 1-2 capsules (500-1000 mg) up to 3 times daily

Preparation Methods:

- Tea: Steep dried root in boiling water for 12-14 min.
- Tincture: Take directly under the tongue or diluted in water.
- Capsules: Take as a dietary supplement with water.

Eucalyptus (Eucalyptus globulus)

Traditional Applications: Eucalyptus has been used in traditional Australian Aboriginal medicine and later in Western medicine for its antiseptic and respiratory benefits. It is commonly used in steam inhalations and topical applications for respiratory issues.

Health Benefits:

- Supports respiratory health
- Provides antiseptic and antibacterial properties
- Helps alleviate congestion and sinus issues
- Reduces inflammation

Recommended Dosage:

- Steam Inhalation: Add a few drops of eucalyptus oil to a bowl of hot water and inhale the steam
- Topical Application: Dilute eucalyptus oil with a carrier oil and apply to the chest or affected area
- Tea: 1 tsp of dried leaves per cup of boiling water, up to 3 times daily

Preparation Methods:

- Steam Inhalation: Inhale steam from hot water with eucalyptus oil.
- Topical Application: Use diluted eucalyptus oil on the skin.
- Tea: Steep dried leaves in boiling water for 10 min.

Evening Primrose (Oenothera biennis)

Traditional Applications: Evening Primrose has been used traditionally by Native Americans and European settlers for its oil, which is believed to help with various conditions such as skin disorders and hormonal imbalances.

Health Benefits:

- Supports hormonal balance
- Eases symptoms of PMS and menopause
- Promotes skin health
- Reduces inflammation

Recommended Dosage:

- Capsules: 1-2 capsules (500-1000 mg) up to 3 times daily
- Oil: 1-2 tsp taken internally or applied topically

Preparation Methods:

- Capsules: Take with water as a dietary supplement.
- Oil: Can be consumed directly or applied to the skin for conditions like eczema or dryness.

False Unicorn Root (Chamaelirium luteum)

Traditional Applications: False Unicorn Root has been used in traditional Native American and folk medicine to support reproductive health, particularly for women. It is known for its use in treating menstrual issues and infertility.

Health Benefits:

- Supports reproductive health
- Alleviates menstrual cramps
- Balances hormones
- May aid in treating infertility

Recommended Dosage:

- Tincture: 1-2 dropperfuls up to 3 times daily
- Decoction: 1-2 tsp of dried root per cup of water, simmered for 20 min, up to 3 times daily

Preparation Methods:

- Tincture: Take directly under the tongue or diluted in water.
- Decoction: Simmer dried root in water for 20 min.

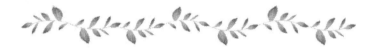

Fennel (Foeniculum vulgare)

Traditional Applications: Fennel has been used in traditional medicine for its digestive benefits and ability to relieve bloating and gas. It is also known for promoting lactation in nursing mothers.

Health Benefits:

- Aids in digestion
- Relieves bloating and gas
- Supports respiratory health
- Promotes lactation

Recommended Dosage:

- Tea: 1-2 tsp of crushed seeds per cup of boiling water, up to 3 times daily
- Tincture: 1-2 dropperfuls up to 3 times daily

Preparation Methods:

- Tea: Steep crushed seeds in boiling water for 12-14 min.

- Tincture: Take directly under the tongue or diluted in water.

Fenugreek (Trigonella foenum-graecum)

Traditional Applications: Fenugreek has been used traditionally in Middle Eastern and Indian medicine for its ability to enhance lactation and manage diabetes. It is also known for its use in treating digestive issues.

Health Benefits:

- Enhances lactation in nursing mothers
- Helps manage blood sugar levels
- Supports digestive health
- Reduces inflammation

Recommended Dosage:

- Capsules: 1-2 capsules (500-1000 mg) up to 3 times daily
- Tea: 1-2 tsp of seeds per cup of boiling water, up to 3 times daily
- Powder: 1-2 tsp added to food or smoothies

Preparation Methods:

- Capsules: Take with water as a dietary supplement.
- Tea: Steep seeds in boiling water for 12-14 min.
- Powder: Add to food or smoothies for nutritional benefits.

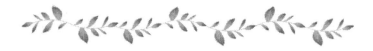

Fig (Ficus carica)

Traditional Applications: Figs have been used since ancient times in Mediterranean and Middle Eastern cultures for their nutritional and medicinal benefits. They are known for aiding digestion and providing a rich source of dietary fiber.

Health Benefits:

- Supports digestive health
- Rich in dietary fiber
- Promotes heart health
- Provides antioxidants

Recommended Dosage:

- Fresh Figs: 2-3 fresh figs daily
- Dried Figs: 2-4 dried figs daily

Preparation Methods:

- Fresh: Eat as a snack or add to salads and desserts.
- Dried: Can be eaten as a snack, added to baked goods, or rehydrated by soaking in water.

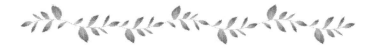

Fireweed (Epilobium angustifolium)

Traditional Applications: Fireweed has been used traditionally by Native Americans and Europeans for its anti-inflammatory properties and to treat various ailments, such as digestive issues and skin conditions.

Health Benefits:

- Reduces inflammation
- Supports digestive health
- Aids in skin healing
- Provides antioxidants

Recommended Dosage:

- Tea: 1-2 tsp of dried leaves per cup of boiling water, up to 3 times daily
- Tincture: 1-2 dropperfuls up to 3 times daily

Preparation Methods:

- Tea: Steep dried leaves in boiling water for 12-14 min.
- Tincture: Take directly under the tongue or diluted in water.

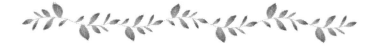

Flax (Linum usitatissimum)

Traditional Applications: Flax has been cultivated for thousands of years for its seeds and fibers. It is used traditionally for its nutritional benefits and to support digestive health.

Health Benefits:

- Rich in omega-3 fatty acids
- Supports digestive health
- Provides dietary fiber
- Helps manage cholesterol levels

Recommended Dosage:

- Ground Flaxseed: 1-2 tbsp daily
- Flaxseed Oil: 1-2 tsp daily

Preparation Methods:

- Ground Flaxseed: Add to smoothies, yogurt, or baked goods.
- Flaxseed Oil: Use in salad dressings or take directly.

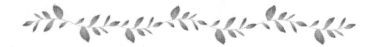

Flaxseed (Linum usitatissimum)

Traditional Applications: Flaxseed is known for its nutritional value and has been used for centuries to support digestive health, provide essential fatty acids, and promote overall well-being.

Health Benefits:

- High in omega-3 fatty acids
- Supports digestive health
- Rich in dietary fiber
- Helps reduce inflammation

Recommended Dosage:

- Whole or Ground Flaxseed: 1-2 tbsp daily
- Flaxseed Oil: 1-2 tsp daily

Preparation Methods:

- Whole or Ground: Add to cereals, smoothies, or baked goods.
- Flaxseed Oil: Use in salad dressings or take directly.

Frankincense (Boswellia sacra)

Traditional Applications: Frankincense has been used for thousands of years in religious ceremonies and traditional medicine, particularly in the Middle East and Africa. It is known for its anti-inflammatory and aromatic properties.

Health Benefits:

- Reduces inflammation
- Supports respiratory health
- Enhances skin health
- Provides stress relief

Recommended Dosage:

- Essential Oil: 1-2 drops in a diffuser or mixed with a carrier oil for topical use
- Resin: Chew a small piece (pea-sized) or use in incense

Preparation Methods:

- Essential Oil: Add to a diffuser, use in massage oils, or mix with lotion for skin application.
- Resin: Burn as incense or chew directly for digestive benefits.

Fumitory (Fumaria officinalis)

Traditional Applications: Fumitory has been used in European traditional medicine for its liver-supporting and detoxifying properties. It is commonly used to treat skin conditions and digestive issues.

Health Benefits:

- Supports liver health
- Aids in detoxification
- Helps treat skin conditions
- Promotes digestive health

Recommended Dosage:

- Tea: 1 tsp of dried herb per cup of boiling water, up to 3 times daily
- Tincture: 1-2 dropperfuls up to 3 times daily

Preparation Methods:

- Tea: Steep dried herb in boiling water for 12-14 min.
- Tincture: Take directly under the tongue or diluted in water.

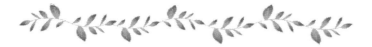

Galangal (Alpinia galanga)

Traditional Applications: Galangal is a staple in Southeast Asian cuisine and traditional medicine. It is known for its warming properties and is used to treat digestive issues, inflammation, and respiratory problems.

Health Benefits:

- Supports digestive health
- Reduces inflammation

- Enhances respiratory health
- Provides antioxidant benefits

Recommended Dosage:

- Fresh Root: 1-2 inches of fresh root, grated or sliced, daily
- Powder: 1-2 tsp daily

Preparation Methods:

- Fresh Root: Add to soups, stews, and teas.
- Powder: Use in cooking or mix with warm water to make tea.

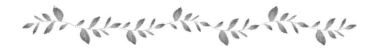

Gambir (Uncaria gambir)

Traditional Applications: Gambir has been used in traditional Chinese and Ayurvedic medicine for its astringent properties. It is commonly used to treat digestive issues, sore throats, and skin conditions.

Health Benefits:

- Supports digestive health
- Treats sore throats
- Promotes skin health
- Provides anti-inflammatory benefits

Recommended Dosage:

- Extract: 1-2 tsp daily
- Tea: 1 tsp of dried leaves per cup of boiling water, up to 3 times daily

Preparation Methods:

- Extract: Mix with water or take directly.
- Tea: Steep dried leaves in boiling water for 12-14 min.

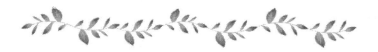

Garlic (Allium sativum)

Traditional Applications: Garlic has been used for its medicinal properties in many cultures around the world, particularly in traditional Chinese and Ayurvedic medicine. It is known for its immune-boosting, antibacterial, and cardiovascular benefits.

Health Benefits:

- Supports cardiovascular health
- Boosts the immune system
- Acts as a natural antibiotic
- Reduces blood pressure

Recommended Dosage:

- Fresh Cloves: 1-2 cloves daily
- Powder: 1/4 to 1/2 tsp daily

Preparation Methods:

- Fresh Cloves: Eat raw, add to cooking, or crush and mix with honey.
- Powder: Use in cooking or mix with warm water for a drink.

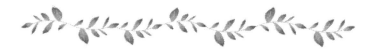

Gentian (Gentiana lutea)

Traditional Applications: Gentian has been used in European herbal medicine for centuries, especially as a digestive tonic. It is known for its bitter properties and is often used to stimulate appetite and aid digestion.

Health Benefits:

- Stimulates appetite
- Aids in digestion
- Supports liver health

- Reduces inflammation

Recommended Dosage:

- Tincture: 1-2 dropperfuls before meals
- Tea: 1 tsp of dried root per cup of boiling water, up to 3 times daily

Preparation Methods:

- Tincture: Take directly under the tongue or dilute in water.
- Tea: Steep dried root in boiling water for 12-14 min.

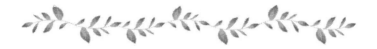

Ginger (Zingiber officinale)

Traditional Applications: Ginger has been widely used in traditional Chinese, Ayurvedic, and other herbal medicines for its warming and anti-nausea properties. It is known to aid digestion, reduce inflammation, and alleviate nausea.

Health Benefits:

- Reduces nausea
- Supports digestive health
- Acts as an anti-inflammatory
- Boosts the immune system

Recommended Dosage:

- Fresh Root: 1-2 inches grated or sliced daily
- Powder: 1/2 to 1 tsp daily

Preparation Methods:

- Fresh Root: Add to teas, soups, or juices.
- Powder: Use in cooking or mix with warm water for a tea.

Ginkgo Biloba (Ginkgo biloba)

Traditional Applications: Ginkgo biloba has been used in traditional Chinese medicine for thousands of years, primarily to enhance cognitive function and improve blood circulation. It is known for its powerful antioxidant properties.

Health Benefits:

- Enhances memory and cognitive function
- Improves blood circulation
- Acts as an antioxidant
- Supports mental clarity and focus

Recommended Dosage:

- Leaf Extract: 1/4 to 1/2 tsp of standardized extract daily
- Tea: 1-2 tsp of dried leaves per cup of boiling water, up to 3 times daily

Preparation Methods:

- Leaf Extract: Take in capsule or liquid form.
- Tea: Steep dried leaves in boiling water for 12-14 min.

Ginseng (Panax ginseng)

Traditional Applications: Ginseng has been a cornerstone in traditional Chinese medicine for centuries. It is used to boost energy, reduce stress, and promote overall vitality and longevity.

Health Benefits:

- Boosts energy and stamina
- Reduces stress and promotes relaxation
- Enhances immune function
- Improves cognitive function

Recommended Dosage:

- Root Powder: 1/4 to 1/2 tsp daily
- Tea: 1-2 slices of dried root per cup of boiling water, up to 3 times daily

Preparation Methods:

- Root Powder: Mix with water, juice, or add to smoothies.
- Tea: Steep dried root slices in boiling water for 12-14 min.

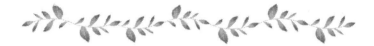

Goldenseal (Hydrastis canadensis)

Traditional Applications: Goldenseal has been widely used in Native American and traditional Western herbal medicine. It is valued for its antimicrobial properties and is often used to treat infections and digestive issues.

Health Benefits:

- Acts as a natural antibiotic
- Supports digestive health
- Boosts immune function
- Reduces inflammation

Recommended Dosage:

- Root Powder: 1/4 to 1/2 tsp daily
- Tincture: 1-2 dropperfuls up to 3 times daily

Preparation Methods:

- Root Powder: Mix with water or juice.
- Tincture: Take directly under the tongue or dilute in water.

Gotu Kola (Centella asiatica)

Traditional Applications: Gotu Kola is a staple in Ayurvedic and traditional Chinese medicine. It is used to improve mental clarity, support wound healing, and promote longevity.

Health Benefits:

- Enhances cognitive function
- Supports wound healing
- Reduces anxiety and stress
- Promotes skin health

Recommended Dosage:

- Leaf Powder: 1/4 to 1/2 tsp daily
- Tea: 1-2 tsp of dried leaves per cup of boiling water, up to 3 times daily

Preparation Methods:

- Leaf Powder: Mix with water, juice, or add to smoothies.
- Tea: Steep dried leaves in boiling water for 12-14 min.

Green Tea (Camellia sinensis)

Traditional Applications: Green tea has been consumed in China and Japan for centuries for its health benefits. It is used to promote longevity, boost energy, and improve mental alertness.

Health Benefits:

- Rich in antioxidants
- Boosts metabolism and aids in weight loss
- Enhances brain function and alertness
- Supports heart health

Recommended Dosage:

- Tea: 1 tsp of dried leaves per cup of boiling water, up to 3 times daily

Preparation Methods:

- Tea: Steep dried leaves in boiling water for 2-3 min. Avoid oversteeping to prevent bitterness.

Hawthorn (Crataegus monogyna)

Traditional Applications: Hawthorn has been used in traditional European herbal medicine for centuries, particularly for heart-related ailments. It is known to improve cardiovascular health and circulation.

Health Benefits:

- Supports cardiovascular health
- Improves blood circulation
- Acts as an antioxidant
- Reduces blood pressure

Recommended Dosage:

- Berry Extract: 1/4 to 1/2 tsp daily
- Tea: 1-2 tsp of dried berries per cup of boiling water, up to 3 times daily

Preparation Methods:

- Berry Extract: Take in capsule or liquid form.
- Tea: Steep dried berries in boiling water for 12-14 min.

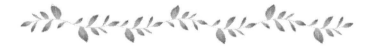

Holy Basil (Ocimum sanctum)

Traditional Applications: Holy Basil, also known as Tulsi, is revered in Ayurvedic medicine for its adaptogenic properties. It is used to reduce stress, support immune function, and promote overall wellness.

Health Benefits:

- Reduces stress and anxiety

- Supports immune function
- Acts as an antioxidant
- Promotes respiratory health

Recommended Dosage:

- Leaf Powder: 1/4 to 1/2 tsp daily
- Tea: 1-2 tsp of dried leaves per cup of boiling water, up to 3 times daily

Preparation Methods:

- Leaf Powder: Mix with water, juice, or add to smoothies.
- Tea: Steep dried leaves in boiling water for 5-10 min.

Horsetail (Equisetum arvense)

Traditional Applications: Horsetail has been used for centuries in traditional European and Chinese medicine. It is valued for its diuretic properties and ability to support bone health.

Health Benefits:

- Promotes bone health and supports bone density
- Acts as a diuretic, aiding in fluid retention and urinary issues
- Supports wound healing
- Rich in silica, promoting hair, skin, and nail health

Recommended Dosage:

- Tea: 1-2 tsp of dried herb per cup of boiling water, up to 3 times daily
- Tincture: 1/2 to 1 tsp, up to 3 times daily

Preparation Methods:

- Tea: Steep dried herb in boiling water for 12-14 min.
- Tincture: Take in liquid form, mix with water or juice if desired.

Hops (Humulus lupulus)

Traditional Applications: Hops have been traditionally used in European herbal medicine for their calming effects. They are commonly used to promote sleep and alleviate anxiety.

Health Benefits:

- Promotes relaxation and reduces anxiety
- Supports healthy sleep patterns
- Acts as a digestive aid
- Contains antioxidant and anti-inflammatory properties

Recommended Dosage:

- Tea: 1-2 tsp of dried flowers per cup of boiling water, up to 3 times daily
- Tincture: 1/2 to 1 tsp, up to 3 times daily

Preparation Methods:

- Tea: Steep dried flowers in boiling water for 12-14 min.
- Tincture: Take in liquid form, mix with water or juice if desired.

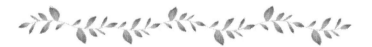

Jiaogulan (Gynostemma pentaphyllum)

Traditional Applications: Jiaogulan, known as "Southern Ginseng" in traditional Chinese medicine, is used for its adaptogenic and longevity-promoting properties.

Health Benefits:

- Acts as an adaptogen, reducing stress and fatigue
- Supports cardiovascular health
- Boosts immune function
- Contains antioxidant properties

Recommended Dosage:

- Tea: 1-2 tsp of dried leaves per cup of boiling water, up to 3 times daily
- Capsule: 500-1000 mg daily

Preparation Methods:

- Tea: Steep dried leaves in boiling water for 5-10 min.
- Capsule: Take as directed on the package.

Juniper (Juniperus communis)

Traditional Applications: Juniper berries have been used in traditional medicine for their diuretic properties and to support digestive health. They are also used in culinary applications and for making gin.

Health Benefits:

- Acts as a diuretic, aiding in urinary tract health
- Supports digestive health
- Contains antioxidant and anti-inflammatory properties
- May help manage blood sugar levels

Recommended Dosage:

- Tea: 1 tsp of crushed berries per cup of boiling water, up to 3 times daily
- Tincture: 1/2 to 1 tsp, up to 3 times daily

Preparation Methods:

- Tea: Steep crushed berries in boiling water for 12-14 min.
- Tincture: Take in liquid form, mix with water or juice if desired.

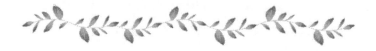

Kava Kava (Piper methysticum)

Traditional Applications: Kava Kava has been used for centuries in the Pacific Islands for its calming and relaxing properties. It is traditionally consumed in social and ceremonial contexts to promote relaxation and sociability.

Health Benefits:

- Promotes relaxation and reduces anxiety
- Supports restful sleep
- Alleviates symptoms of stress
- Acts as a muscle relaxant

Recommended Dosage:

- Tea: 1-2 tsp of dried root per cup of water, up to 3 times daily
- Tincture: 1/2 to 1 tsp, up to 3 times daily

Preparation Methods:

- Tea: Simmer dried root in water for 12-14 min, then strain.
- Tincture: Take in liquid form, mix with water or juice if desired.

Kudzu (Pueraria lobata)

Traditional Applications: Kudzu has been used in traditional Chinese medicine for its cooling and detoxifying properties. It is often used to treat alcohol dependency and to alleviate symptoms of hangovers.

Health Benefits:

- Supports detoxification, particularly from alcohol
- Alleviates symptoms of headaches and hangovers
- Promotes cardiovascular health
- Contains anti-inflammatory properties

Recommended Dosage:

- Tea: 1-2 tsp of dried root per cup of boiling water, up to 3 times daily
- Capsule: 500-1000 mg daily

Preparation Methods:

- Tea: Steep dried root in boiling water for 12-14 min.
- Capsule: Take as directed on the package.

Lavender (Lavandula angustifolia)

Traditional Applications: Lavender has been used in traditional European and Mediterranean medicine for its calming and soothing properties. It is often used to promote relaxation and alleviate anxiety and insomnia.

Health Benefits:

- Promotes relaxation and reduces anxiety
- Supports restful sleep
- Alleviates headaches and migraines
- Contains anti-inflammatory and antimicrobial properties

Recommended Dosage:

- Tea: 1-2 tsp of dried flowers per cup of boiling water, up to 3 times daily
- Tincture: 1/2 to 1 tsp, up to 3 times daily

Preparation Methods:

- Tea: Steep dried flowers in boiling water for 12-14 min.
- Tincture: Take in liquid form, mix with water or juice if desired.

Lemon Balm (Melissa officinalis)

Traditional Applications: Lemon Balm has been used in traditional European herbal medicine for its calming and uplifting properties. It is often used to alleviate anxiety, promote sleep, and improve digestive health.

Health Benefits:

- Promotes relaxation and reduces anxiety
- Supports restful sleep
- Improves digestive health
- Contains antiviral and antioxidant properties

Recommended Dosage:

- Tea: 1-2 tsp of dried leaves per cup of boiling water, up to 3 times daily
- Tincture: 1/2 to 1 tsp, up to 3 times daily

Preparation Methods:

- Tea: Steep dried leaves in boiling water for 12-14 min.
- Tincture: Take in liquid form, mix with water or juice if desired.

Lemon Verbena (Aloysia citrodora)

Traditional Applications: Lemon Verbena has been used in traditional Mediterranean and South American herbal medicine for its refreshing lemon scent and flavor. It is often used to aid digestion and relieve stress.

Health Benefits:

- Promotes relaxation and reduces anxiety
- Aids in digestion and relieves bloating
- Contains anti-inflammatory and antioxidant properties
- Supports respiratory health

Recommended Dosage:

- Tea: 1-2 tsp of dried leaves per cup of boiling water, up to 3 times daily
- Tincture: 1/2 to 1 tsp, up to 3 times daily

Preparation Methods:

- Tea: Steep dried leaves in boiling water for 12-14 min.
- Tincture: Take in liquid form, mix with water or juice if desired.

Licorice (Glycyrrhiza glabra)

Traditional Applications: Licorice has been used in traditional Chinese and Ayurvedic medicine for its sweet flavor and health benefits. It is often used to soothe sore throats and support digestive and respiratory health.

Health Benefits:

- Soothes sore throats and coughs
- Supports digestive health
- Contains anti-inflammatory and immune-boosting properties
- Helps manage stress and adrenal fatigue

Recommended Dosage:

- Tea: 1-2 tsp of dried root per cup of boiling water, up to 3 times daily
- Tincture: 1/2 to 1 tsp, up to 3 times daily

Preparation Methods:

- Tea: Simmer dried root in water for 12-14 min, then strain.
- Tincture: Take in liquid form, mix with water or juice if desired.

Linden Flower (Tilia cordata)

Traditional Applications: Linden Flower has been traditionally used in European and Native American medicine for its calming and anti-inflammatory properties. It is often used to treat colds, coughs, fever, anxiety, and insomnia.

Health Benefits:

- Reduces anxiety and promotes relaxation
- Alleviates symptoms of colds and respiratory infections
- Acts as an anti-inflammatory
- Induces sweating to reduce fever

Recommended Dosage:

- Tea: 1-2 tsp of dried Linden flowers per cup of boiling water, steep for 10-15 min, up to 3 times daily
- Tincture: 1-2 droppersful, up to 3 times daily

Preparation Methods:

- Tea: Steep dried Linden flowers in boiling water for 10-15 min.
- Tincture: Take as directed on the product label.
- Capsules: Take as directed on the product label.

Maca (Lepidium meyenii)

Traditional Applications: Maca has been used for centuries in traditional Peruvian medicine as a natural energy booster and hormone balancer. It is often consumed to enhance stamina, endurance, and fertility.

Health Benefits:

- Enhances energy and stamina
- Supports hormonal balance

- Improves mood and mental clarity
- Boosts fertility and sexual health

Recommended Dosage:

- Powder: 1-3 tsp daily, added to smoothies or foods
- Capsule: 500-1000 mg daily

Preparation Methods:

- Powder: Add to smoothies, oatmeal, or baked goods.
- Capsule: Take as directed on the package.

Marshmallow Root (Althaea officinalis)

Traditional Applications: Marshmallow Root has been used in traditional European and Middle Eastern medicine for its soothing and demulcent properties. It is commonly used to treat coughs, sore throats, and digestive issues.

Health Benefits:

- Soothes sore throats and coughs
- Supports digestive health
- Contains anti-inflammatory properties
- Promotes skin health and healing

Recommended Dosage:

- Tea: 1-2 tsp of dried root per cup of boiling water, up to 3 times daily
- Tincture: 1/2 to 1 tsp, up to 3 times daily

Preparation Methods:

- Tea: Simmer dried root in water for 12-14 min, then strain.
- Tincture: Take in liquid form, mix with water or juice if desired.

Meadowsweet (Filipendula ulmaria)

Traditional Applications: Meadowsweet has been used in traditional European medicine for its anti-inflammatory and pain-relieving properties. It is often used to treat headaches, fevers, and digestive issues.

Health Benefits:

- Relieves pain and inflammation
- Reduces fever
- Supports digestive health
- Contains anti-ulcer properties

Recommended Dosage:

- Tea: 1-2 tsp of dried flowers per cup of boiling water, up to 3 times daily
- Tincture: 1/2 to 1 tsp, up to 3 times daily

Preparation Methods:

- Tea: Steep dried flowers in boiling water for 12-14 min.
- Tincture: Take in liquid form, mix with water or juice if desired.

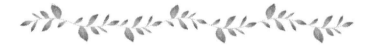

Milk Thistle (Silybum marianum)

Traditional Applications: Milk Thistle has been used in traditional European and Chinese medicine to support liver health and detoxification. It is commonly used to treat liver and gallbladder disorders.

Health Benefits:

- Supports liver health and detoxification
- Protects against liver damage
- Contains antioxidant and anti-inflammatory properties

- Promotes healthy skin

Recommended Dosage:

- Extract: 1-3 tsp of milk thistle extract daily
- Capsule: 1-2 capsules of standardized extract daily

Preparation Methods:

- Extract: Add to water or juice and consume.
- Capsule: Take as directed on the package.

Moringa (Moringa oleifera)

Traditional Applications: Moringa, known as the "miracle tree," has been used in traditional African and Indian medicine for its nutrient-rich leaves and seeds. It is used to boost energy, support the immune system, and improve overall health.

Health Benefits:

- Rich in vitamins, minerals, and antioxidants
- Boosts energy and stamina
- Supports immune health
- Promotes healthy skin and hair

Recommended Dosage:

- Powder: 1-2 tsp of moringa powder daily
- Capsule: 1-2 capsules daily

Preparation Methods:

- Powder: Add to smoothies, soups, or teas.
- Capsule: Take as directed on the package.

Mucuna Pruriens (Velvet Bean)

Traditional Applications: Mucuna Pruriens has been used in traditional Ayurvedic medicine for its neuroprotective and mood-enhancing properties. It is commonly used to support mental health and improve libido.

Health Benefits:

- Supports mental health and cognitive function
- Enhances mood and reduces anxiety
- Boosts libido and sexual health
- Contains antioxidant properties

Recommended Dosage:

- Powder: 1-2 tsp of mucuna powder daily
- Capsule: 1-2 capsules daily

Preparation Methods:

- Powder: Add to smoothies, teas, or foods.
- Capsule: Take as directed on the package.

Mullein (Verbascum thapsus)

Traditional Applications: Mullein has been used in traditional European and Native American medicine for respiratory health. It is commonly used to treat coughs, colds, and bronchitis.

Health Benefits:

- Soothes respiratory issues
- Reduces inflammation

- Acts as an expectorant
- Supports ear health

Recommended Dosage:

- Tea: 1-2 tsp of dried leaves per cup of boiling water, up to 3 times daily
- Tincture: 1/2 to 1 tsp, up to 3 times daily

Preparation Methods:

- Tea: Steep dried leaves in boiling water for 12-14 min.
- Tincture: Take in liquid form, mix with water or juice if desired.

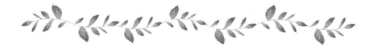

Neem (Azadirachta indica)

Traditional Applications: Neem has been used in traditional Indian and Ayurvedic medicine for its antimicrobial and anti-inflammatory properties. It is used to support skin health, detoxify the body, and boost the immune system.

Health Benefits:

- Supports skin health and treats acne
- Detoxifies the body
- Enhances immune function
- Acts as an anti-inflammatory and antimicrobial agent

Recommended Dosage:

- Powder: 1/2 to 1 tsp of neem powder daily
- Capsule: 1-2 capsules daily

Preparation Methods:

- Powder: Add to smoothies, teas, or foods.
- Capsule: Take as directed on the package.

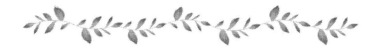

Nettle (Urtica dioica)

Traditional Applications: Nettle has been used in traditional European and Native American medicine for its nutritive and anti-inflammatory properties. It is used to treat allergies, support joint health, and improve overall wellness.

Health Benefits:

- Reduces allergy symptoms
- Supports joint health and reduces inflammation
- Promotes urinary health
- Rich in vitamins and minerals

Recommended Dosage:

- Tea: 1-2 tsp of dried leaves per cup of boiling water, up to 3 times daily
- Tincture: 1/2 to 1 tsp, up to 3 times daily

Preparation Methods:

- Tea: Steep dried leaves in boiling water for 12-14 min.
- Tincture: Take in liquid form, mix with water or juice if desired.

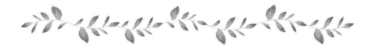

Nutmeg (Myristica fragrans)

Traditional Applications: Nutmeg has been used in traditional Chinese and Indian medicine for its digestive and anti-inflammatory properties. It is used to treat digestive issues, improve sleep, and enhance cognitive function.

Health Benefits:

- Aids digestion and relieves nausea
- Improves sleep quality
- Enhances cognitive function

- Contains anti-inflammatory and antioxidant properties

Recommended Dosage:

- Powder: 1/4 to 1/2 tsp of nutmeg powder daily
- Essential Oil: 1-2 drops, diluted in a carrier oil

Preparation Methods:

- Powder: Add to teas, foods, or desserts.
- Essential Oil: Use topically, diluted in a carrier oil, or diffuse for aromatherapy.

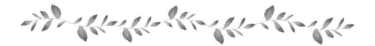

Olive Leaf (Olea europaea)

Traditional Applications: Olive leaf has been used in Mediterranean and Middle Eastern traditional medicine for its immune-boosting and cardiovascular benefits. It is commonly used to treat infections, support heart health, and reduce inflammation.

Health Benefits:

- Enhances immune function
- Supports cardiovascular health
- Reduces inflammation
- Antioxidant properties

Recommended Dosage:

- Tea: 1-2 tsp of dried leaves per cup of boiling water, up to 3 times daily
- Extract: 1/4 to 1/2 tsp of olive leaf extract, up to 3 times daily

Preparation Methods:

- Tea: Steep dried leaves in boiling water for 12-14 min.
- Extract: Take in liquid form, mix with water or juice if desired.

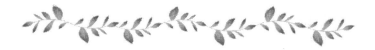

Oregano (Origanum vulgare)

Traditional Applications: Oregano has been used in traditional European and Mediterranean medicine for its antimicrobial and digestive benefits. It is used to treat respiratory and gastrointestinal issues and to support overall immune health.

Health Benefits:

- Antimicrobial properties
- Supports respiratory health
- Aids digestion
- Enhances immune function

Recommended Dosage:

- Tea: 1-2 tsp of dried leaves per cup of boiling water, up to 3 times daily
- Oil: 1-2 drops of oregano oil, diluted in a carrier oil

Preparation Methods:

- Tea: Steep dried leaves in boiling water for 12-14 min.
- Oil: Use topically, diluted in a carrier oil, or take internally with guidance.

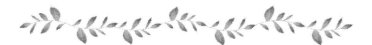

Passionflower (Passiflora incarnata)

Traditional Applications: Passionflower has been used in traditional Native American and European medicine for its calming and sedative effects. It is commonly used to treat anxiety, insomnia, and nervous disorders.

Health Benefits:

- Reduces anxiety and stress
- Improves sleep quality
- Calms nervous system
- Anti-inflammatory properties

Recommended Dosage:

- Tea: 1-2 tsp of dried flowers per cup of boiling water, up to 3 times daily
- Tincture: 1-2 dropperfuls, up to 3 times daily

Preparation Methods:

- Tea: Steep dried flowers in boiling water for 12-14 min.
- Tincture: Take in liquid form, mix with water or juice if desired.

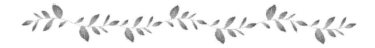

Peppermint (Mentha x piperita)

Traditional Applications: Peppermint has been used in traditional European and Middle Eastern medicine for its digestive and cooling properties. It is commonly used to treat indigestion, headaches, and respiratory issues.

Health Benefits:

- Aids digestion and relieves nausea
- Eases headaches and migraines
- Supports respiratory health
- Provides a cooling sensation and reduces muscle pain

Recommended Dosage:

- Tea: 1-2 tsp of dried leaves per cup of boiling water, up to 3 times daily
- Oil: 1-2 drops of peppermint oil, diluted in a carrier oil

Preparation Methods:

- Tea: Steep dried leaves in boiling water for 12-14 min.
- Oil: Use topically, diluted in a carrier oil, or inhale for aromatherapy.

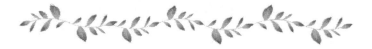

Prickly Pear Cactus (Opuntia ficus-indica)

Traditional Applications: Prickly pear cactus has been used in traditional Mexican and Native American medicine for its ability to regulate blood sugar levels and support digestive health. It is also known for its anti-inflammatory properties.

Health Benefits:

- Regulates blood sugar levels
- Supports digestive health
- Reduces inflammation
- Provides antioxidants

Recommended Dosage:

- Juice: 1/2 to 1 cup daily
- Powder: 1-2 tsp daily, mixed in water or juice

Preparation Methods:

- Juice: Extract juice from the cactus pads and consume fresh.
- Powder: Use dried and powdered cactus pads, mix with water or juice.

Psyllium (Plantago ovata)

Traditional Applications: Psyllium has been used in traditional Indian and Ayurvedic medicine for its high fiber content, which helps regulate digestion and promote bowel health. It is commonly used as a natural laxative.

Health Benefits:

- Promotes bowel regularity
- Supports digestive health
- Helps manage cholesterol levels
- Aids in weight management

Recommended Dosage:

- Whole Husks: 1-2 tbsp mixed in water, up to 3 times daily
- Powder: 1-2 tsp mixed in water, up to 3 times daily

Preparation Methods:

- Whole Husks: Mix with water, juice, or smoothies and consume immediately.
- Powder: Mix with water or juice, stir well, and drink immediately.

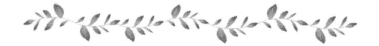

Red Clover (Trifolium pratense)

Traditional Applications: Red clover has been used in traditional European and Native American medicine for its blood-purifying properties and to support women's health. It is often used to treat menopausal symptoms and skin conditions.

Health Benefits:

- Supports women's health and hormone balance
- Purifies blood
- Promotes skin health
- Provides anti-inflammatory benefits

Recommended Dosage:

- Tea: 1-2 tsp of dried flowers per cup of boiling water, up to 3 times daily
- Tincture: 1-2 dropperfuls, up to 3 times daily

Preparation Methods:

- Tea: Steep dried flowers in boiling water for 12-14 min.
- Tincture: Take in liquid form, mix with water or juice if desired.

Red Raspberry Leaf (Rubus idaeus)

Traditional Applications: Red raspberry leaf has been used in traditional European and Native American medicine to support women's reproductive health, particularly during pregnancy and childbirth. It is known for its ability to strengthen the uterus.

Health Benefits:

- Supports reproductive health
- Strengthens the uterus
- Reduces menstrual cramps
- Provides vitamins and minerals

Recommended Dosage:

- Tea: 1-2 tsp of dried leaves per cup of boiling water, up to 3 times daily
- Capsules: 1-2 capsules, up to 3 times daily

Preparation Methods:

- Tea: Steep dried leaves in boiling water for 12-14 min.
- Capsules: Take with water as directed.

Reishi Mushroom (Ganoderma lucidum)

Traditional Applications: Reishi mushroom has been used for thousands of years in traditional Chinese medicine to promote longevity, enhance the immune system, and reduce stress. It is often referred to as the "mushroom of immortality."

Health Benefits:

- Boosts the immune system
- Reduces stress and fatigue
- Supports liver health
- Provides anti-inflammatory and antioxidant properties

Recommended Dosage:

- Capsules: 1-2 capsules, 2-3 times daily
- Tea: 1-2 cups daily, using 1 tsp of dried mushroom per cup of water

Preparation Methods:

- Capsules: Take with water as directed.
- Tea: Simmer dried reishi slices in water for at least 30 min, strain, and drink.

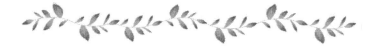

Rhodiola (Rhodiola rosea)

Traditional Applications: Rhodiola has been used in traditional Russian and Scandinavian medicine for centuries to enhance physical and mental endurance, combat fatigue, and improve resilience to stress.

Health Benefits:

- Enhances mental and physical performance
- Reduces fatigue
- Supports stress resilience
- Improves mood

Recommended Dosage:

- Capsules: 1-2 capsules, 1-2 times daily
- Tincture: 1-2 dropperfuls, up to 3 times daily

Preparation Methods:

- Capsules: Take with water as directed.
- Tincture: Take in liquid form, mix with water or juice if desired.

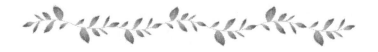

Rosemary (Salvia rosmarinus)

Traditional Applications: Rosemary has been used in Mediterranean traditional medicine for its memory-enhancing properties and to support digestion. It is also commonly used in culinary applications.

Health Benefits:

- Enhances memory and concentration
- Supports digestive health
- Provides antioxidant and anti-inflammatory benefits
- Improves circulation

Recommended Dosage:

- Tea: 1-2 tsp of dried leaves per cup of boiling water, up to 3 times daily
- Essential Oil: 2-3 drops diluted in carrier oil for topical use or aromatherapy

Preparation Methods:

- Tea: Steep dried leaves in boiling water for 12-14 min.
- Essential Oil: Dilute in carrier oil for massage or add to a diffuser for aromatherapy.

Saffron (Crocus sativus)

Traditional Applications: Saffron has been used in traditional Persian and Ayurvedic medicine for its mood-enhancing properties and to support digestion and menstrual health. It is also valued as a culinary spice.

Health Benefits:

- Enhances mood and alleviates depression
- Supports digestive health
- Relieves menstrual discomfort
- Provides antioxidant benefits

Recommended Dosage:

- Tea: A few strands per cup of boiling water, 1-2 times daily
- Capsules: 1 capsule, up to 2 times daily

Preparation Methods:

- Tea: Steep a few strands in boiling water for 5-10 min.
- Capsules: Take with water as directed.

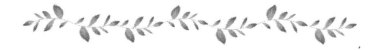

Sage (Salvia officinalis)

Traditional Applications: Sage has been used for centuries in traditional European medicine for its antiseptic and anti-inflammatory properties. It has been commonly used to treat digestive issues, sore throats, and to enhance memory.

Health Benefits:

- Improves cognitive function and memory
- Supports digestive health
- Provides anti-inflammatory and antioxidant benefits
- Helps relieve sore throats and coughs

Recommended Dosage:

- Tea: 1-2 tsp of dried leaves per cup of boiling water, up to 3 times daily
- Tincture: 1-2 dropperfuls, 2-3 times daily

Preparation Methods:

- Tea: Steep dried leaves in boiling water for 12-14 min.
- Tincture: Take in liquid form, mix with water or juice if desired.

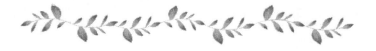

Saw Palmetto (Serenoa repens)

Traditional Applications: Saw palmetto has been used in traditional Native American medicine for its benefits to urinary and reproductive health. It is particularly well-known for supporting prostate health in men.

Health Benefits:

- Supports prostate health
- Reduces urinary tract symptoms
- Balances hormone levels
- Provides anti-inflammatory properties

Recommended Dosage:

- Capsules: 1-2 capsules, 1-2 times daily
- Extract: 1-2 tsp of liquid extract, up to 3 times daily

Preparation Methods:

- Capsules: Take with water as directed.
- Extract: Take in liquid form, mix with water or juice if desired.

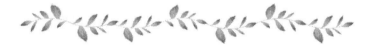

Schisandra (Schisandra chinensis)

Traditional Applications: Schisandra has been used in traditional Chinese medicine for centuries as an adaptogen to improve stamina and mental clarity. It is known as a "five-flavor berry" due to its complex taste profile.

Health Benefits:

- Enhances stamina and endurance
- Supports liver function
- Reduces stress and fatigue
- Improves mental clarity and focus

Recommended Dosage:

- Berries: 1-2 tbsp of dried berries, up to 3 times daily
- Tincture: 1-2 dropperfuls, 2-3 times daily

Preparation Methods:

- Berries: Eat dried berries as a snack or steep in boiling water for tea.
- Tincture: Take in liquid form, mix with water or juice if desired.

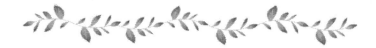

Skullcap (Scutellaria lateriflora)

Traditional Applications: Skullcap has been used in traditional Native American and Chinese medicine for its calming properties and to treat insomnia, anxiety, and nervous tension.

Health Benefits:

- Reduces anxiety and nervous tension
- Supports restful sleep
- Provides anti-inflammatory benefits
- Relieves muscle spasms

Recommended Dosage:

- Tea: 1-2 tsp of dried leaves per cup of boiling water, up to 3 times daily
- Tincture: 1-2 dropperfuls, 2-3 times daily

Preparation Methods:

- Tea: Steep dried leaves in boiling water for 12-14 min.
- Tincture: Take in liquid form, mix with water or juice if desired.

Slippery Elm (Ulmus rubra)

Traditional Applications: Slippery elm has been used by Native American tribes for its soothing and healing properties, especially for sore throats, coughs, and digestive issues. The inner bark is known for its mucilaginous texture, which helps coat and soothe irritated tissues.

Health Benefits:

- Soothes sore throats and coughs
- Alleviates digestive discomfort
- Supports healing of the gastrointestinal tract
- Provides anti-inflammatory benefits

Recommended Dosage:

- Powder: 1-2 tsp of powdered bark, up to 3 times daily
- Lozenges: 1-2 lozenges, as needed

Preparation Methods:

- Tea: Mix powdered bark with hot water to create a soothing tea.
- Lozenges: Dissolve slowly in the mouth to soothe throat irritation.

Solomon's Seal (Polygonatum biflorum)

Traditional Applications: Solomon's Seal has been used in traditional medicine to support joint health, heal wounds, and balance bodily fluids. It is known for its ability to help with ligament and tendon injuries.

Health Benefits:

- Supports joint and tendon health
- Promotes healing of wounds and bruises
- Balances bodily fluids and helps with hydration
- Reduces inflammation

Recommended Dosage:

- Tincture: 1-2 dropperfuls, 2-3 times daily
- Decoction: 1-2 cups of decoction, up to 3 times daily

Preparation Methods:

- Tincture: Take in liquid form, mix with water or juice if desired.
- Decoction: Simmer the roots in water for 20-30 min to make a decoction.

Spearmint (Mentha spicata)

Traditional Applications: Spearmint has been widely used in traditional medicine for its digestive and respiratory benefits. It is often used to soothe upset stomachs, reduce nausea, and freshen breath.

Health Benefits:

- Soothes digestive issues and reduces nausea
- Supports respiratory health
- Freshens breath and supports oral health
- Provides a calming and refreshing effect

Recommended Dosage:

- Tea: 1-2 tsp of dried leaves per cup of boiling water, up to 3 times daily
- Fresh Leaves: Chew on a few fresh leaves, as needed

Preparation Methods:

- Tea: Steep dried leaves in boiling water for 5-10 min.
- Fresh Leaves: Use fresh leaves in salads, beverages, or chew directly.

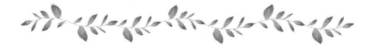

St. John's Wort (Hypericum perforatum)

Traditional Applications: St. John's Wort has been used in traditional European medicine to treat a variety of ailments, including depression, anxiety, and nerve pain. It is known for its mood-lifting properties.

Health Benefits:

- Supports mental health and alleviates depression
- Reduces anxiety and stress
- Provides relief from nerve pain
- Offers anti-inflammatory benefits

Recommended Dosage:

- Capsules: 1-2 capsules, 2-3 times daily
- Tincture: 1-2 dropperfuls, 2-3 times daily

Preparation Methods:

- Capsules: Take with water as directed.
- Tincture: Take in liquid form, mix with water or juice if desired.

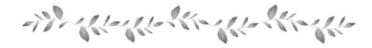

Stinging Nettle (Urtica dioica)

Traditional Applications: Stinging nettle has been used in traditional European and Native American medicine for its anti-inflammatory and diuretic properties. It is commonly used to treat arthritis, urinary issues, and seasonal allergies.

Health Benefits:

- Reduces inflammation and pain from arthritis
- Supports urinary health
- Alleviates symptoms of seasonal allergies
- Provides essential vitamins and minerals

Recommended Dosage:

- Tea: 1-2 tsp of dried leaves per cup of boiling water, up to 3 times daily
- Capsules: 1-2 capsules, up to 3 times daily

Preparation Methods:

- Tea: Steep dried leaves in boiling water for 5-10 min.
- Capsules: Take with water as directed.

Thyme (Thymus vulgaris)

Traditional Applications: Thyme has been used in traditional medicine for its antimicrobial and respiratory benefits. It is often used to treat coughs, bronchitis, and sore throats.

Health Benefits:

- Supports respiratory health and relieves coughs
- Provides antimicrobial and antifungal benefits
- Promotes digestive health
- Reduces inflammation

Recommended Dosage:

- Tea: 1 tsp of dried leaves per cup of boiling water, up to 3 times daily
- Tincture: 1-2 dropperfuls, up to 3 times daily

Preparation Methods:

- Tea: Steep dried leaves in boiling water for 5-10 min.
- Tincture: Take in liquid form, mix with water or juice if desired.

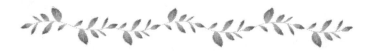

Tulsi (Ocimum sanctum)

Traditional Applications: Tulsi, also known as Holy Basil, is revered in Ayurvedic medicine for its adaptogenic properties. It is used to reduce stress, support respiratory health, and promote overall wellness.

Health Benefits:

- Reduces stress and anxiety
- Supports respiratory health
- Enhances immune function
- Provides antioxidant benefits

Recommended Dosage:

- Tea: 1-2 tsp of dried leaves per cup of boiling water, up to 3 times daily
- Capsules: 1-2 capsules, up to 3 times daily

Preparation Methods:

- Tea: Steep dried leaves in boiling water for 5-10 min.
- Capsules: Take with water as directed.

Turmeric (Curcuma longa)

Traditional Applications: Turmeric has been used in traditional Indian and Chinese medicine for its anti-inflammatory and antioxidant properties. It is commonly used to treat digestive issues, joint pain, and skin conditions.

Health Benefits:

- Reduces inflammation and pain
- Supports digestive health
- Provides antioxidant benefits
- Promotes skin health

Recommended Dosage:

- Powder: 1 tsp of turmeric powder, up to 3 times daily
- Capsules: 1-2 capsules, up to 3 times daily

Preparation Methods:

- Tea: Mix turmeric powder with hot water and a dash of black pepper.
- Capsules: Take with water as directed.

Valerian (Valeriana officinalis)

Traditional Applications: Valerian has been used for centuries in traditional European medicine to promote relaxation and sleep. It is commonly used to treat insomnia, anxiety, and muscle tension.

Health Benefits:

- Promotes relaxation and improves sleep quality
- Reduces anxiety and stress
- Relieves muscle tension and spasms
- Supports overall nervous system health

Recommended Dosage:

- Tea: 1 tsp of dried root per cup of boiling water, up to 3 times daily
- Tincture: 1-2 dropperfuls, up to 3 times daily

Preparation Methods:

- Tea: Steep dried root in boiling water for 12-14 min.
- Tincture: Take in liquid form, mix with water or juice if desired.

White Willow Bark (Salix alba)

Traditional Applications: White willow bark has been used in traditional European medicine as a natural pain reliever and anti-inflammatory agent. It is often used to treat headaches, arthritis, and muscle pain.

Health Benefits:

- Provides natural pain relief
- Reduces inflammation and swelling
- Supports joint health
- Alleviates headaches and muscle pain

Recommended Dosage:

- Tea: 1-2 tsp of dried bark per cup of boiling water, up to 3 times daily
- Capsules: 1-2 capsules, up to 3 times daily

Preparation Methods:

- Tea: Steep dried bark in boiling water for 12-14 min.
- Capsules: Take with water as directed.

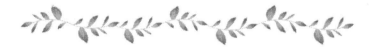

Wormwood (Artemisia absinthium)

Traditional Applications: Wormwood has been used in traditional European and Chinese medicine for its digestive and antimicrobial properties. It is commonly used to treat digestive disorders, intestinal parasites, and as a tonic for overall health.

Health Benefits:

- Supports digestive health and relieves digestive disorders
- Provides antimicrobial and antifungal benefits
- Helps eliminate intestinal parasites
- Acts as a tonic for overall health

Recommended Dosage:

- Tea: 1/2 to 1 tsp of dried leaves per cup of boiling water, up to 3 times daily
- Tincture: 1/2 to 1 dropperful, up to 3 times daily

Preparation Methods:

- Tea: Steep dried leaves in boiling water for 5-10 min.
- Tincture: Take in liquid form, mix with water or juice if desired.

Yarrow (Achillea millefolium)

Traditional Applications: Yarrow has been used in traditional European medicine for its wound-healing and anti-inflammatory properties. It is often used to treat wounds, fevers, and digestive issues.

Health Benefits:

- Promotes wound healing and reduces bleeding
- Reduces inflammation and fever
- Supports digestive health
- Alleviates menstrual cramps

Recommended Dosage:

- Tea: 1-2 tsp of dried leaves per cup of boiling water, up to 3 times daily
- Tincture: 1-2 dropperfuls, up to 3 times daily

Preparation Methods:

- Tea: Steep dried leaves in boiling water for 12-14 min.
- Tincture: Take in liquid form, mix with water or juice if desired.

BOOK 2: THE LOST HERBAL REMEDIES GUIDE

Chapter 1: Introduction to Ancient Remedies

1.1 Holistic Approach to Health

The holistic approach to health has been a fundamental aspect of ancient herbal remedies, focusing on the interconnectedness of mind, body, and spirit to achieve overall wellness. This interconnectedness is at the core of ancient practices, which emphasize balance and harmony in all aspects of life.

Ancient healers believed that true health could only be attained by addressing the whole person, not just the physical symptoms of an ailment. They understood that the mind, body, and spirit are intricately linked and must be in harmony for optimal health to be achieved. This holistic approach meant that treatments not only targeted physical symptoms but also addressed emotional, mental, and spiritual well-being.

In ancient times, healers recognized the importance of balance in all aspects of life. This balance extended beyond the individual to encompass the relationship between the individual and the environment. Holistic health was seen as a state of equilibrium between the individual and their surroundings, including nature, society, and the spiritual realms.

Herbal remedies played a significant role in maintaining this balance and promoting overall well-being. Ancient healers used herbs not only for their physical healing properties but also for their ability to restore harmony within the body and mind. The use of herbs in conjunction with other healing modalities, such as meditation, prayer, and energy work, was a common practice to address the interconnected nature of health.

The holistic approach to health also recognized the importance of prevention rather than just treatment. Ancient healers understood that maintaining balance and harmony in the body was key to preventing illness and promoting longevity. By incorporating herbal remedies into their daily routines, individuals could support their overall health and well-being.

Today, the holistic approach to health is gaining recognition for its effectiveness in promoting wellness and preventing disease. Many people are turning to ancient herbal remedies as a natural and sustainable way to support their health. By incorporating herbs into their diets, using herbal supplements, and exploring holistic healing modalities, individuals are rediscovering the interconnectedness of mind, body, and spirit in achieving optimal health.

In conclusion, the holistic approach to health emphasized in ancient herbal remedies serves as a valuable guide for achieving overall wellness. By recognizing the interconnected nature of mind, body, and spirit, individuals can cultivate balance and harmony in their lives. Incorporating herbal remedies into daily routines can support this balance and promote optimal health. The ancient wisdom of holistic healing reminds us of the importance of addressing all aspects of health to achieve true well-being.

1.2 Introduction to Herbal Medicine Practices

An overview of herbal medicine reveals the rich historical and cultural roots it has in various ancient civilizations. The evolution of herbal practices over time has shaped their role in maintaining health and treating ailments. Understanding the significance of herbs in traditional medicine can provide valuable insights into holistic approaches to wellness and inspire a deeper appreciation for these natural remedies.

Ancient civilizations across the globe, from the Egyptians and Greeks to the Chinese and Native Americans, recognized the healing properties of herbs. The knowledge and practices surrounding herbal medicine were passed down through generations, forming a vital part of these cultures. The use of herbs was intertwined with spiritual beliefs, community rituals, and everyday healthcare practices, reflecting a holistic view of health that considered the interconnectedness of the mind, body, and spirit.

In ancient Egypt, medicinal herbs were used in various forms, including ointments, teas, and poultices, to treat a wide range of ailments. The Ebers Papyrus, an ancient Egyptian medical document dating back to around 1550 BCE, contains references to over 700 herbal remedies. These remedies targeted conditions such as digestive issues, skin conditions, and respiratory infections, highlighting the Egyptians' advanced understanding of herbal pharmacology.

The Greeks, particularly Hippocrates, the father of Western medicine, emphasized the importance of diet, exercise, and herbal treatments in maintaining health. Hippocrates believed in the power of nature to heal, advocating for a balance between the four humors (blood, phlegm, yellow bile, and black bile) to achieve well-being. The use of herbs such as garlic, chamomile, and mint in Greek medicine showcased the diverse range of botanical remedies available to ancient practitioners.

In China, traditional herbal medicine has a history dating back thousands of years, with a strong emphasis on balancing the body's energy, or "qi." The principles of Traditional Chinese Medicine (TCM) revolve around the concept of yin and yang, opposing forces that must be in harmony for optimal health. Chinese herbalists prescribed combinations of herbs tailored to individual patients based on their unique constitution and health needs, highlighting the personalized approach of traditional herbal medicine.

Native American healing traditions also incorporated a deep connection to the natural world, with a focus on using herbs native to the land for medicinal purposes. Plants such as echinacea, goldenseal, and sage were revered for their healing properties and used in ceremonies and remedies to address various health issues. The Native American approach to herbal medicine emphasized the importance of respecting and honoring the plants, viewing them as allies in promoting wellness.

As herbal medicine practices evolved over time, they adapted to changing societal norms, technological advancements, and scientific discoveries. The Renaissance period in Europe saw a resurgence of interest in herbal remedies, with botanists and herbalists like John Gerard and Nicholas Culpeper documenting the medicinal properties of plants. The development of pharmacology and modern medicine eventually led to the standardization and regulation of herbal preparations, shaping the integration of herbal remedies into contemporary healthcare systems.

In the present day, the resurgence of interest in herbal medicine reflects a growing awareness of the benefits of natural remedies and the limitations of conventional pharmaceuticals. Herbal supplements, teas, tinctures, and essential oils are widely available, offering a holistic approach to health that complements conventional treatments. The popularity of herbal remedies in addressing issues such as stress, sleep disorders, and immune support underscores their relevance in modern healthcare practices.

Exploring the roots of herbal medicine in ancient civilizations provides a valuable perspective on the role of herbs in maintaining health and treating ailments. The diverse cultural traditions and historical practices surrounding herbal remedies offer a wealth of knowledge that can inspire individuals to incorporate natural remedies into their daily lives. By understanding the evolution of herbal medicine and its enduring value, we can embrace the holistic approach to wellness that has stood the test of time.

Historical Overview of Herbal Medicine

In ancient times, herbal medicine was a cornerstone of healing practices across various civilizations, laying the foundation for the utilization of herbs in the treatment of ailments. The historical overview of herbal medicine showcases a rich tapestry of knowledge, innovation, and influential figures that have shaped the evolution of herbal remedies to the present day.

Herbal medicine dates back to prehistoric times when early humans discovered the healing properties of plants through trial and error. Ancient civilizations such as the Egyptians, Greeks, Romans, Chinese, and Indigenous cultures around the world developed sophisticated herbal practices based on observation and experimentation. These early healers documented their findings and passed down their knowledge through oral traditions and written records, establishing a legacy that continues to influence modern herbal medicine.

One of the key milestones in the historical development of herbal medicine is the compilation of medicinal plants and their uses in texts such as the Ebers Papyrus in ancient Egypt and the works of Hippocrates in ancient Greece. These written records served as foundational texts that guided generations of healers in the application of herbal remedies. As knowledge spread across continents through trade and exploration, herbal practices merged and diversified, leading to the globalization of herbal medicine.

Influential figures throughout history have significantly contributed to the advancement of herbal medicine. The contributions of Dioscorides, a Greek physician and pharmacologist, are immortalized in his work "De Materia Medica," a comprehensive herbal encyclopedia that cataloged hundreds of medicinal plants. Avicenna, an influential Persian polymath, furthered the understanding of herbal medicine in the Islamic Golden Age with his seminal work "The Canon of Medicine."

The Renaissance period witnessed a revival of interest in herbal medicine, with figures like Nicholas Culpeper in England and Paracelsus in Switzerland challenging traditional medical practices and advocating for the accessibility of herbal remedies to the general population. The 19th and 20th centuries saw the scientific validation of herbal medicine through pharmacological research, leading to the standardization and commercialization of herbal products.

Understanding the historical context of herbal medicine provides insight into the enduring efficacy and relevance of traditional remedies. By delving into the past, we can appreciate the wisdom of ancient healers and honor their legacy by integrating traditional herbal practices with modern healthcare approaches. Embracing the historical overview of herbal medicine not only enriches our understanding of natural healing methods but also empowers us to explore the diverse benefits of herbal remedies in promoting holistic health and wellness in the present era.

Cultural Significance of Herbal Practices

Exploring the cultural importance of herbal practices in various societies, this subsection delves into how different cultures have utilized herbs for healing and spiritual purposes.

Ancient herbal practices hold a significant place in the cultural fabric of societies around the world. The utilization of herbs for healing and spiritual purposes dates back centuries and has been a cornerstone of many cultures. Native American tribes, for instance, have a rich tradition of using herbs such as sage, sweetgrass, and cedar in spiritual ceremonies to cleanse and purify spaces. These rituals not only treat physical ailments but also aim to restore harmony within individuals and communities.

In Chinese culture, herbal medicine has a long history intertwined with philosophical concepts such as Yin and Yang, Qi energy, and the Five Elements. Chinese herbal practices focus on restoring balance within the body to promote health and prevent illness. The cultural significance of these practices is deeply rooted in the belief that harmony between nature and the body is essential for well-being.

Ayurveda, an ancient healing system from India, incorporates herbs into its treatments to bring balance to the body's doshas—Vata, Pitta, and Kapha. The cultural importance of Ayurvedic herbs lies in their ability to not only address physical ailments but also nurture the mind and spirit. The practice of Ayurveda is deeply connected to spiritual beliefs and the concept of holistic health, where the interplay of the physical, mental, and spiritual realms is crucial.

In African traditional medicine, herbal remedies play a vital role in healing and maintaining overall well-being. The cultural significance of herbs in African societies is evident in rituals and ceremonies where specific plants are used to invoke protection, healing, and spiritual guidance. These practices highlight the interconnectedness between the natural world, ancestral wisdom, and the health of individuals.

The utilization of herbs in different cultural practices underscores the universal belief in the healing power of nature and the interconnectedness of all living beings. By understanding the cultural significance of herbal practices, we not only gain insight into diverse healing traditions but also appreciate the profound wisdom passed down through generations.

As we delve deeper into the cultural significance of herbal practices, it becomes evident that the utilization of herbs transcends mere physical healing—it encompasses spiritual, emotional, and communal aspects that contribute to a holistic approach to well-being. Embracing and honoring these cultural traditions can enrich our understanding of herbal remedies and inspire us to incorporate them into our own lives for overall health and harmony.

Modern Applications of Traditional Herbal Remedies

Throughout history, herbal remedies have played a significant role in maintaining health and treating ailments. Modern advancements have allowed for the adaptation and integration of traditional herbal practices into contemporary healthcare, showcasing the relevance and sustainability of these ancient remedies in the modern era.

Modern Applications of Traditional Herbal Remedies:

In today's healthcare landscape, there has been a notable resurgence of interest in traditional herbal remedies as people seek natural and holistic alternatives to conventional medicine. The bridge between ancient practices and modern applications is becoming increasingly evident as more research supports the effectiveness of these time-honored remedies.

One key aspect of the modern application of traditional herbal remedies is their utilization in conjunction with conventional medical approaches. Integrative medicine, which combines traditional practices with modern healthcare techniques, has gained popularity and recognition for its ability to provide comprehensive and individualized care to patients.

Moreover, the growing body of scientific evidence supporting the efficacy of certain herbs has led to their incorporation into mainstream medical practices. Herbal supplements, derived from ancient knowledge, are being used to complement traditional treatments for various health conditions, offering patients a more well-rounded approach to wellness.

Additionally, traditional herbal remedies are being adapted to meet the needs of the modern world. From herbal teas to essential oils, these natural products are being integrated into daily routines to promote overall well-being. Many individuals are also exploring the benefits of herbal remedies as a preventive measure, incorporating them into their lifestyles to support their immune systems and overall health.

It is worth noting that modern applications of traditional herbal remedies are not meant to replace conventional medical treatments but rather to complement them. By embracing the wisdom of our ancestors and combining it with the advancements of modern science, individuals can experience the best of both worlds in their healthcare journey.

In conclusion, the utilization of traditional herbal remedies in modern healthcare is a testament to the enduring value of ancient knowledge. By understanding and incorporating these practices into our lives, we can embrace a holistic approach to health that honors the wisdom of the past while embracing the innovations of the present. Let us continue to explore the benefits of herbal remedies and discover the ways in which they can enhance our overall well-being.

1.3 Importance of Ancient Herbal Traditions

In exploring the importance of ancient herbal traditions, it becomes evident that these practices hold significant value in the contemporary world, offering a wealth of benefits that resonate with individuals seeking holistic health and wellness. The preservation and integration of these traditions are crucial in fostering a harmonious balance between the ancient wisdom and modern healthcare practices.

Ancient herbal traditions are rooted in centuries of wisdom, emphasizing the profound connections between nature, the human body, and spiritual well-being. These traditions recognize the intimate interplay between mind, body, and spirit, viewing health as a holistic concept that requires balance and harmony in all aspects of life. By understanding and embracing these ancient practices, individuals can embark on a journey towards overall wellness that encompasses not just physical health, but mental and spiritual vitality as well.

The relevance of ancient herbal traditions in today's world lies in their ability to complement and enhance modern healthcare practices. While advancements in medical science have undoubtedly revolutionized the field of healthcare, ancient herbal remedies offer a natural and gentle approach to healing that resonates with individuals seeking alternative or complementary treatments. The rich history of herbal medicine from various ancient civilizations serves as a testament to the enduring efficacy of these practices, providing a foundation upon which modern healthcare can build and innovate.

Preserving ancient knowledge and traditions is essential in ensuring that the wisdom of our ancestors is not lost to time. Efforts to document, catalog, and pass down herbal knowledge through oral traditions, written records, and modern documentation are invaluable in maintaining the integrity and authenticity of these practices. By preserving ancient wisdom, we not only honor the legacy of our forebearers but also pave the way for future generations to benefit from the timeless wisdom of herbal remedies.

The integration of traditional herbal practices with modern medical approaches represents a harmonious synergy between the ancient and the contemporary. Collaborations between herbalists, traditional healers, and modern healthcare practitioners showcase the potential for bridging the gap between ancient wisdom and modern science. Through successful case studies and partnerships, the integration of traditional herbal practices into mainstream healthcare systems has demonstrated positive outcomes for patients, highlighting the complementary nature of these approaches in promoting holistic wellness.

The benefits of ancient herbal traditions in today's world are manifold, offering a diverse range of advantages that contribute to holistic health and well-being. From the use of herbs for physical healing to the incorporation of spiritual practices for emotional and mental balance, ancient herbal traditions provide a comprehensive approach to health that addresses the multifaceted nature of human wellness. By embracing these traditions, individuals can harness the power of nature and ancient wisdom to cultivate a lifestyle that nurtures the body, mind, and spirit.

In conclusion, the importance of ancient herbal traditions in the modern era cannot be overstated. These practices offer a wealth of benefits that resonate with individuals seeking holistic health and wellness, emphasizing the interconnectedness of mind, body, and spirit in achieving overall well-being. By preserving and integrating ancient herbal traditions with modern practices, we honor the wisdom of our ancestors and pave the way for a healthier and more balanced future. It is through the exploration and incorporation of these ancient remedies that we truly discover the lost treasures of herbal medicine.

Preserving Ancient Wisdom

Preserving ancient herbal knowledge and practices is essential to maintain the richness of traditional remedies and ensure their availability for future generations. Efforts to safeguard this wisdom encompass various methods, including oral traditions, written records, and modern documentation.

Oral traditions play a significant role in passing down herbal knowledge from one generation to the next. Through storytelling, folklore, and teachings, elders and herbalists transmit valuable information about the properties and uses of different herbs. These verbal exchanges not only preserve ancient wisdom but also foster a sense of community and cultural identity.

In addition to oral traditions, written records have been pivotal in documenting herbal remedies throughout history. Ancient texts, manuscripts, and scrolls have served as repositories of herbal knowledge, detailing the uses, preparations, and dosages of various medicinal plants. By safeguarding these written records, scholars and practitioners can access and study the wealth of information left by our predecessors.

Furthermore, modern documentation techniques have revolutionized the preservation of ancient herbal wisdom. With advancements in technology, herbalists and researchers can now create comprehensive databases, digital archives, and research papers that catalog the effectiveness and safety of herbal treatments. This integration of traditional knowledge with contemporary tools ensures that ancient remedies remain relevant and applicable in today's healthcare practices.

By combining oral traditions, written records, and modern documentation, the collective effort to preserve ancient herbal wisdom becomes a collaborative endeavor that transcends time and cultural boundaries. It is through these preservation methods that the holistic approach to health and healing, rooted in ancient practices, continues to thrive and provide valuable insights for current and future generations.

Embracing and supporting these preservation efforts not only honors the traditions of our ancestors but also empowers individuals to explore the benefits of herbal remedies in their daily lives. By recognizing the importance of preserving ancient wisdom, we contribute to the longevity and sustainability of herbal traditions, ensuring that their significance endures for years to come.

Integrating Traditional and Modern Practices

The integration of traditional herbal practices with modern medical approaches is a pivotal step towards bridging ancient wisdom with contemporary healthcare. Collaboration between these two realms is essential for the advancement and preservation of herbal remedies.

Throughout history, traditional herbal practices have played a significant role in promoting well-being and treating various ailments. As modern medicine continues to evolve, there is a growing recognition of the value that ancient herbal traditions bring to the table. By integrating these practices with modern medical approaches, a harmonious balance can be achieved, leading to improved health outcomes and holistic wellness.

One of the key aspects of integrating traditional and modern practices is the acknowledgment of the strengths of both systems. Traditional herbal practices often focus on natural remedies and preventive care, emphasizing the body's intrinsic ability to heal. On the other hand, modern medicine provides advanced diagnostic tools, evidence-based treatment options, and specialized care.

Successful collaborations between traditional herbalists and modern healthcare providers have resulted in innovative treatment approaches that draw from the best of both worlds. By combining the wisdom of ancient herbal traditions with the scientific advancements of modern medicine, practitioners can offer patients a comprehensive and personalized approach to healthcare.

Case studies have illustrated the benefits of integrating traditional and modern practices. For example, incorporating herbal remedies alongside conventional treatments for chronic conditions has shown promising results in managing symptoms and improving overall quality of life. Additionally, the use of herbal supplements to complement traditional therapies has been found to enhance efficacy and reduce side effects.

By fostering a collaborative environment between traditional healers, medical professionals, researchers, and policymakers, the integration of herbal practices with modern healthcare can be further enhanced. Education and training programs that promote interdisciplinary cooperation and mutual respect between different healing modalities are crucial in this process.

Ultimately, the integration of traditional herbal practices with modern medical approaches offers a holistic and patient-centered approach to healthcare. It empowers individuals to explore diverse treatment options and encourages a deeper understanding of the interconnectedness between ancient wisdom and contemporary science. Through this harmonious integration, individuals can reap the benefits of both worlds, leading to improved health outcomes and overall well-being.

Benefits of Ancient Herbal Traditions Today

Ancient herbal traditions have stood the test of time for a reason, offering a wealth of benefits that continue to be relevant in today's world. The contemporary advantages of these practices extend beyond mere physical health, contributing to holistic well-being and wellness in the modern era.

One significant benefit of ancient herbal traditions in today's context is their ability to address not only physical ailments but also mental and emotional well-being. The interconnectedness of mind, body, and spirit emphasized in these traditions aligns with the holistic approach to health, promoting a balanced and harmonious state of being. By incorporating herbal remedies into daily routines, individuals can tap into a more comprehensive and sustainable approach to overall wellness.

Furthermore, the cultural significance of herbal practices offers a window into diverse societies' healing and spiritual beliefs. Exploring these cultural connections can foster a deeper understanding of different traditions and promote a sense of unity and respect for various cultural practices. By embracing and integrating these diverse herbal traditions, individuals can enrich their own health practices while honoring the wisdom of ancient cultures.

The integration of traditional herbal practices with modern medical approaches showcases the adaptability and effectiveness of herbal remedies in contemporary healthcare. Successful collaborations and case studies highlight the synergies between traditional knowledge and modern advancements, demonstrating how ancient herbal wisdom can complement and enhance current medical practices.

Moreover, the preservation of ancient herbal knowledge is crucial in ensuring that these valuable traditions are passed down through generations. Efforts to document and share this knowledge, whether through oral traditions, written records, or modern documentation, play a vital role in safeguarding these practices for the future.

In conclusion, the benefits of ancient herbal traditions today extend far beyond their initial uses. By incorporating these practices into daily life, individuals can experience holistic health benefits, gain insight into diverse cultural practices, and contribute to the preservation and integration of valuable ancient knowledge. Embracing these traditions not only promotes personal well-being but also honors the richness and sustainability of ancient herbal remedies.

Chapter 2: Fundamentals of Ancient Herbalism

2.1 Understanding Ancient Herbal Wisdom

In the realm of ancient herbalism, the foundations rest not just on the herbs themselves but on deep-seated principles and philosophies that have weathered the passage of time. These principles have shaped how cultures across the globe perceive the natural world and our relationship with it, particularly in the context of healing and wellness. Understanding these time-honored wisdoms not only provides insight into past practices but also offers valuable lessons that can be integrated into our modern lives.

At the core of ancient herbal wisdom is the principle of holistic health. This concept emphasizes the interconnectedness of body, mind, and spirit, advocating for a comprehensive approach to wellness that transcends the physical aspects of healing. Ancient herbalists understood that true health encompasses emotional and spiritual well-being, and that herbs possess qualities that can support all dimensions of human health. This holistic approach contrasts sharply with the compartmentalized view often seen in modern medicine, reminding us of the importance of addressing the root causes of illness rather than merely treating symptoms.

The philosophy of interconnectedness extends beyond the individual to encompass the whole ecosystem. Ancient herbal practices are grounded in the belief that humans are an integral part of the natural world and that maintaining harmony with our environment is essential for health. This perspective is echoed in sustainable practices today, highlighting the relevance of ancient wisdom in addressing contemporary challenges such as environmental degradation and climate change.

Another foundational philosophy of ancient herbalism is the Doctrine of Signatures. This fascinating concept suggests that herbs reveal their use through their shape, color, and form. For example, a liverwort plant, which somewhat resembles a liver, was traditionally used to treat liver ailments. While modern science may not always support these direct correlations, the Doctrine of Signatures reflects the intuitive ways in which ancient peoples understood and classified the natural world. It reminds us of the importance of observation and intuition in discovering the healing properties of plants.

The role of herbalists in ancient societies was not just that of healers but also educators, spiritual guides, and stewards of herbal knowledge. They were respected figures who passed down their understanding of plants and their uses through generations. The spiritual and cultural significance of herbal practices was profound, with many herbs being used in rituals and ceremonies to promote spiritual health and connection with the divine. This spiritual aspect of herbalism is an area where modern practices often diverge, yet it offers a rich vein of knowledge for those seeking a deeper, more holistic connection to their healing practices.

In recent years, there has been a growing interest in integrating ancient herbal wisdom with modern science. This integration has led to the validation of many traditional remedies through clinical research, demonstrating the effectiveness of herbs in treating various conditions. For instance, the anti-inflammatory properties of turmeric, long used in Ayurvedic medicine, have been supported by numerous scientific studies. Such case studies not only validate ancient practices but also open up new avenues for the development of herbal medicines based on traditional knowledge.

The ongoing relevance of ancient herbal wisdom in our contemporary world cannot be overstated. In an era where many are seeking sustainable, natural alternatives to conventional medicine, the principles and practices of ancient herbalism offer valuable insights. The emphasis on holistic health, the interconnectedness of humans and nature, and the integration of spiritual well-being into healing practices are particularly resonant today.

Moreover, the sustainable practices inherent in traditional herbalism, such as mindful harvesting and respect for natural cycles, provide a blueprint for environmentally sustainable living. These practices encourage us to reconsider our relationship with the natural world, advocating for a more respectful, balanced approach that benefits both our health and the health of our planet.

In conclusion, the wisdom of ancient herbalism holds timeless lessons for modern society. By understanding and applying these foundational principles and philosophies, we can foster a more holistic, sustainable approach to health and wellness. Encouraging the integration of ancient wisdom with modern science not only enriches our understanding of herbal medicine but also supports the broader movement towards sustainable, environmentally conscious living. As we continue to explore and appreciate the depths of ancient herbal practices, we open ourselves to a wealth of knowledge that can enhance our health, our communities, and our world.

Principles of Traditional Herbal Wisdom

Ancient herbal practices are guided by a profound understanding of the natural world and our place within it. Central to these practices is the principle of holistic health, which views the body, mind, and spirit as interconnected and interdependent. This holistic approach emphasizes the importance of maintaining balance and harmony within the individual and between the individual and their environment. By addressing not just the physical symptoms of an ailment but also its emotional, spiritual, and environmental aspects, ancient herbalism seeks to restore the whole person to a state of well-being.

- **Holistic Health:** Emphasizes treating the whole person, rather than focusing solely on symptoms. This approach considers the emotional, spiritual, and physical aspects of health, advocating for a balanced lifestyle that integrates herbal remedies as a part of overall wellness.
- **Interconnectedness of Body, Mind, and Spirit:** Ancient herbalism teaches that our physical health is deeply connected to our mental and spiritual states. By nurturing all aspects of ourselves, we can achieve a healthier and more balanced life.
- **Herbs for Balance and Harmony:** The use of herbs in ancient practices is not just about treating specific ailments but also about maintaining balance and harmony within the body and with nature. Herbs are chosen not only for their medicinal properties but also for their ability to align with the individual's unique constitution and the energetic qualities of their surroundings.

This holistic and interconnected view of health and healing is not merely a historical curiosity but remains relevant and powerful in our modern world. By embracing these ancient principles, we can learn to live more harmoniously with ourselves and our environment, leading to greater health and happiness.

Philosophies of Ancient Herbal Practices

Ancient herbalism is deeply rooted in philosophies that reflect an understanding of the natural world and its profound connection to human health and wellness. Among these, the Doctrine of Signatures stands out as a prime example. This philosophy posits that herbs resembling various parts of the body can be used to treat ailments related to those body parts. For instance, a liverwort plant, due to its liver-like shape, was traditionally used for liver issues. Even without modern scientific methods, ancient herbalists discerned the potential healing properties of plants through careful observation of their shapes, colors, and environments.

The role of herbalists in ancient societies was both pivotal and revered. These individuals were not merely caregivers but were often considered wise sages who held the knowledge of the natural world and its intricate relationship with human health. They served as the community's healers, teachers, and often spiritual guides, emphasizing the holistic approach to wellness that included physical, mental, and spiritual health.

Furthermore, the spiritual and cultural significance of herbal practices cannot be overstated. Many cultures believed in the sacred character of plants and their divine origin. For example, several indigenous traditions consider plants to be teachers or spirit allies that can offer healing beyond the physical realm. The act of gathering and preparing herbs was, and in some places still is, accompanied by rituals and prayers, underscoring the respectful relationship between humans and the natural world.

These ancient philosophies highlight a holistic approach to life and wellness, where the interconnectedness of body, mind, spirit, and nature is recognized and honored. They remind us of the wisdom held in the natural world and encourage a respectful and mindful approach to utilizing its resources. In a modern context, these principles can inspire a more integrated approach to health that values the balance and harmony inherent in nature and within ourselves.

Integrating Ancient Wisdom with Modern Science

- The integration of ancient herbal wisdom with modern science offers a compelling testament to the enduring value of traditional practices. As we delve into this synthesis, we find numerous instances where the efficacy of time-honored remedies gains validation from contemporary scientific research. This convergence not only illuminates the depth of ancient knowledge but also paves the way for innovative approaches to holistic health care.

- **Case Studies of Validation:** Various studies have played pivotal roles in bridging the gap between ancient herbal traditions and modern pharmacology. For instance, the anti-inflammatory properties of turmeric, long celebrated in Ayurvedic medicine, have been substantiated through clinical research, highlighting its potential in treating conditions like arthritis and other inflammatory disorders. Similarly, the antiviral effects of elderberry, a staple in traditional European folk medicine, have been confirmed in studies assessing its efficacy in mitigating flu symptoms.

- **Scientific Endorsement of Traditional Methods:** The scientific community's growing acknowledgment of herbal medicine's value is evident in the increasing number of peer-reviewed publications and funded research projects focused on traditional botanical remedies. This endorsement extends beyond validating specific herbs to appreciating the holistic frameworks within which these remedies were used, recognizing the importance of treating the individual as a whole rather than focusing solely on symptom management.

Relevance and Sustainability: The resurgence of interest in herbal medicine, bolstered by scientific validation, underscores its relevance in today's health care landscape. Beyond efficacy, the appeal of herbal remedies often lies in their sustainability and accessibility, presenting a low-impact, cost-effective alternative to conventional pharmaceuticals. Moreover, the integration of traditional wisdom with scientific rigor offers a pathway to developing more personalized and preventive health care strategies, aligning with contemporary trends towards natural and sustainable wellness practices.

This synergy between ancient wisdom and modern science not only validates the past but also offers a hopeful vision for the future of health care, one that is inclusive, holistic, and sustainable.

2.2 Traditional Herbal Practices

In the realm of ancient herbalism, the knowledge and methods employed by our ancestors were not only aimed at treating physical ailments but also at nurturing a holistic balance between the body, mind, and spirit. This harmonious approach is evident in the traditional practices of preparing and using herbal infusions, poultices, and decoctions. Each method, endowed with its unique properties and benefits, offers a glimpse into the depth and breadth of ancient herbal wisdom.

Herbal Infusions and Their Benefits

Herbal infusions, often simply referred to as herbal teas, are among the most accessible and commonly used herbal remedies. The simplicity of steeping dried or fresh herbs in hot water belies the profound healing potential contained within. The process of making an herbal infusion involves pouring boiling water over the herb(s) and allowing them to steep for a period, typically between 5 to 15 minutes. This method is particularly well-suited for extracting the healing properties of delicate parts of plants, such as leaves, flowers, and fine stems, ensuring that the essential oils and therapeutic constituents are not destroyed by boiling.

The benefits of herbal infusions are wide-ranging and depend on the herbs used. For instance, a chamomile infusion is renowned for its calming and soothing properties, making it an excellent remedy for stress and insomnia. Meanwhile, peppermint tea is celebrated for its digestive benefits and its ability to relieve headaches. Incorporating these infusions into one's daily regimen can support overall well-being, promote relaxation, and aid in the maintenance of various bodily systems.

The Use of Poultices in Traditional Healing

Poultices represent another cornerstone of traditional herbal medicine, utilized for their direct and potent healing effects on the body. They involve the application of herbs (fresh, dried, or powdered) directly onto the skin, often combined with a moistening agent to form a paste. This paste is then typically spread onto a cloth and applied to the affected area, allowing the active constituents of the herbs to penetrate the skin and exert their therapeutic effects.

Historically, poultices have been used to treat a wide array of conditions, including wounds, bruises, infections, and various skin conditions. For example, a poultice made from crushed plantain leaves can be a powerful remedy for insect bites and stings, thanks to its anti-inflammatory and antimicrobial properties. Similarly, a mustard poultice has been traditionally used to alleviate chest congestion and stimulate circulation. The direct application method employed in poultices ensures that the healing properties of the herbs are concentrated on the area of the body that requires attention, providing targeted relief.

Decoctions: Preparation and Uses

Decoctions are another vital practice in ancient herbalism, especially suited for extracting the medicinal properties from the tougher parts of plants, such as roots, bark, and hard seeds. The process involves simmering the plant material in water for an extended period, usually between 15 to 30 minutes, allowing the active compounds to be drawn out into the liquid. This method ensures a more potent remedy, ideal for addressing more serious or deep-seated ailments.

The uses of decoctions are as varied as the plants themselves. For example, a decoction made from ginger root is a well-known remedy for digestive issues, nausea, and to boost the immune system. On the other hand, a decoction from willow bark, which contains salicin (a precursor to aspirin), has long been used to relieve pain and reduce inflammation.

Each of these traditional practices — herbal infusions, poultices, and decoctions — embodies the ancient wisdom of herbalists who understood the profound connection between the natural world and human health. By incorporating these practices into modern life, we continue a centuries-old tradition of healing and nurturing the body in a natural, gentle manner. Moreover, these practices encourage a more sustainable and conscious approach to health, emphasizing the importance of understanding and respecting the plants that offer their healing properties.

In conclusion, the ancient practices of preparing and utilizing herbal remedies offer invaluable insights into the holistic approach to health that characterized traditional herbal medicine. By learning and applying these methods in our daily lives, we not only honor the wisdom of our ancestors but also open ourselves to a world of natural healing and balance. Whether through the calming ritual of brewing an herbal infusion, the targeted healing provided by poultices, or the potent relief offered by decoctions, the legacy of ancient herbalism continues to enrich our modern lives, reminding us of the enduring power and relevance of nature's pharmacy.

2.3 Tools and Techniques of Ancient Herbalists

In the realm of ancient herbalism, the knowledge and skills of early herbalists were deeply intertwined with the natural world, showcasing a profound understanding of the environment's rhythm and how to harness the healing powers of plants. Their expertise, passed down through generations, is a testament to the enduring legacy of traditional herbal remedies. This section delves into the tools and techniques employed by ancient herbalists, offering valuable insights into their practices, which continue to influence modern herbalism today.

Harvesting Techniques Ancient herbalists were adept at identifying and collecting the right herbs at optimal times, a practice crucial for ensuring the maximum efficacy of the plants used in remedies. They adhered to specific:

- **Seasonal Guidelines:** Understanding that plants' medicinal properties vary with the seasons, they meticulously followed natural cycles, harvesting roots in early spring or late autumn when the plant's energy is concentrated below ground, leaves and stems when the plant is in full growth, and flowers and fruits at their peak.
- **Lunar Cycles:** Many believed that the phases of the moon affected the potency of plants. Herbs were often harvested during certain lunar phases to maximize their healing properties, with the full moon being a particularly auspicious time for collection.
- **Ethical Practices:** Sustainability was inherent to their approach. They harvested with respect, taking only what was needed and leaving enough for the plant to continue to grow, ensuring that natural habitats were preserved for future generations.

Drying and Storing Herbs Once harvested, the herbs needed to be preserved to retain their medicinal qualities. Ancient herbalists developed effective methods for drying and storing herbs:

- **Drying Methods:** Herbs were typically air-dried in a shaded, well-ventilated area to prevent mold and maintain their essential oils. Some were hung in bunches, while others were spread out on screens or straw mats.
- **Storing Techniques:** Proper storage was paramount to prevent decay and loss of potency. Dried herbs were kept in containers made of materials that "breathed," such as clay pots or wooden boxes, in a cool, dark place. This helped in maintaining their effectiveness for use in remedies throughout the year.

Preparation of Herbal Remedies The core of ancient herbalism was the preparation of remedies. Herbalists possessed a diverse repertoire of techniques to create healing concoctions:

- **Teas and Infusions:** Simple yet effective, teas were made by steeping herbs in hot water. This method was particularly used for delicate parts of the plant, such as leaves and flowers, to extract their medicinal properties.
- **Decoctions:** For tougher plant parts like roots, bark, and seeds, decoctions were prepared by gently boiling the materials to extract their active compounds.
- **Tinctures and Extracts:** Alcohol or vinegar was used as solvents to create tinctures and extracts, allowing for a concentrated and longer-lasting remedy. These were especially valued for their ease of storage and potent efficacy.
- **Poultices and Salves:** Fresh or rehydrated herbs were often applied directly to the skin as poultices for localized healing. Additionally, salves were made by infusing herbs in oils or fats, creating a soothing balm for wounds and irritations.

Holistic Approach and Customization Ancient herbalists viewed healing as a holistic process, considering the individual's physical, emotional, and spiritual needs. They tailored their remedies to the person, not just the ailment, a practice that required deep knowledge of both the patient and the plants. This personalized approach is a hallmark of ancient herbalism, emphasizing the practitioner's role as a healer and guide.

Integration with Modern Practices Today, the principles and techniques of ancient herbalism are being revisited and integrated with modern scientific research, validating the effectiveness of many traditional remedies. The tools and methods of ancient herbalists, though simple, were grounded in a profound understanding of nature and its cycles. Modern herbalists continue to draw on this rich tradition, combining ancient wisdom with contemporary science to promote wellness and healing.

As we rediscover these ancient practices, the relevance of traditional herbalism in today's world becomes increasingly apparent. Its emphasis on sustainability, personalization, and harmony with nature offers valuable insights for addressing modern health challenges. By learning from the past, we can forge a future where the ancient art of herbalism continues to enrich our lives, offering natural and holistic pathways to health and well-being.

Traditional Harvesting Methods

Herbal harvesting is a practice deeply rooted in understanding the intricate cycles of nature and the plants themselves. Ancient herbalists developed methods that were not only effective but also sustainable, ensuring that plant populations thrived for future generations. A fundamental aspect of these methods was the timing of harvesting, which varied depending on the type of herb and its intended use.

- **Best Times for Harvesting:** The optimal time for harvesting herbs largely depends on the specific parts of the plant being used. For leaves, the best time is usually just before the plant flowers, when the concentration of beneficial compounds is at its peak. Flowers should be picked as soon as they open, while roots are generally harvested in the fall when the plant's energy has retreated underground. Seeds, on the other hand, should be collected when they are mature and dry.

- **Respecting Natural Cycles:** Ancient herbalists paid close attention to the lunar and seasonal cycles, believing that these natural rhythms could affect the quality and potency of herbal remedies. For instance, some traditions hold that roots are best harvested under a waning moon, as it is thought that the earth's energy is drawing inward, concentrating the plant's medicinal properties.
- **Sustainable Practices:** Sustainability was an integral part of traditional harvesting methods. Herbalists would take care not to overharvest, often leaving behind a portion of the plant or its seeds to ensure regrowth. In some cases, they would also plant seeds from the harvested herbs to aid in the regeneration of the plant population.

These traditional methods reflect a profound respect for nature and its cycles, emphasizing the interconnectedness of all living things. By adopting these practices, modern herbal enthusiasts can continue to enjoy the benefits of herbal remedies while honoring the ancient wisdom that has preserved these traditions through the ages.

Techniques for Drying and Storing Herbs

Drying and storing herbs properly is crucial to preserving their medicinal qualities and ensuring their longevity. Ancient herbalists developed a variety of techniques to achieve this, many of which are still used today due to their effectiveness. Understanding these methods allows contemporary enthusiasts and practitioners to maintain the potency of herbal remedies.

Drying Methods:

- **Air Drying:** Perhaps the most traditional method, air drying involves hanging bunches of herbs in a well-ventilated, dark, and dry place. This method is best suited for herbs with long stems and is remarkably effective for preserving both the herbs' potency and their color.
- **Screen Drying:** For smaller herbs or individual leaves, laying them out on a screen encourages even air circulation around each piece, facilitating a quicker drying process. This method is favorable in humid climates where air drying may be slower.
- **Dehydrator Drying:** Using a dehydrator can be a more controlled method for drying herbs, allowing for precise temperature regulation which is essential for preserving delicate compounds in certain herbs that might be sensitive to heat.

Storing Techniques:

- **Glass Jars:** Once dried, herbs should be stored in airtight glass jars. Clear jars need to be kept in dark places as light can degrade the quality of the herbs. Alternatively, amber or other colored glass jars can be used to protect the contents from light, making it easier to store them in visible locations.

- **Labeling:** Proper labeling is crucial. Include the name of the herb and the date of storage. Herbs tend to lose their potency over time, so it's important to use them within one to three years.
- **Conditions:** Ideally, herbs should be stored in a cool, dry place away from direct sunlight, moisture, and heat. These conditions help to ensure that the herbs retain their medicinal properties for as long as possible.

Incorporating these traditional methods into modern practices not only honors the wisdom of ancient herbalists but also maximizes the effectiveness of herbal remedies prepared at home. By preserving herbs effectively, we maintain a direct link to the natural world and its healing powers.

Methods of Preparing Herbal Remedies

Throughout history, ancient herbalists have employed a variety of methods to prepare herbal remedies, each tailored to harness the unique healing properties of plants. These techniques, ranging from the simplicity of teas to the complexity of tinctures and ointments, encapsulate the essence of traditional herbal wisdom.

- **Teas and Infusions**: One of the simplest and most common methods for preparing herbal remedies is through teas or infusions. This involves steeping herbs in hot water to extract their therapeutic properties. The process typically requires a tablespoon of dried herbs or a handful of fresh herbs per cup of boiling water, steeped for about 5-10 minutes. Teas are particularly effective for herbs that act on the digestive system or provide relaxation.
- **Tinctures**: Tinctures are concentrated herbal extracts made by soaking herbs in alcohol or vinegar. The alcohol extracts active ingredients from the plants, resulting in a potent remedy that can be administered in small doses. To make a tincture, fill a jar with herbs, cover them with alcohol, and let the mixture sit for 4-6 weeks, shaking it daily. After straining the herbs, the liquid can be stored in a dark bottle for use.
- **Poultices**: For localized ailments, poultices offer a direct way to apply herbs to the skin. This involves creating a paste from fresh or dried herbs, which is then applied to the affected area. Poultices can reduce inflammation, soothe pain, or draw out infections.
- **Ointments**: Combining herbs with a base like beeswax or oil creates ointments that can be applied to the skin. This method is suitable for delivering herbs that promote wound healing or offer relief from skin conditions.

These methods exemplify the versatility and ingenuity of ancient herbalists, whose practices continue to inspire modern herbal medicine. By following their guidance, one can craft effective remedies that embody the healing power of nature.

Chapter 3: Historical Remedies and Their Modern Relevance

3.1 Comparative Studies on Ancient and Modern Uses

The exploration into the intersection of historical and modern uses of herbal remedies opens a fascinating chapter in the narrative of medicine. Herbal remedies, deeply rooted in the annals of history, have found their way into the contemporary era, bridging millennia of human innovation and understanding of natural medicine. This comparative study serves not only as a testament to the enduring legacy of herbal practices but also as a guidepost for their continued relevance in modern healthcare.

Historically, herbal remedies were the cornerstone of medical practices across various civilizations. From the ancient Egyptians to the Greek, Chinese, and Indian cultures, herbs were not only used for their direct healing properties but also played a significant role in religious, ceremonial, and daily life. These early uses were based largely on empirical observations and the herbal knowledge was passed down through generations. For instance, the Ebers Papyrus, an ancient Egyptian text, lists a myriad of herbal recipes, illustrating the extensive use of plants like aloe vera, garlic, and juniper for healing purposes. Similarly, in ancient China, the Huangdi Neijing presented a comprehensive system of medicine where herbs were categorized based on their therapeutic actions.

Fast forward to the modern era, the essence of these ancient practices has permeated contemporary medicine, albeit through a more scientific lens. The transition from traditional to modern use of herbal remedies is underscored by rigorous scientific research and clinical trials aimed at validating their efficacy. Today, many herbal remedies are incorporated into modern pharmacology; for instance, the use of willow bark extract, a precursor to aspirin, and the antimalarial properties derived from the bark of the Cinchona tree, are prime examples of ancient wisdom manifesting in modern medicine.

This juxtaposition reveals both similarities and differences in the application of herbal remedies. The core similarity lies in the intrinsic therapeutic value attributed to plants, a belief that has remained unchanged despite the passage of time. However, the method of application and integration into healthcare systems marks a stark difference. Modern methodologies involve standardized dosages, controlled conditions, and a greater understanding of active compounds, a shift from the more holistic and less precise methods of ancient times.

The evolution of herbal practices is marked by several key factors. Advancements in science and technology have played a pivotal role, allowing for a deeper understanding of the biochemical mechanisms behind herbal remedies. This scientific backing has led to increased credibility and acceptance of herbal medicine in mainstream healthcare. Additionally, cultural shifts towards more sustainable and natural living have propelled herbal remedies into the limelight, as people seek alternatives to synthetic drugs and their associated side effects. The global exchange of knowledge, facilitated by technological advancements, has also enabled a cross-cultural fusion of herbal practices, enriching the global compendium of herbal medicine.

Despite their proven benefits, integrating traditional herbal remedies into modern medical practices is not without challenges. Standardization remains a significant hurdle, given the natural variability of plant compounds. Furthermore, the cultural nuances of medical practices can influence the perception and acceptance of herbal remedies in different regions. However, the potential benefits of this integration, including the holistic approach to healing and the sustainability of natural resources, offer compelling reasons to overcome these challenges.

In conclusion, the comparative study of ancient and modern uses of herbal remedies highlights a dynamic and evolving field of medicine. The enduring legacy of herbal practices is a testament to their intrinsic value and efficacy. As science continues to unveil the mechanisms behind these ancient remedies, their integration into contemporary medicine promises a more holistic, sustainable, and culturally inclusive approach to healthcare. Encouraging the exploration and adoption of herbal remedies not only pays homage to the wisdom of our ancestors but also paves the way for a future where natural and conventional medicine converge for the betterment of human health.

Historical Use of Herbal Remedies

The annals of history are replete with the myriad ways in which herbs have been employed for healing purposes. These practices, deeply embedded in the cultural fabric of ancient civilizations, offer a window into the resourcefulness and ingenuity of our ancestors in their quest for health and wellness.

- **Egyptian Civilization**: Ancient Egyptians are renowned for their sophisticated use of herbal remedies, a practice meticulously documented in the Ebers Papyrus, dating back to 1550 BC. Herbs such as garlic, used for its broad-spectrum antimicrobial properties, and aloe vera, prized for its healing and soothing capabilities, were staples in their medicinal arsenal.

- **Chinese Tradition**: In China, the use of herbs is a cornerstone of Traditional Chinese Medicine (TCM), a system of health and wellness that has persisted for thousands of years. The Shen Nong Ben Cao Jing, an ancient Chinese text, catalogues hundreds of medicinal plants and their uses, emphasizing the importance of balance and harmony between the body and nature.
- **Indian Ayurveda**: Similarly, Ayurveda, the traditional system of medicine in India, incorporates a vast pharmacopeia of herbal remedies. Plants like turmeric, with its anti-inflammatory properties, and ashwagandha, known for its adaptogenic effects, are just a few examples of how herbs play a pivotal role in Ayurvedic healing practices.

These cultures developed and maintained their herbal practices through careful observation of the natural world, passed down through generations. The holistic approach taken by these ancient systems—viewing the body as an interconnected whole—underscores a profound understanding of the human body and its relationship with nature. This historical use of herbal remedies, deeply rooted in tradition and empirical knowledge, lays the foundation for their continued relevance and application in modern times, encouraging us to explore and possibly reincorporate these age-old practices into our contemporary health and wellness paradigms.

Modern Applications of Ancient Remedies

In the realm of contemporary medicine, the utilization of ancient herbal remedies has seen a remarkable transition. This evolution from traditional to modern applications is not only a testament to the enduring value of herbal knowledge but also highlights the growing interest in integrating natural therapies into mainstream healthcare. Scientific research and clinical trials have played a pivotal role in this transformation, offering validation and a deeper understanding of how these ancient remedies can be harnessed today.

One of the most compelling aspects of this modern application is the scientific community's increased focus on the potential benefits of herbal remedies. For instance, studies on St. John's Wort have provided substantial evidence of its effectiveness in treating mild to moderate depression, mirroring its historical use for mood disorders. Similarly, the anti-inflammatory properties of turmeric, long celebrated in Ayurvedic medicine, have been substantiated through rigorous clinical research, underscoring its potential in treating conditions like arthritis and digestive disorders.

Furthermore, the transition of some herbal remedies into pharmaceuticals exemplifies their modern relevance. The development of drugs from willow bark extract, which has a rich history of use dating back to ancient civilizations for pain relief, into aspirin, one of the most widely used medications worldwide, is a prime example of this.

However, this journey from ancient to contemporary medicine has not been without challenges. Standardization of herbal extracts, ensuring consistent dosages and purity, remains a significant hurdle. Moreover, integrating these remedies within a regulatory framework that balances traditional knowledge with scientific scrutiny continues to be an ongoing process.

In essence, the modern applications of ancient herbal remedies represent a convergence of historical wisdom and scientific exploration. This integration not only validates the time-honored practices but also opens new avenues for sustainable and holistic approaches to healthcare. As research continues to evolve, the promise of these ancient remedies in addressing modern health challenges becomes increasingly evident, encouraging a broader acceptance and integration into contemporary medicinal practices.

Evolution of Herbal Practices

The evolution of herbal practices is a fascinating journey through history, shaped by scientific advancements, cultural shifts, and the increased global exchange of knowledge. Initially, herbal remedies were developed through empirical observation and the traditional knowledge passed down through generations. These practices were deeply rooted in the cultural contexts of various civilizations, each with their own methodologies for harvesting, preparing, and applying herbal remedies.

Over time, the advent of scientific methodologies introduced a new dimension to the understanding and application of herbal medicine. The Renaissance period marked a significant shift as scholars began to study and document the medicinal properties of plants systematically. This period laid the groundwork for modern pharmacology by linking the chemical properties of herbs to their therapeutic effects.

The 19th and 20th centuries saw further evolution with the isolation of active compounds from plants, leading to the development of pharmaceuticals. For instance, the discovery of salicylic acid from willow bark paved the way for the synthesis of aspirin, one of the most widely used medications today. This era underscored the shift from traditional herbal preparations to standardized pharmaceutical drugs, highlighting the scientific validation of some ancient remedies.

In recent decades, there has been a cultural shift towards holistic and natural approaches to health, driven by concerns over the synthetic nature and side effects of conventional drugs. This has culminated in a resurgence of interest in herbal medicine, not only as an alternative but as a complementary practice alongside modern medicine. The global exchange of knowledge, facilitated by digital communication, has played a crucial role in this resurgence. People around the world have unprecedented access to a wealth of information on herbal traditions from various cultures, contributing to a more integrated and holistic approach to health.

The evolution of herbal practices reflects a continuum from empirical, tradition-based approaches to scientifically validated methods. It is a testament to the enduring value and relevance of herbal remedies, bridging ancient wisdom with modern scientific insight.

3.2 Case Studies on Traditional Remedies

Herbal remedies have been an essential part of human health care for thousands of years, predating recorded history and forming the backbone of traditional medicines across the world. This invaluable legacy of herbal knowledge has been passed down through generations, offering modern society a rich tapestry of ancient wisdom to explore, validate, and incorporate into contemporary healing practices. In this context, several traditional remedies stand out for their historical significance, enduring relevance, and the scientific interest they have garnered in recent years.

Case Study: Aloe Vera in Ancient Egypt

Aloe Vera, often referred to as the "plant of immortality" in ancient Egyptian texts, has been a cornerstone of herbal medicine for thousands of years. The historical use of this succulent plant in Egyptian culture extends far beyond mere decoration; it was deeply integrated into their daily life, health, and even the afterlife rituals. Aloe Vera's gel, extracted from the leaf's interior, was primarily used for its healing properties, particularly in treating wounds, burns, and skin conditions. Historical records indicate that both Cleopatra and Nefertiti attributed their renowned beauty to this plant, utilizing it as a part of their skincare regimens.

The preparation methods in ancient times were straightforward yet effective. The Aloe leaves were carefully cut and the potent gel was directly applied to the skin or mixed with other natural ingredients to create soothing ointments. This method ensured the preservation of the bioactive compounds responsible for the plant's therapeutic effects.

Fast forward to modern day, scientific research has substantiated many of the traditional uses of Aloe Vera, confirming its efficacy as a natural remedy. Studies have demonstrated its antimicrobial, anti-inflammatory, and healing properties, making it a valuable ingredient in contemporary skincare and health products. Notably, research supports its use in accelerating wound healing, improving skin hydration, and reducing the severity of conditions like psoriasis and dermatitis.

The enduring value of Aloe Vera, from the sandy plains of ancient Egypt to the modern laboratory, exemplifies the timeless relevance of herbal remedies. Its journey through time highlights the importance of integrating traditional knowledge with contemporary scientific validation, offering a holistic approach to well-being that is both sustainable and effective.

Case Study: Turmeric in Ayurvedic Medicine

Turmeric, a vibrant yellow spice, has been a cornerstone of Ayurvedic medicine for thousands of years, esteemed for its anti-inflammatory and healing properties. Its active compound, curcumin, is credited with much of its medicinal value, offering anti-inflammatory, antioxidant, and potential anti-cancer effects. Historically, turmeric was used in Ayurveda to treat a broad range of ailments, from pain and inflammation to digestive issues and wounds.

The method of preparation and use varied, often involving the creation of pastes for topical application or the ingestion of turmeric in various forms, such as teas or powders, to address internal issues. The holistic approach of Ayurvedic medicine emphasizes balance within the body, with turmeric serving as a key element in promoting health and wellness.

Modern research supports many of these traditional uses, with studies demonstrating curcumin's potential to alleviate symptoms of arthritis, reduce the risk of heart disease, and even combat certain forms of cancer. However, curcumin's bioavailability is a noted challenge, prompting the development of various strategies, including the use of adjuvants like piperine, to enhance absorption.

Despite the need for further research, the enduring use of turmeric in both traditional and contemporary practices underscores its significance. Its widespread acceptance in the dietary supplement market, as well as its incorporation into modern medical studies, attests to the blend of ancient wisdom with modern science, offering promising avenues for holistic health solutions and the potential for new therapeutic applications.

Case Study: Willow Bark in Ancient Greece

Willow bark, often referred to as nature's aspirin, has a rich history dating back to ancient Greek medicine. The use of willow bark for its analgesic properties was well documented by Hippocrates, who advised his patients to chew on willow bark or drink willow bark tea to reduce fever and alleviate pain. This practice was based on the recognition of the bark's therapeutic effects, which stem from its active compound, salicin. When ingested, salicin is metabolized into salicylic acid, a precursor of the active ingredient in modern aspirin, acetylsalicylic acid.

The significance of willow bark in ancient Greece extends beyond its use in pain relief. It was part of a broader pharmacopeia that integrated natural remedies into holistic approaches to health and wellness. This integration underscores the ancient Greeks' understanding of the natural world's potential to heal, a concept that continues to resonate in modern herbal medicine.

In recent years, scientific studies have reinforced the historical use of willow bark as an effective natural remedy. Research has confirmed its analgesic and anti-inflammatory properties, making it a viable option for treating headaches, lower back pain, and osteoarthritis. These studies often involve standardized extracts of willow bark, ensuring consistent dosages of salicin, which validate the analgesic properties observed by the ancients.

The continued relevance of willow bark in modern herbal medicine is a testament to the enduring value of traditional remedies. It exemplifies how ancient wisdom, when examined through the lens of contemporary science, can offer sustainable alternatives to synthetic medications. This aligns with a growing interest in natural and holistic approaches to health, encouraging individuals to explore and possibly incorporate herbal remedies like willow bark into their wellness routines.

The Continuity and Evolution of Herbal Wisdom

These case studies exemplify the continuity of herbal wisdom from ancient times to the present day, underlining the enduring value and relevance of traditional remedies. The journey from empirical use, based on observation and experience, to scientific validation highlights the dynamic evolution of herbal practices influenced by advancements in science, cultural exchanges, and the global movement towards integrative health approaches.

Despite the tremendous advances in medicine, the interest in and respect for these ancient remedies persist, driven by their natural origin, fewer side effects, and the growing body of scientific research validating their efficacy. Challenges such as standardization, quality control, and ensuring the sustainable use of these natural resources are focal points for contemporary herbal practice and research.

In integrating traditional remedies with modern medical practices, a holistic approach to health that respects the wisdom of the past while leveraging scientific advancements presents a promising path forward. This synthesis not only enhances the therapeutic arsenal available to practitioners and patients alike but also honors the rich heritage of herbal medicine that has been a bedrock of human health care through the ages.

3.3 Evaluating the Efficacy of Ancient Remedies Today

In the quest to meld the wisdom of ancient herbal practices with the precision of contemporary science, a fascinating journey unfolds—one that evaluates the efficacy of time-honored remedies through the lens of modern scientific methodologies. This exploration not only honors the heritage of traditional medicine but also seeks to substantiate its value in today's health paradigm, emphasizing an integrative approach to healing.

Scientific Research on Herbal Remedies

Remarkable strides have been made in the scientific investigation of herbal remedies, with numerous studies illuminating the biological mechanisms through which these natural healers exert their effects. For instance, curcumin, the active component in turmeric, has been extensively studied for its anti-inflammatory, antioxidant, and anticarcinogenic properties. Similarly, ginkgo biloba, used for centuries to enhance cognitive function, has been subjected to clinical trials that examine its impact on dementia and memory impairment. These studies not only validate the therapeutic benefits of these herbs but also pave the way for their incorporation into conventional treatment protocols.

Challenges in Validating Ancient Practices

Despite the promising insights gained from scientific research, several challenges persist in validating the efficacy of ancient remedies. One of the primary hurdles is the inherent variability of natural products, which can lead to inconsistencies in potency and effectiveness. Additionally, the lack of standardized extraction methods and dosages complicates the process of scientific validation. Cultural differences in medical practices and the subjective interpretation of healing also pose significant challenges, necessitating a nuanced approach to the evaluation of traditional remedies.

Integrating Traditional and Modern Medicine

The integration of traditional remedies into modern medical practices represents an exciting frontier in healthcare. This holistic approach acknowledges the value of ancient wisdom while leveraging the advancements of contemporary science to offer a more comprehensive and personalized treatment paradigm. For example, the incorporation of St. John's Wort, a herb known for its antidepressant properties, into treatment plans for mild to moderate depression exemplifies the potential of this synergy. Similarly, the use of acupuncture alongside conventional pain management strategies offers a compelling illustration of how traditional and modern practices can complement each other to enhance patient outcomes.

The Role of Ethnobotany and Ethnopharmacology

Ethnobotany and ethnopharmacology play critical roles in bridging the gap between traditional knowledge and scientific validation. By documenting the medicinal uses of plants within indigenous cultures, researchers can identify promising candidates for further scientific investigation. This not only enriches our understanding of plant-based medicine but also supports the conservation of biodiversity and the protection of indigenous knowledge.

Future Directions

Looking ahead, the future of evaluating the efficacy of ancient remedies is ripe with potential. Advances in pharmacognosy, pharmacology, and biotechnology hold the promise of unlocking new therapeutic discoveries from the ancient pharmacopeia. Moreover, the growing interest in personalized medicine and the increasing acceptance of integrative health practices underscore the relevance of traditional remedies in addressing the complex health challenges of the modern world.

Conclusion

As we continue to evaluate the efficacy of ancient remedies through the rigorous lens of modern science, we are reminded of the profound wisdom embedded in traditional practices. This synthesis of the old and the new not only validates the enduring value of herbal remedies but also expands our therapeutic arsenal, offering new avenues for healing and well-being. By embracing the richness of our global heritage and the advancements of contemporary research, we pave the way for a more inclusive and holistic approach to health, one that honors the past while innovating for the future.

Scientific Research on Herbal Remedies

In recent years, the scientific community has taken a renewed interest in the study of traditional herbal remedies, a pursuit that has yielded fascinating results. Clinical trials and laboratory research have begun to shed light on the efficacy of herbs used by ancient cultures, providing a scientific basis for their continued use in modern medicine.

One notable study focused on the effectiveness of ginger in reducing nausea and vomiting during pregnancy. Researchers found that ginger was as effective as vitamin B6, a commonly recommended treatment, in reducing symptoms without significant side effects, echoing ancient Chinese and Ayurvedic practices that have used ginger for gastrointestinal discomfort.

Another significant area of research has been the anti-inflammatory and antioxidant properties of turmeric. Curcumin, the active compound in turmeric, has been extensively studied for its potential in treating chronic conditions such as arthritis, heart disease, and Alzheimer's. Studies have shown that curcumin can reduce markers of inflammation and oxidative stress, offering support for its use as a therapeutic agent, much like it has been used in Ayurvedic medicine for centuries.

The antiviral properties of Echinacea, a remedy long used by Native American tribes for a variety of ailments, have also been confirmed by scientific research. Clinical trials have demonstrated that Echinacea can reduce the duration and severity of the common cold, providing a modern validation of its traditional use.

These studies represent just a fraction of the ongoing research into herbal remedies. The findings not only validate the wisdom of ancient herbal practices but also highlight the potential for these natural compounds to complement modern medicine. As scientific inquiry continues to unravel the complexities of plant-based therapeutics, the integration of herbal remedies into contemporary healthcare offers a promising bridge between traditional wisdom and scientific validation, underscoring their relevance in today's medical landscape.

Challenges in Validating Ancient Practices

The pursuit of integrating ancient herbal remedies into modern medical practices faces a myriad of challenges, chief among them issues of standardization, variability of natural products, and cultural differences in medical approaches. Each of these factors presents a unique set of obstacles that researchers and practitioners must navigate to validate the efficacy of traditional remedies scientifically.

- **Standardization**: One of the significant hurdles in the scientific validation of herbal remedies is the lack of standardization. Unlike synthetic pharmaceuticals, which have precise, quantifiable active ingredients, herbal remedies are complex mixtures of many components. This complexity complicates the process of creating standardized doses and formulations, making it challenging to ensure consistency in the strength and composition of herbal products. As a result, comparing study outcomes or replicating successful treatments can be difficult, undermining the reliability of herbal remedies in the eyes of the medical community.
- **Variability of Natural Products**: The variability in the potency and composition of herbal materials adds another layer of complexity. Factors such as the plant's growing conditions, harvest time, and storage methods can significantly impact the chemical makeup of the final herbal product. This inherent variability makes it hard to predict the efficacy and safety of herbal treatments, posing a challenge to their clinical validation and acceptance.
- **Cultural Differences in Medical Approaches**: Furthermore, the integration of traditional herbal practices into modern medicine is complicated by cultural differences in medical philosophies. While Western medicine typically focuses on treating specific symptoms or diseases,

many traditional herbal practices take a more holistic approach, considering the patient's overall physical and mental well-being. Bridging these differing perspectives requires not only scientific validation of herbal remedies but also a cultural understanding and appreciation of traditional medical systems.

Navigating these challenges is crucial for the scientific community to unlock the full potential of ancient herbal remedies, ensuring their safe and effective integration into contemporary medicine. By addressing these issues, we can pave the way for a more holistic and inclusive approach to healthcare, combining the best of both worlds.

Integrating Traditional and Modern Medicine

The integration of traditional remedies into modern medical practices signifies a groundbreaking blend of ancient wisdom and contemporary scientific knowledge. This fusion not only acknowledges the value of historical herbal practices but also enhances the efficacy and scope of modern healthcare solutions.

Benefits of Integrating Traditional and Modern Medicine

1. **Comprehensive Healthcare Approach**: Combining traditional herbal remedies with modern medicine offers a more holistic approach to healthcare. This integration addresses not only the physical symptoms of a disease but also its underlying causes, recognizing the interconnectedness of the body, mind, and environment.

2. **Enhanced Patient Outcomes**: Utilizing herbal remedies alongside conventional treatments can lead to improved patient outcomes. For instance, certain herbs may reduce the side effects of chemotherapy, increase its efficacy, or alleviate pain and discomfort in palliative care, thereby improving the quality of life for patients.

3. **Sustainability**: Many traditional remedies are derived from renewable plant sources, making them more environmentally sustainable than some synthetic drugs. Integrating these practices encourages the use of natural, biodegradable resources and supports conservation efforts.

4. **Cultural Sensitivity**: Integrating traditional medicine respects and preserves indigenous knowledge and cultural heritage. This approach fosters a healthcare system that is sensitive to the cultural context of patients, promoting inclusivity and accessibility.

5. **Cost-Effectiveness**: In many cases, herbal remedies offer a cost-effective alternative to pharmaceutical drugs, especially for chronic conditions. This accessibility can make healthcare more affordable and attainable for a broader segment of the population.

Conclusion

The integration of traditional remedies into modern medical practices presents an exciting frontier in healthcare. By acknowledging the value of ancient wisdom and subjecting it to scientific scrutiny, we can unlock potent and sustainable healthcare solutions that respect cultural traditions and are accessible to all. This blending of worlds not only enriches our medical toolkit but also ensures a comprehensive, holistic approach to wellness that is both effective and respectful of the earth and its cultures.

Chapter 4: Lost and Lesser-Known Herbs

4.1 Rediscovering Forgotten Herbs

Herbal remedies have been a cornerstone of traditional medicine for centuries, offering a wealth of health benefits that modern science is only beginning to understand. In the quest for improved health and wellness, there is a growing interest in revisiting the wisdom of the past, particularly the use of forgotten and lesser-known herbs. These plants, once integral to daily life and healing practices, have gradually fallen out of favor due to various factors. This exploration seeks to unearth the historical significance of these herbs, understand the reasons behind their decline, and inspire a resurgence in their use.

Historical Significance of Forgotten Herbs

The use of herbs in medicine and daily life dates back thousands of years, with early civilizations relying on the natural world for healing and sustenance. These plants were not only used for their medicinal properties but also held cultural and spiritual significance. For example, ancient texts and archaeological findings reveal the extensive use of herbs such as Silphium, used for its contraceptive properties in ancient Libya, and Lovage, a key culinary and medicinal herb in medieval Europe. These herbs played crucial roles in their respective societies, from enhancing the flavors of meals to providing remedies for common ailments.

In many cultures, the knowledge of herbal remedies was passed down through generations, embedding these plants deeply into the fabric of daily life. Healers, often women, were the custodians of this knowledge, using herbs to treat wounds, prevent diseases, and maintain health. The historical significance of these herbs extends beyond their practical applications, reflecting the interconnection between humans and nature and the reliance on the environment for survival and well-being.

Reasons for Decline in Use

The decline in the use of many once-popular herbs can be attributed to several factors. The advent of modern medicine, with its focus on synthetic drugs and quick fixes, has led to a diminished interest in traditional herbal remedies. As societies industrialized and became more urbanized, the direct connection to nature and the knowledge of local flora diminished. Additionally, the globalization of food and medicine has resulted in a homogenization of healing practices, with a focus on a narrow range of commercially viable herbs, neglecting the rich diversity of local plant life.

Changes in medical practices and regulations have also played a role in the decline of some herbs. With the rise of evidence-based medicine, herbs that could not be easily standardized or lacked scientific research to support their efficacy were sidelined. Furthermore, some herbs fell out of use due to concerns over safety and potential side effects, especially when not used correctly or in combination with modern pharmaceuticals.

Current Research and Interest

Despite these challenges, there is a rekindled interest in forgotten and lesser-known herbs, fueled by a growing body of scientific research and a desire to return to more natural and sustainable practices. Researchers are beginning to uncover the pharmacological properties of these plants, validating traditional uses and discovering new applications. For example, studies on the herb Ashwagandha, long used in Ayurvedic medicine for its stress-reducing properties, have shown promising results in clinical trials.

Ethnobotanical research, exploring the relationship between people and plants, has also contributed to the revival of interest in these herbs. By documenting traditional uses and knowledge, scientists and herbalists are working to ensure that this wisdom is not lost but rather integrated into modern practices. This research is not only about preserving history but also about expanding the toolkit available for health and wellness, offering potential alternatives and complements to conventional medicine.

The rise of the internet and social media has played a significant role in the resurgence of interest in herbal remedies. Online communities and platforms have made it easier for people to share knowledge, experiences, and recipes, bridging the gap between traditional knowledge and modern users. This democratization of information has empowered individuals to explore and experiment with herbal remedies, fostering a culture of curiosity and self-care.

In conclusion, the rediscovery of forgotten and lesser-known herbs represents an exciting frontier in the intersection of history, culture, and medicine. These plants, with their rich historical significance and untapped potential, offer a tangible link to the past and a promising resource for the future. By revisiting the wisdom of our ancestors and integrating it with modern scientific understanding, we can expand our approaches to health and wellness, embracing the diversity and sustainability of the natural world. As interest and research continue to grow, these once-forgotten herbs are poised to regain their rightful place in the pantheon of natural remedies, enriching our lives and healing practices.

4.2 Revival Recipes for Lesser-Known Herbs

In the pursuit of reviving the heritage and wisdom of using lesser-known herbs, it becomes essential to blend traditional knowledge with modern culinary and health practices. This section unveils a collection of practical recipes and methods designed to reintegrate forgotten herbs into our daily lives. These preparations not only honor the timeless traditions from which they originate but are also adapted to suit contemporary tastes and lifestyle needs.

1. NETTLE TEA

Ingredients:

- Fresh or dried nettle leaves
- Water

Steps:

1 Use gloves to handle and rinse fresh nettle leaves.
2 Steep 1-2 tablespoons of leaves in hot water for 10-15 minutes.
3 Strain and serve.

Usage Tips: Nettle tea is nutrient-rich and historically consumed for its benefits to the kidneys and urinary tract.

2. DANDELION ROOT DIGESTIVE TONIC

Ingredients:

- Dried dandelion root
- Water
- Honey (optional)

Steps:

1 Simmer 1 teaspoon of dried dandelion root in a cup of water for 15-20 minutes.
2 Strain and add honey to taste if desired.

Usage Tips: Dandelion root is traditionally used to support liver function and digestion.

3. MUGWORT DREAM PILLOW

Ingredients:

- Dried mugwort
- Fabric
- Needle and thread

Steps:

1 Fill a small fabric pillow with dried mugwort leaves.
2 Sew the pillow shut.
3 Place it under your pillow.

Usage Tips: Mugwort is valued for inducing vivid dreams and supporting sleep.

4. NETTLE PESTO

Ingredients:

- Fresh nettle leaves (blanched)
- Garlic
- Pine nuts
- Parmesan cheese
- Olive oil
- Salt
- Pepper

Steps:

1 Blanch fresh nettle leaves to remove stinging properties.
2 Blend all ingredients in a food processor until smooth.

Usage Tips: Nettle pesto can be used as a nutritious alternative to basil in pasta dishes, sandwiches, and as a dip.

5. DANDELION SALAD

Ingredients:

- Tender dandelion greens
- Cherry tomatoes
- Goat cheese

- Olive oil
- Balsamic vinegar
- Salt
- Pepper

Steps:

1 Wash the dandelion greens thoroughly.
2 Toss greens with cherry tomatoes, goat cheese, olive oil, balsamic vinegar, salt, and pepper.

Usage Tips: Dandelion leaves add a bitter, peppery flavor that complements the creamy goat cheese and sweet balsamic dressing.

6. HERBAL INFUSED OILS

Ingredients:

- Dried herbs of your choice (e.g., mugwort, lavender)
- Carrier oil (e.g., olive, almond)

Steps:

1 Fill a jar with dried herbs.
2 Cover herbs with carrier oil, ensuring they are fully submerged.
3 Place the jar in a sunny spot for 4-6 weeks, shaking occasionally.
4 Strain the oil.

Usage Tips: Use the infused oil for massage, in bathwater, or as a moisturizer.

7. NETTLE SOUP

Ingredients:

- Fresh nettle leaves
- Onion
- Garlic
- Potatoes
- Vegetable broth
- Olive oil
- Salt
- Pepper

Steps:

1 Blanch nettle leaves to remove stinging properties.
2 Sauté onion and garlic in olive oil until soft.
3 Add diced potatoes and vegetable broth, and bring to a boil.
4 Add nettle leaves and simmer until potatoes are tender.

5 Blend until smooth and season with salt and pepper.

Usage Tips: Nettle soup is a nutritious and warming dish, perfect for spring when nettles are in season.

8. DANDELION ROOT COFFEE

Ingredients:

- Dried dandelion root
- Water
- Milk or cream (optional)
- Sweetener (optional)

Steps:

1 Roast dried dandelion root in the oven until dark brown.
2 Grind roasted roots to a fine powder.
3 Simmer 1-2 teaspoons of the powder in a cup of water for 10 minutes.
4 Strain and add milk or cream and sweetener if desired.

Usage Tips: Dandelion root coffee is a caffeine-free alternative to regular coffee, with a rich, earthy flavor.

9. MUGWORT INCENSE STICKS

Ingredients:

- Dried mugwort
- Incense stick bases
- Essential oil (optional)

Steps:

1 Grind dried mugwort into a fine powder.
2 Mix the powder with a small amount of water to form a paste.
3 Coat incense stick bases with the paste.
4 Allow the sticks to dry completely.
5 Add a few drops of essential oil if desired.

Usage Tips: Mugwort incense can be burned to cleanse spaces and promote relaxation and vivid dreams.

10. NETTLE AND DANDELION SMOOTHIE

Ingredients:

- Fresh nettle leaves (blanched)

- Fresh dandelion leaves
- Banana
- Apple
- Lemon juice
- Water or coconut water

Steps:

1 Blanch nettle leaves to remove stinging properties.
2 Combine all ingredients in a blender.
3 Blend until smooth.

Usage Tips: This smoothie is a detoxifying and nutrient-packed drink, great for a healthy start to the day.

Safety and Dosage Guidelines

While exploring the rich world of herbal remedies, it is crucial to adhere to safety and dosage guidelines to ensure beneficial and safe use. Here are some considerations:

- **Consult with a healthcare provider** before incorporating significant amounts of any herb into your diet, especially if you are pregnant, nursing, or have existing health conditions.
- **Start with small doses** to observe how your body reacts to a new herb.
- **Research potential interactions** between herbs and medications you are currently taking.
- **Harvest responsibly** if foraging wild herbs, ensuring correct identification and sustainable practices.

Reviving the use of lesser-known herbs in our daily routines invites us to reconnect with the earth's natural bounty and the ancient wisdom of our ancestors. By weaving these traditional recipes and their modern adaptations into our lives, we open ourselves up to a world of natural flavors, healing properties, and sustainable living practices. This journey not only enriches our personal health and well-being but also fosters a deeper appreciation for the intricate relationships between humans and plants. As we continue to explore and revive these lost remedies, we contribute to the preservation of herbal heritage and empower ourselves with the knowledge to care for our health naturally.

Traditional Recipes

In the realm of herbal remedies, the art of incorporating lesser-known herbs into daily life has a rich history. One emblematic recipe that has stood the test of time is the "Herbal Tonic for Vitality." Historically used to invigorate and rejuvenate, this tonic embodies the essence of herbal tradition, blending the unique properties of herbs that may not be widely recognized today.

Herbal Tonic for Vitality Recipe:

- **Ingredients**:
    - 1 teaspoon of dried mugwort (Artemisia vulgaris)
    - 1 teaspoon of dried vervain (Verbena officinalis)
    - 1 teaspoon of dried nettle leaves (Urtica dioica)
    - 500ml of boiling water
- **Instructions**:

1. Combine the dried mugwort, vervain, and nettle leaves in a teapot or a heat-resistant container.
    2. Pour the boiling water over the herbs and cover the container. Allow it to steep for about 10-15 minutes. This allows the water to become infused with the medicinal properties of the herbs.
    3. Strain the mixture to remove the herbs. The resulting tonic can be consumed warm or cold.
    4. For added benefits and flavor, a teaspoon of honey or lemon juice can be added to taste.

This tonic, grounded in historical usage, was often recommended for its purported benefits in boosting energy and supporting overall well-being. Each herb was selected for its specific properties; mugwort for its ability to stimulate and support digestion, vervain as a nervine tonic, and nettle for its rich mineral content and rejuvenating properties.

In integrating such traditional recipes into contemporary life, it's essential to embrace the historical context and recognize the blend of art and science that ancient herbalists practiced. This approach not only honors the past but also opens a window to a more holistic and nature-connected lifestyle.

Modern Adaptations

In the journey of bringing traditional herbal remedies into the modern era, adapting ancient recipes for contemporary use is both an art and a necessity. This evolution allows us to incorporate the wisdom of the past into our fast-paced lives, ensuring these valuable plants do not fade into obscurity. The key to this adaptation lies in understanding the essence of each herb's benefits and finding innovative ways to include them in daily routines.

- **Herbal Infusions and Teas**: Many traditional recipes start with simple teas or infusions. Modern adaptations can retain the simplicity of this method while introducing these drinks as a regular part of one's wellness routine. For instance, a calming tea made from lesser-known herbs like lemon balm or passionflower can be prepared in advance and enjoyed chilled as a refreshing and therapeutic summer beverage.

- **Culinary Uses**: Integrating herbs into daily meals not only enhances flavor but also boosts nutritional value. Herbs such as lovage, with its celery-like taste, can be incorporated into soups and stews. Meanwhile, sweet herbs like stevia can naturally sweeten dishes without the need for processed sugars.
- **Topical Applications**: The modern adaptations of herbal salves and ointments for skin and body care offer a direct connection to traditional uses while catering to contemporary desires for natural and sustainable beauty products. Herbs with anti-inflammatory properties, such as comfrey or yarrow, can be infused into oils to create soothing balms.

The adaptation of traditional herbal recipes to fit modern lifestyles not only preserves these ancient practices but also underscores the timeless relevance of herbal remedies. By creatively integrating these herbs into our daily lives, we honor our heritage and embrace a more natural and holistic approach to health.

4.3 Modern Applications of Historical Herbs

In the realm of herbal remedies, the resurgence of historical herbs presents a bridge between the past and present, weaving the rich tapestry of traditional medicine into the fabric of contemporary health practices. As we delve into the modern applications of these long-forgotten botanicals, a new world of potential benefits and scientific understanding unfolds, illuminating the path for integrating these ancient wonders into our daily wellness routines.

Historical herbs, once staples in the apothecaries and healing rituals of ancient civilizations, are now being re-evaluated under the rigorous lens of modern science. Studies have begun to validate what traditional healers have known for centuries - these plants possess potent pharmacological properties capable of addressing a wide array of modern ailments. From anti-inflammatory and antimicrobial effects to stress reduction and immune support, the potential health benefits of rediscovered herbs are vast and varied. Research exploring the efficacy of herbs like Ashwagandha for stress relief, Turmeric for its anti-inflammatory properties, and St. John's Wort for depression showcases the intersection of ancient wisdom and contemporary science.

The integration of historical herbs into modern health and wellness practices is not merely about consuming these plants as supplements. It is about understanding their multifaceted roles in holistic health. For instance, incorporating herbal elements into dietary routines, embracing herbal teas for their therapeutic benefits, and utilizing herbal extracts in skincare regimens exemplify the versatile use of these botanicals. Moreover, the principles of sustainable sourcing and ethical cultivation of these herbs underscore the importance of environmental stewardship and social responsibility in the herbal supplement industry.

Yet, the journey of integrating these ancient plants into contemporary life does not come without challenges. The variability in the quality of herbal products, the need for standardized dosages, and the scarcity of comprehensive clinical trials are hurdles that must be navigated carefully. Educating consumers about the importance of consulting healthcare providers before embarking on herbal treatments ensures informed decisions are made, safeguarding against potential drug-herb interactions and side effects.

Inspiring stories of individuals and communities successfully incorporating historical herbs into their health practices serve as beacons of possibility. From athletes utilizing adaptogenic herbs to enhance physical performance and recovery, to individuals battling chronic illnesses finding relief in the ancient remedies, these success stories highlight the transformative power of integrating historical herbs into modern wellness paradigms.

In conclusion, the revival and integration of historical herbs into contemporary health and wellness practices represent a confluence of tradition and innovation. As scientific research continues to unravel the mysteries of these ancient botanicals, their incorporation into modern life holds the promise of enhanced health and wellness. By embracing the wisdom of the past and harnessing the scientific advancements of the present, we pave the way for a future where holistic and integrative health practices are accessible to all.

Current Scientific Understanding

The resurgence of interest in traditional herbal remedies has been paralleled by an increase in scientific research aimed at understanding the pharmacological properties and potential health benefits of these plants. Studies have begun to unveil the scientific basis behind the efficacy of many herbs that were once staples in ancient healing practices but had fallen into obscurity.

For instance, research into the **herb Ginkgo biloba**, long revered for its memory-enhancing properties, has shown it contains powerful antioxidants that may help protect nerve cells and improve blood circulation to the brain. Similarly, **St. John's Wort**, used for centuries to combat depression, has been scientifically validated for its antidepressant properties, attributed to the active compounds hypericin and hyperforin which appear to impact neurotransmitter activity.

Another lesser-known herb, **Ashwagandha**, has been the subject of numerous studies due to its adaptogenic properties, which help the body withstand stress. Research suggests that its bioactive compounds, including withanolides, may significantly reduce cortisol levels and thus potentially aid in stress management and anxiety reduction.

Moreover, the **Turmeric** root, a staple in ancient medicine for its anti-inflammatory properties, has been substantiated through research to contain curcumin, a compound that can modulate the inflammatory processes within the body. This finding supports its traditional use and opens up possibilities for its application in chronic inflammation and pain management.

These examples underscore the importance of integrating traditional knowledge with modern scientific inquiry. By doing so, it becomes possible to not only validate the historical uses of these herbs but also to unlock potentially groundbreaking applications in contemporary medicine. Such research not only enriches our understanding of herbal pharmacology but also emphasizes the relevance of these ancient remedies in addressing modern health challenges.

Integrating Historical Herbs into Modern Practices

The reintegration of historical herbs into modern health and wellness practices represents a bridge between ancient wisdom and contemporary science. As we delve deeper into the pharmacological properties and potential health benefits of these plants, we find compelling reasons to incorporate them into our daily routines.

Herbal Medicine: One of the most direct applications is in the realm of herbal medicine, where these plants are utilized for their therapeutic properties. For instance, adaptogenic herbs, once used by ancient cultures to increase resilience to stress, are finding their place in modern herbal formulations to support the body's stress response system. Herbs like Ashwagandha and Rhodiola, scarcely known a few decades ago, are now staples in health food stores, backed by scientific studies affirming their efficacy.

Nutrition: In nutrition, forgotten herbs are making a comeback as superfoods. Moringa, often referred to as the "miracle tree," was used in ancient India and Africa to combat malnutrition. Today, it's celebrated for its high vitamin and mineral content, making it a valuable addition to smoothies, teas, and supplements aiming to boost overall health and wellness.

Alternative Therapies: Beyond ingestion, these herbs are also being incorporated into alternative therapies such as aromatherapy and massage. Essential oils derived from once-overlooked plants are now prized for their ability to promote relaxation, enhance mood, and even improve cognitive function. Lavender and peppermint are two prominent examples, with studies supporting their use in reducing anxiety and alleviating headache pain, respectively.

The integration of historical herbs into these facets of modern life not only offers a broader spectrum of tools for improving health and wellness but also reinforces the importance of biodiversity and the conservation of plant species. As we continue to validate the benefits of these plants through scientific research, their role in enhancing our quality of life becomes ever more apparent, encouraging a holistic approach to health that honors the wisdom of the past while embracing the innovations of the present.

Case Studies and Success Stories

In the realm of herbal remedies, the revival of ancient practices is not just a trend but a testament to the enduring wisdom of traditional medicine. Among the notable examples of this revival is the story of a small community in the rural areas of Vermont, where the use of *Valeriana officinalis*, commonly known as valerian, has transformed the health and wellness practices of the local population. Historically used for its sedative and calming effects, valerian root had fallen out of favor in the community due to the availability of synthetic alternatives. However, a local herbalist, inspired by ethnobotanical research highlighting the plant's efficacy in treating mild anxiety and sleep disorders, began cultivating valerian in her garden. She shared her harvest and knowledge with the community, leading to a resurgence in its use. The outcomes were significant, with many reporting improved sleep patterns and reduced anxiety levels, demonstrating the practical applications of this historical herb in a modern context.

Another success story comes from the southwestern United States, where the native herb *Eriodictyon californicum*, or Yerba Santa, was traditionally used by indigenous tribes for respiratory health. Recent scientific studies have validated its anti-inflammatory and expectorant properties, sparking interest among herbal practitioners. A group of herbal medicine enthusiasts, in collaboration with local indigenous communities, initiated workshops to teach people how to utilize Yerba Santa for treating colds and allergies. These workshops have not only led to improved respiratory health in the region but also fostered a deeper appreciation and respect for indigenous knowledge and practices.

These case studies underscore the potential of integrating historical herbs into contemporary health and wellness practices. They highlight not just the therapeutic benefits of these plants but also the importance of preserving and respecting traditional knowledge. As we continue to explore the vast pharmacopeia of the natural world, stories like these serve as powerful reminders of the relevance and sustainability of herbal remedies in our modern lives.

Chapter 5: Ancient Cultivation and Harvesting Techniques

5.1 Traditional Cultivation Methods

The traditional methods used to cultivate herbs are not just agricultural practices; they are a testament to the deep connection our ancestors had with the earth and its bounty. These methods, having stood the test of time, offer not only a window into the past but a potential path forward for sustainable and effective herbal cultivation.

Soil Preparation and Planting

Central to traditional herbal cultivation is the meticulous preparation of soil, a process that ensures the land is fertile and conducive to plant growth. Ancient methods relied heavily on natural and organic practices, with crop rotation being a fundamental technique. By alternating the types of crops grown in each area of land, our ancestors promoted soil health, reducing the risk of soil depletion and pest build-up. This method ensured that the soil remained rich in nutrients, which is essential for the growth of robust herbal plants.

Companion planting was another technique widely used in traditional herb cultivation. This method involves planting different crops in close proximity for pest control, pollination, providing habitat for beneficial insects, maximizing use of space, and increasing crop productivity. For example, the planting of marigolds alongside herbs to deter pests naturally without the use of synthetic chemicals.

Natural fertilization methods were also integral to soil preparation. Composting, the process of converting organic waste into rich soil, was commonly used. This not only provided a natural source of nutrients for the plants but also promoted soil moisture retention, crucial for the growth of healthy herbs.

Watering and Maintenance

The challenge of watering and maintaining an herb garden was met with innovative solutions that mimicked natural ecosystems. Ancient herbalists often utilized natural irrigation methods such as the use of small waterways or channels that allowed water to flow gently and directly to the roots of plants. This method, akin to the modern technique of drip irrigation, ensured that plants received an adequate amount of water without wastage.

Maintaining plant health was a cornerstone of traditional herbal cultivation, with a strong emphasis on preventing issues before they arose. This preventative approach included practices such as mulching, which helped retain soil moisture and regulate temperature, and the selection of resilient plant varieties well-suited to local conditions. Without synthetic chemicals, the health of the herb garden relied on the balance and health of the ecosystem, illustrating a holistic approach to plant care.

Pest Control and Disease Management

Pest control and disease management in traditional herb cultivation were handled with an understanding of the natural environment and a preference for balance rather than domination. Herbalists often employed natural remedies, such as planting pest-deterring plants or employing biological control agents like insects that prey on herb pests.

One of the most fascinating aspects of traditional pest management was the use of botanical preparations made from other plants. For instance, neem oil, derived from the seeds of the neem tree, has been used for centuries to control pests naturally. These methods reflect a deep understanding of nature's interconnected systems, where every solution is sourced directly from the environment.

The concept of 'pests' was also seen through a different lens, with a greater tolerance for non-destructive insects, recognizing their role in the broader ecosystem. This symbiotic relationship between plants and insects encouraged a biodiversity that is often lacking in modern agriculture.

5.2 Harvesting Techniques from Ancient Texts

The practice of harvesting herbs is as ancient as the cultivation of these plants themselves. Throughout history, various cultures have developed specialized techniques, documented in numerous ancient texts, to ensure the efficacy and potency of herbal remedies. These methods, refined through generations, highlight the deep connection between humans and the natural world, offering modern herbalists insights into sustainable and effective practices.

Timing of Harvest

The timing of the harvest is crucial for maximizing the medicinal properties of herbs. Ancient texts often emphasize the importance of considering both the time of day and the phase of the plant's lifecycle. For instance, it is commonly advised to harvest leaves and flowers in the morning after the dew has evaporated but before the midday sun diminishes their essential oils. Roots, on the other hand, are typically harvested in the late afternoon or early evening when the plant's energy is concentrated below ground.

The phase of the moon was also considered influential, with many cultures preferring to harvest during specific lunar phases to enhance the potency of the plants. The waning moon, for example, was seen as an ideal time for harvesting roots as it was believed that the earth's energy was drawing inward, concentrating the plant's essence.

Harvesting Techniques

The methods of harvesting varied significantly depending on the type of herb and its intended use. Leaves, flowers, seeds, roots, and barks all required different approaches:

- **Hand-Picking**: This method was widely used for delicate flowers and leaves, ensuring minimal damage and preserving their vital energies. It allowed for selective harvesting, where only the most vibrant and healthy parts of the plant were chosen.
- **Cutting**: For herbs with tougher stems or those that needed to be harvested in bunches, sharp knives or sickles were used. The angle and height of the cut were carefully considered to promote regrowth and sustain the health of the plant.
- **Gathering**: Seeds and some types of flowers were gathered by shaking or tapping the plant, allowing the ripe seeds to fall naturally. This technique ensured that only seeds at the peak of their maturity were collected.

The tools used in harvesting were often made from natural materials such as stone, bone, or wood, believed to maintain the harmony between the plant and its environment. Metals were chosen carefully, with some traditions favoring iron for its grounding properties and others preferring bronze or copper for their association with Venus, the planet often linked to plants and fertility.

Post-Harvest Handling

Once harvested, the careful handling of herbs was essential to preserve their qualities. Ancient texts provide detailed instructions on cleaning, drying, and storing herbs:

- **Cleaning**: Herbs were gently shaken or brushed to remove dirt and insects, avoiding washing with water unless absolutely necessary to prevent the loss of essential oils.
- **Drying**: The drying process was crucial and varied depending on the herb. Many traditions used airy, shaded spaces to slow-dry herbs, preserving their color and potency. Hanging bundles upside down was a common practice, allowing the essential oils to concentrate in the leaves and flowers.
- **Storing**: Proper storage was essential for maintaining the efficacy of herbs. Ancient herbalists recommended using containers made of natural materials such as clay, wood, or glass, and storing them in cool, dark places. Herbs were often categorized and stored according to their properties, ensuring ease of access and preventing cross-contamination of their energetic qualities.

The knowledge of these ancient practices provides a window into the past, revealing the sophisticated understanding our ancestors had of the natural world. By studying and revitalizing these time-tested techniques, modern herbalists can not only ensure the potency of their remedies but also contribute to the preservation of herbal traditions and the environment.

Integrating these practices requires a deep respect for nature and an understanding of the delicate balance within ecosystems. It encourages a sustainable approach to herbalism that values the health of both the plant and the planet. As we continue to face environmental challenges, the wisdom contained in ancient texts becomes not just a tool for personal health, but a blueprint for ecological stewardship.

By embracing the lessons of the past, we can cultivate a future where the healing power of plants is accessible to all, ensuring the continuity of knowledge for generations to come. This is not just about preserving tradition for tradition's sake; it's about recognizing the inherent value of these practices and their relevance in a modern context. As we move forward, let us do so with the understanding that ancient wisdom, when applied thoughtfully, can lead to innovative solutions that address both our health and the health of our planet.

5.3 Insights from Historical Herbal Practices

Delving into historical herbal practices offers more than just practical cultivation techniques; it provides a philosophy of balance, sustainability, and respect for nature. These ancient methods, developed over generations, highlight a deep understanding of ecological balance and the vital role of herbs in both human and environmental health.

Integration into Daily Life

Herbal cultivation was not merely an agricultural activity but a way of life integrated into the daily routines and cultural practices of ancient communities. Herbs were cultivated not just for their medicinal properties but also for their spiritual, culinary, and aromatic qualities. This integration underscores the versatile role of herbs in ancient societies and their significance beyond mere utility.

Lessons for Modern Herbalists

Modern herbalists can draw valuable lessons from traditional cultivation methods, particularly in terms of sustainability and ecological awareness. By adopting practices such as crop rotation, companion planting, and natural pest management, contemporary herbal cultivation can benefit from increased biodiversity, soil health, and resilience against climate change.

Moreover, these traditional techniques encourage a deeper connection with the plants we cultivate, fostering an appreciation for the intricate relationships within ecosystems. Such an approach is not only beneficial for the environment but also for the cultivation of herbs with potent medicinal properties, as stressors such as pests and diseases are managed in harmony with nature rather than through force.

Preserving Traditional Knowledge

The preservation of traditional herbal knowledge is crucial for the continuation of these sustainable practices. By documenting ancient techniques and adapting them to modern contexts, we can ensure that this wisdom is not lost but rather evolves and grows with us. Strategies for preserving this knowledge include the creation of herbal cultivation communities, both online and in-person, and the integration of traditional methods into contemporary agricultural education.

In closing, the exploration of traditional methods used to cultivate herbs illuminates a path forward that honors our heritage while promoting sustainability and health. By embracing these ancient practices, we not only pay homage to our ancestors but also contribute to a more balanced and sustainable future.

Soil Preparation and Planting

The traditional methods of preparing soil and planting herbs are deeply rooted in practices that harmonize with nature's rhythms and cycles. These techniques, honed over countless generations, offer valuable insights into sustainable cultivation methods that modern herbalists and gardeners can adopt to nurture their gardens.

- **Crop Rotation:** This ancient agricultural practice involves alternating the types of crops grown in a particular area with each season or year. By rotating different herbs and plants, the soil maintains its fertility, reducing the need for synthetic fertilizers. Crop rotation helps in managing soil nutrients and minimizing the buildup of pests and diseases, ensuring a healthy, vibrant garden.
- **Companion Planting:** This method involves planting different herbs close to each other to mutually benefit their growth, health, and flavor. Companion planting is based on the understanding that certain plants can improve the growth environment for others by attracting beneficial insects, providing shade, or enhancing soil nutrients. For instance, planting basil near tomatoes not only improves the flavor of the tomatoes but also repels pests. Such symbiotic relationships between plants enhance biodiversity and contribute to a resilient ecosystem within the garden.
- **Natural Fertilization:** Enriching the soil with natural fertilizers is essential for healthy herb cultivation. Traditional methods include the use of compost, animal manure, green manures (cover crops), and mineral powders to supply essential nutrients to the soil. These natural fertilizers improve soil structure, water retention, and microbial activity, leading to robust plant growth without the adverse environmental impact associated with chemical fertilizers.

Implementing these age-old methods of soil preparation and planting can significantly enhance the health and yield of herb gardens. Encouraging a return to these practices not only sustains the environment but also reconnects us with the wisdom of our ancestors, fostering a deeper appreciation for the natural world and its cycles.

Watering and Maintenance

In the realm of traditional herb cultivation, the practices surrounding watering and maintaining herb gardens are fundamental to the vitality and efficacy of the plants. Ancient methodologies often employed natural irrigation techniques that harmonized with the local ecosystem, ensuring that plants received the optimal amount of water without depleting resources or introducing harmful substances into the environment.

One prevalent method was the use of rainwater harvesting systems, where rainwater was collected and stored during wet seasons to be utilized during drier periods. This technique not only provided a sustainable water source but also ensured that the water was free from the chemicals often found in municipal water supplies, maintaining the purity of the herbs.

In addition to responsible watering practices, maintaining the health of herb gardens without synthetic chemicals was a cornerstone of ancient horticulture. Cultivators turned to a variety of organic means to enrich the soil and protect plants from pests and diseases. Composting, the process of turning organic waste into nutrient-rich soil, was a common method to naturally fertilize herb gardens. This practice supported healthy plant growth and strengthened the plants' natural defenses.

Moreover, the ancients implemented biological pest control methods, introducing beneficial insects that prey on harmful pests into the garden. This form of natural pest management reduced the need for chemical interventions, preserving the integrity of the herbs. Companion planting, another age-old technique, involved growing certain plants together to mutually benefit from each other's properties, such as natural pest repellants or soil nutrients enhancers, fostering a healthy and thriving herb garden.

These time-honored watering and maintenance practices underscore the wisdom of ancient herbalists, who embraced the principles of sustainability and ecological balance. By studying and reviving these methods, modern herbalists can cultivate herb gardens that are not only productive but also environmentally responsible.

Pest Control and Disease Management

In ancient herbal cultivation, managing pests and diseases was paramount to ensuring a bountiful and healthy harvest. Without the modern convenience of synthetic chemicals, ancient herbalists relied on a deep understanding of nature and its cycles to protect their gardens from harm. Here are some traditional methods employed by these wise cultivators:

- **Companion Planting:** Many ancient cultures practiced companion planting, a method where specific plants are grown near each other for mutual benefit. For instance, marigolds were often planted alongside herbs to deter pests with their strong scent. This method not only reduced pest infestations but also promoted biodiversity in the garden.
- **Natural Predators:** Encouraging the presence of natural predators was another strategy. Birds, ladybugs, and other beneficial insects were attracted to the garden to feed on common pests. This natural form of pest control helped maintain the ecological balance and reduced the need for intervention.

- **Crop Rotation:** Rotating crops was a common practice to prevent the depletion of soil nutrients and the build-up of pathogens and pests. By changing the location of herbs each season, ancient farmers could break the life cycle of pests and diseases, keeping their soil healthy and productive.
- **Botanical Preparations:** Herbalists often prepared botanical sprays and remedies from other plants. Garlic, neem, and chili were commonly used to create natural pesticides. These concoctions were sprayed on crops to deter pests without harming the plants or the ecosystem.
- **Physical Barriers:** Sometimes, physical methods were employed to protect herbs from insects and animals. This included the use of netting or fences, and in some cases, the removal of infected plants to prevent the spread of disease.

These age-old practices demonstrate a profound respect for nature and a deep understanding of ecological balance. They remind us that effective pest and disease management is possible without resorting to harmful chemicals, a lesson that holds great relevance for modern herbalists seeking sustainable ways to nurture their gardens.

Scan the QR code

below to receive your exclusive additional content!

EXCLUSIVE CONTENT INCLUDED

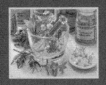

101 EXCLUSIVE VIDEOS BY DR. BARBARA O'NEILL:
Deepen your understanding with hours of invaluable content

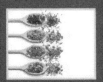

SEASONAL HERBAL TEA BLENDS:
Refreshing and health-boosting recipes for every time of year

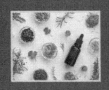

HERBAL COMPATIBILITY CHART:
A practical guide to combining herbs and essential oils for therapeutic benefits

BOOK 3: THE WHOLESOME BARBARA O'NEILL COOKBOOK

Chapter 1: Cooking with Herbs for Health and Flavor

1.1 Enhancing Everyday Meals with Herbs

In the realm of culinary delights, fresh herbs stand out not only for their ability to transform the flavor profile of a dish but also for their numerous nutritional benefits. Incorporating fresh herbs into daily cooking practices can significantly enhance meals, turning even the simplest dish into a symphony of flavors while contributing to overall health and well-being. This section delves into the art and science of integrating herbs into various aspects of daily meal preparation, from main courses to the often-overlooked snacks.

Incorporating Fresh Herbs into Daily Cooking

The first step toward enriching your daily meals with herbs is understanding the importance of freshness. Fresh herbs offer a vibrancy in flavor and a higher content of essential oils, which can diminish in dried forms. When selecting herbs, look for bright, perky leaves without signs of wilting or browning, and ensure to rinse them gently before use.

Proper chopping techniques can also maximize the flavor of herbs. For softer herbs like cilantro or basil, a gentle chop is sufficient to release their aromatic oils without crushing the delicate leaves. Sturdier herbs like rosemary or thyme, however, may require a finer chop to unlock their full flavor potential. Regardless of the herb, always use a sharp knife to avoid bruising the leaves, which can lead to flavor loss.

Storing herbs correctly extends their shelf life and maintains their flavor. Most herbs thrive when stored in the refrigerator, wrapped loosely in a damp paper towel, and placed inside a plastic bag. Some, like basil, are better kept at room temperature with their stems placed in a glass of water.

Pairing herbs with the right ingredients is crucial to achieving harmony in flavors. Here are some classic pairings to get you started:

- Basil pairs wonderfully with tomatoes, garlic, and mozzarella, epitomizing the flavors of Italian cuisine.
- Rosemary enhances the taste of lamb, chicken, and roasted potatoes with its woodsy aroma.
- Cilantro, with its bright and citrusy notes, complements the flavors of Mexican and Thai dishes beautifully.
- Dill, with its delicate feathery leaves, is a natural match for salmon and cucumber, offering a fresh, tangy lift.

Herb-Infused Oils and Vinegars for Flavor Boost

Creating herb-infused oils and vinegars is a simple yet effective way to capture the essence of herbs and infuse meals with complex flavors. Start with a high-quality base — extra virgin olive oil or a neutral oil like grapeseed for oils, and white wine or apple cider vinegar for vinegars. Add your chosen herbs, either singly or in combinations, ensuring they are thoroughly washed and completely dried to prevent spoilage.

For oils, gently heat the oil and herbs to release the flavors, then allow to cool and steep for up to two weeks before straining. For vinegars, no heat is needed; simply combine the vinegar with the herbs and let the mixture steep. Both should be stored in a cool, dark place and can be used to dress salads, marinate meats, or add a finishing touch to dishes.

Creative Uses of Herbs in Appetizers and Snacks

Herbs can transform appetizers and snacks from ordinary to extraordinary with minimal effort. Consider herb-based dips such as a basil pesto or a cilantro chutney, which can be used as spreads on sandwiches or as dips for vegetables and bread. Herbed yogurt, combining plain yogurt with dill, mint, or chives, makes for a refreshing and healthy dip or spread.

For a creative twist on finger foods, incorporate finely chopped herbs into cheese balls or mix them into the dough of savory pastries for an added layer of flavor. Even popcorn can be elevated with a sprinkle of finely chopped herbs like rosemary or thyme, combined with a touch of sea salt and melted butter.

Herbs offer a world of possibilities when it comes to enhancing the flavor and nutritional value of everyday meals. By incorporating fresh herbs into your cooking, you not only elevate the taste of your dishes but also imbibe the myriad health benefits these culinary gems have to offer. From the simple act of chopping and adding herbs to a dish, creating infused oils and vinegars, to the more creative endeavors of crafting herb-based dips and spreads, the opportunities to incorporate herbs into your culinary repertoire are endless. As you experiment with different herbs and combinations, you'll not only develop a deeper appreciation for their individual flavors but also for the remarkable ways in which they can transform your cooking.

1.2 Mastering Herbal Seasoning Blends

The art of creating and using herbal seasoning blends is an integral part of cooking that not only enhances the flavor of food but also incorporates the health benefits of herbs into our daily diet. Mastering the craft of making these blends allows for a personalized cooking experience, offering a unique touch to every dish. This guide provides a comprehensive look into the basics of formulating your own herbal seasoning blends, employing them in various culinary applications, and tips for drying and storing herbs to ensure they retain their vibrant flavors.

Crafting Custom Herb Blends for Various Cuisines

Crafting your own herb blends begins with understanding the flavor profiles of different herbs and how they can complement each other. Here are steps to create custom blends suited to various cuisines:

- **Identify the Cuisine's Flavor Profile:** Each cuisine has its unique palette. For instance, Italian cuisine often utilizes basil, oregano, and rosemary, while Mediterranean dishes might favor combinations of mint, dill, and thyme.
- **Select Your Herbs:** Choose fresh or dried herbs that align with the cuisine's flavor profile. Fresh herbs will provide a more vibrant flavor, whereas dried herbs offer convenience and a more concentrated taste.
- **Experiment with Ratios:** Start with equal amounts of each herb and adjust based on your taste preference. Some herbs have stronger flavors and may need to be used more sparingly.
- **Mix and Match:** Don't be afraid to experiment. Additions like garlic powder, onion powder, or even citrus zest can add an extra dimension to your blend.

Using Herbal Rubs and Marinades for Meat and Vegetables

Herbal rubs and marinades infuse meats and vegetables with robust flavors. Here's how to utilize your herb blends effectively:

- *Prepare Your Base:* For rubs, mix your herb blend with a bit of oil to help it adhere to the food. For marinades, combine your blend with oil and an acid (like vinegar or lemon juice) to not only flavor but also tenderize the meat.
- *Application:* Generously apply rubs directly onto the surface of meats or vegetables. For marinades, ensure that the food is fully submerged and allowed to soak for at least an hour, or overnight for more profound flavor.
- *Cooking:* Remember that fresh herbs may burn at high temperatures, so consider adding them towards the end of the cooking process, especially when grilling or roasting.

Tips for Drying and Storing Herbs for Maximum Flavor

Drying and storing herbs correctly is crucial for preserving their essence and potency. Here are techniques to ensure your herbs remain flavorful:

- Drying Herbs:
  - *Air Drying:* Bundle the herbs and hang them upside down in a warm, dry, and well-ventilated area away from direct sunlight. This method works best for herbs with low moisture content.
  - *Oven Drying:* Place herb leaves on a baking sheet and dry in an oven set to the lowest possible temperature. Keep the oven door slightly open to allow moisture to escape. Check frequently to prevent burning.
  - *Dehydrator:* If you have a dehydrator, follow the manufacturer's instructions for drying herbs. This method is more controlled and can yield consistent results.
- Storing Dried Herbs:
  - *Airtight Containers:* Store dried herbs in airtight containers away from light and heat. Glass jars with tight-fitting lids are ideal.
  - *Labeling:* Always label your containers with the name of the herb and the date it was dried.
  - *Usage:* Dried herbs are best used within a year. To test their potency, crush a small amount in your hand and smell. If the aroma is weak, it's time to replace them.

By understanding these fundamentals, you can begin to explore the vast and flavorful world of herbal seasoning blends. Whether it's crafting a unique blend to capture the essence of a cuisine, infusing meats and vegetables with aromatic rubs and marinades, or preserving the vibrant flavors of herbs through proper drying and storage, the possibilities are endless. Embrace the journey of experimenting with herbs and discover the transformative power they can bring to your culinary creations.

1.3 Herbal Cooking Techniques

Herbal cooking techniques offer a delightful opportunity to enrich both the flavor and nutritional value of everyday meals. Incorporating herbs into your culinary practices not only elevates the taste of dishes but also enhances the dietary benefits, contributing to a healthier lifestyle. Here, we delve into several methods for weaving herbs into your cooking, ranging from infusions in soups and stews to baking and crafting herb-based sauces and dressings. Embrace these techniques to infuse your meals with an extra layer of flavor and health.

Infusing Herbs into Soups and Stews

Infusing herbs into soups and stews is a classic method that instills depth and complexity into these comforting dishes. The key is to select the right herbs that complement the flavor profile of your dish. Herbs like bay leaves, thyme, and rosemary are robust and can withstand longer cooking times, releasing their flavors gradually, making them perfect for stews and broths. Meanwhile, delicate herbs like parsley, cilantro, or basil should be added towards the end of the cooking process to preserve their vibrant color and fresh flavor.

- Timing is Crucial: For hardy herbs, add them early in the cooking process. Delicate herbs should be stirred in just before serving.
- Whole vs. Chopped: Adding herbs in their whole form (like bay leaves) makes them easier to remove before serving, whereas chopped herbs can disperse more flavor throughout the dish.
- Experiment with Blends: Don't hesitate to experiment with combinations, such as herbes de Provence or Italian seasoning, to discover new flavor profiles.

Baking with Herbs: Breads, Pastries, and More

Baking with herbs can transform the simplest bread, pastry, or savory dish into something extraordinary. Herbs like rosemary, sage, and thyme pair wonderfully with baked goods, offering a hint of garden freshness and aroma.

- **Incorporating Herbs into Doughs:** Mix finely chopped herbs into bread or pastry doughs for an aromatic twist.
- **Creating Herb-Infused Glazes:** Brush breads or pastries with an herb-infused oil or butter before baking to add a flavorful crust.
- **Pairing with Ingredients:** Consider the compatibility of the herb flavors with your other ingredients. For instance, basil pairs well with tomato-based recipes, while dill complements dairy-based dishes.

Incorporating fresh herbs into baking can transform the ordinary into the extraordinary, infusing breads, pastries, and savory items with delightful and unique flavors. Herbs bring not only a burst of flavor but also a touch of nutritional benefits, making each baked good not just a treat to the palate but also a boon to health.

Herb-Based Sauces and Dressings

Incorporating fresh herbs into sauces and dressings not only amplifies the flavor profile of dishes but also infuses them with a plethora of health benefits. Creating herb-based sauces and dressings from scratch is a simple yet profound way to elevate everyday meals into culinary delights that tantalize the taste buds and nourish the body.

- **Basic Herb-Based Sauce Recipe**: To craft a basic herb sauce, you'll need a handful of fresh herbs, such as basil, parsley, or cilantro, blended with olive oil, garlic, lemon juice, and salt to taste. This sauce pairs wonderfully with grilled meats, roasted vegetables, or as a vibrant dressing for salads.
- **Herb-Infused Dressings:** For a refreshing salad dressing, whisk together vinegar (balsamic or apple cider vinegar works well), extra virgin olive oil, minced fresh herbs of your choice, a touch of honey or maple syrup for sweetness, and salt and pepper. This concoction can transform a simple green salad into an irresistible dish.
- **Balancing Flavors:** Understanding the flavor profile of herbs is key to creating balanced sauces and dressings. Robust herbs like rosemary and thyme pair well with hearty dishes such as roasted meats and stews, while delicate herbs like mint and dill complement lighter fare like seafood and salads.
- **Health Benefits**: Fresh herbs are not only flavor powerhouses but also packed with antioxidants and beneficial nutrients. Incorporating herb-based sauces and dressings into your diet can aid in digestion, boost immune function, and contribute to overall health.
- **Pairing with Dishes:** To maximize the culinary experience, consider the main components of your dish when selecting an herb-based sauce or dressing. For example, a minty yogurt dressing is

a perfect complement to spicy dishes, offering a cooling contrast, while a chimichurri sauce made with parsley and cilantro can elevate grilled steaks or vegetables.

- ***Storage Tips:*** Fresh herb-based sauces and dressings are best enjoyed soon after preparation to preserve their vibrant flavors and health benefits. However, they can be stored in an airtight container in the refrigerator for a few days. For extended storage, consider freezing the sauce in ice cube trays for easy, portion-sized use in future meals.

Exploring the art of making herb-based sauces and dressings allows home cooks to unleash their creativity in the kitchen, turning simple ingredients into exquisite, healthful culinary creations. Whether drizzling over a salad, marinating a piece of meat, or using as a dip for fresh vegetables, these herb-infused condiments are sure to impress and delight.

Chapter 2: Nutrition and Herbal Use in The Kitchen

2.1 Understanding the Health Benefits of Culinary Herbs

Culinary herbs have been at the heart of traditional cooking and natural medicine for centuries, celebrated for their aromatic flavors and myriad health benefits. These plant-derived wonders are not only essential for culinary purposes but also boast impressive nutritional profiles, rich in vitamins, minerals, and bioactive compounds that contribute significantly to overall health and well-being. Understanding the health benefits of common culinary herbs unveils a holistic approach to nutrition, where food not only satisfies taste buds but also nourishes the body and supports its vital functions.

The Nutrient Profiles of Common Culinary Herbs

Culinary herbs not only add flavor and aroma to our meals but are also powerhouses of nutrition, packed with an array of vitamins, minerals, and beneficial compounds. By incorporating common herbs such as parsley, basil, and thyme into our diets, we can significantly enhance the nutritional value of our meals.

- **Parsley**, often relegated to the role of a plate garnish, is a nutrient-dense herb worth incorporating more frequently into our diets. It is an excellent source of Vitamin K, essential for bone health, and contains high levels of other vitamins (A and C), which serve for immune function and eyes. Additionally, parsley provides flavonoids like luteolin, which possess antioxidant properties to protect against cellular damage.

- **Basil** is another culinary gem, celebrated not only for its aromatic presence in dishes but also for its rich nutrient profile. Basil contains vitamin K, manganese, iron and vitamin A. Its standout feature, however, is the array of essential oils it contains, such as eugenol, citronellol, and linalool, which have anti-inflammatory and antibacterial properties. Questi composti mostrano il significato del basilico oltre il suo uso culinario.

- **Thyme** offers more than its delightful flavor; it's a source of Vitamin C, Vitamin A, iron, and manganese. Thyme contains thymol, an essential oil with powerful antioxidant and antimicrobial activities. This not only makes thyme a great addition to the diet for its role in preventing diseases but also highlights its historical use in medicinal practices.

Incorporating these herbs into daily meals can significantly contribute to health maintenance and disease prevention. Whether used fresh or dried, they provide a convenient, low-calorie method to enhance both the flavor profile and nutritional content of dishes. Encouraging the exploration of these and other culinary herbs can inspire a deeper appreciation for the natural abundance of nutrients available to us, promoting a lifestyle that values both flavor and well-being.

Antioxidant Properties of Herbs and Their Health Benefits

Antioxidants play a crucial role in maintaining our health by protecting our bodies from oxidative stress, which can damage cells and has been linked to various chronic diseases. Culinary herbs are rich sources of antioxidants, making them not just flavorful additions to our meals but also powerful allies in our quest for wellness.

The antioxidant properties of herbs come from a diverse range of compounds they contain, including flavonoids, phenolic acids, and essential oils. These compounds scavenge free radicals, thereby reducing oxidative stress and protecting the body against inflammation, heart disease, and certain types of cancer.

- **Rosemary** is renowned for its high antioxidant content, attributed mainly to compounds like carnosic acid and rosmarinic acid. Research suggests that rosemary may help protect against cognitive decline and brain aging, thanks to its potent antioxidant properties.
- **Oregano** is another herb that packs a powerful antioxidant punch, often used in Italian and Mediterranean cuisine. It contains thymol and carvacrol, two antioxidants that have been shown to fight bacteria in addition to reducing oxidative stress.
- **Thyme** is rich in thymol, a compound with antioxidant properties that may also have antibacterial and antifungal abilities. Thyme's antioxidants can help support the immune system and promote overall health.
- **Sage** contains a variety of antioxidants, including rosmarinic acid, which has been studied for its potential to improve brain function and memory. Sage's antioxidant content may also offer protective benefits against certain types of cancer.
- **Parsley** is not just a garnish; it's a nutritional powerhouse rich in vitamins A, C, and K, and it boasts a high antioxidant content, particularly luteolin, which has been studied for its potential to prevent certain diseases.
- **Basil** offers a unique range of antioxidants, including water-soluble flavonoids like vicenin and orientin. These compounds have been shown to protect cell structures as well as chromosomes from radiation and oxygen-based damage.

Incorporating these herbs into daily meals not only enhances flavor but also contributes significantly to our antioxidant intake, offering protection against the harmful effects of oxidative stress. By understanding and utilizing the antioxidant properties of herbs, we can better support our body's natural defenses, promote long-term health, and enjoy the rich flavors these herbs bring to our culinary creations.

Herbs for Digestive Health and Detoxification

Digestive health is a cornerstone of overall well-being, and detoxification plays a key role in maintaining this delicate balance. A variety of herbs, celebrated for their culinary uses, also possess remarkable properties that support digestion and aid in the body's natural detoxification processes. Among these, ginger, peppermint, and fennel stand out for their potent effects.

- **Ginger**: Renowned for its potent anti-inflammatory and antioxidant properties, ginger has been used for centuries to alleviate gastrointestinal distress. It is effective in stimulating saliva, bile, and gastric enzymes, facilitating more efficient digestion and absorption of nutrients. Ginger also eases motion sickness and nausea, making it a valuable ally in maintaining digestive comfort. Furthermore, its ability to promote sweating helps to detoxify the body by eliminating toxins through the skin.

- **Peppermint:** Peppermint is not only refreshing but also possesses antispasmodic properties that can relax the digestive system's muscles, reducing symptoms of irritable bowel syndrome (IBS) such as bloating and abdominal pain. The active compound, menthol, aids in the natural flow of bile from the liver to the gallbladder, contributing to the digestion of fats and the detoxification process.

- **Fennel:** With a licorice-like flavor, fennel seeds are traditionally used to treat flatulence and promote digestion due to their anti-inflammatory and antispasmodic properties. Fennel can soothe the digestive tract, alleviate bloating, and facilitate the removal of toxins from the body. It also supports the liver's function in detoxification, enhancing overall digestive health.

Incorporating these herbs into daily diets not only enriches flavors but also provides a natural, gentle way to support digestive health and detoxification. Whether used in cooking, consumed as tea, or taken as supplements, ginger, peppermint, and fennel offer accessible options to nurture the body from within, underscoring the powerful link between herbal nutrition and digestive well-being.

2.2 Herbs as Nutritional Supplements

The exploration of herbs as nutritional supplements opens a vast landscape of natural health maintenance and enhancement. These gifts from nature not only add flavor to our cuisine but also offer significant health benefits when incorporated into our daily routines. From superfood herbs like spirulina and chlorella to more common herbs turned into supplements, such as ginger and turmeric, the range of options for bolstering health through herbal supplementation is wide and varied.

Using Herbal Supplements for Daily Health Maintenance

In the quest for optimal health and well-being, incorporating herbal supplements into daily routines has emerged as a powerful strategy. These natural allies offer a host of benefits, from boosting immune function to enhancing mental clarity, all while aligning with a holistic approach to health.

Benefits of Herbal Supplements Herbal supplements, derived from plants used for their therapeutic properties, provide a concentrated source of nutritional and medicinal benefits. They can:

- **Boost Immunity:** Herbs like echinacea and elderberry are celebrated for their ability to enhance the immune response, helping the body to ward off colds and other infections.
- **Reduce Inflammation:** Ingredients such as turmeric, rich in curcumin, offer potent anti-inflammatory properties, beneficial for reducing the risk of chronic diseases.
- **Support Digestive Health:** Supplements like peppermint and ginger can soothe the digestive tract, alleviate nausea, and improve nutrient absorption.
- **Enhance Mental Well-being:** Adaptogenic herbs like ashwagandha and rhodiola help the body to manage stress more effectively, supporting overall mental health.

Choosing High-Quality Supplements Not all herbal supplements are created equal. To ensure maximum benefit and safety, it's crucial to select products that meet the following criteria:

- **Purity and Authenticity:** Look for supplements that contain no artificial additives and are verified for the presence of the stated herbal ingredients.
- **Standardization:** Choose products that are standardized to contain a specific amount of active ingredients, ensuring consistent potency.
- **Quality Assurance:** Opt for brands that undergo third-party testing and adhere to good manufacturing practices (GMP).

Recommended Dosages The appropriate dosage of an herbal supplement can vary significantly depending on the specific herb and the individual's health needs. It's advisable to start with the lowest suggested dose and observe how your body responds. Consulting with a healthcare professional, particularly for those with pre-existing conditions or taking other medications, is always recommended to avoid any potential interactions.

Incorporating herbal supplements into daily routines represents a proactive step towards nurturing one's health. By choosing high-quality products and adhering to recommended dosages, individuals can harness the therapeutic powers of herbs to support their journey towards optimal wellness.

Superfood Herbs: Spirulina, Chlorella, and More

In the realm of natural health and nutrition, superfood herbs like spirulina and chlorella have garnered significant attention for their remarkable nutrient profiles and wide-ranging health benefits. These algae-based supplements are not only rich in vitamins and minerals but also in proteins and antioxidants, making them a powerhouse of nutrition.

Spirulina, a blue-green algae, is celebrated for its high protein content, encompassing all essential amino acids making it a complete protein source. It is an excellent source of B vitamins, particularly B12, making it a valuable supplement for vegetarians and vegans. Spirulina is also rich in iron, magnesium, and trace minerals, alongside potent antioxidants like phycocyanin, which has been studied for its antioxidant and anti-inflammatory effects. Incorporating spirulina into the diet can be as simple as adding a teaspoon of the powder to smoothies, juices, or even water. Its mildly savory taste also complements soups and salads.

Chlorella, another green algae, is highly regarded for its detoxifying properties, especially its ability to bind with heavy metals and facilitate their removal from the body. It is a robust source of chlorophyll, the pigment responsible for its deep green color, which is a catalyst for blood detoxification and renewal. Chlorella also supports a healthy immune system and promotes skin health. Similar to spirulina, it can be consumed in powder or tablet form. It's easily blended into smoothies or taken as a dietary supplement to boost daily nutritional intake.

Both spirulina and chlorella have been shown to support cardiovascular health, enhance energy levels, and promote a healthy immune response. They stand out as superfoods not only because of their dense nutrient content but also because of their potential to support overall well-being and prevent chronic diseases.

Incorporating these superfood herbs into one's diet can be an easy and effective way to bolster health. However, it's important to source high-quality products to ensure purity and efficacy. Starting with small doses and gradually increasing as tolerated can help minimize digestive discomfort, allowing the body to adjust to the high concentration of nutrients found in these powerful algae.

Herbal Powders and Extracts: How to Use Them

In the realm of nutritional wellness, herbal powders and extracts have emerged as powerful adjuncts, offering a concentrated dose of nature's finest healing and nourishing properties. Their versatility and potency make them invaluable tools for anyone looking to enrich their diet with the essence of herbal goodness.

Herbal Powders: These are made by finely grinding dried herbs into a powder. This form retains most of the herb's nutritional content, making it an efficient way to consume herbs that might otherwise be difficult to integrate into your diet. For instance, moringa leaf powder, known for its rich iron and vitamin content, can easily be added to smoothies, soups, or teas. The key advantage of powders is their ease of incorporation into daily meals, allowing you to boost the nutritional value of your food without altering its taste significantly.

Herbal Extracts: Extracts are concentrated forms of herbs, typically obtained by processing the herbs with a solvent like water or alcohol to isolate their active compounds. Extracts can be found in liquid form or further processed into powders. They offer a more potent dose of the herb's beneficial properties than you might get from consuming the plant in its natural form. For example, turmeric extract, rich in the anti-inflammatory compound curcumin, can be more effective in smaller doses than the spice itself. Extracts can be added to water, teas, or even taken directly, depending on the concentration and the desired effect.

Using Herbal Powders and Extracts in Recipes: Incorporating these potent forms of herbs into your diet is surprisingly simple and can significantly enhance the nutritional value of your meals. Here are a few suggestions to get you started:

- **Smoothies**: A teaspoon of matcha powder, spirulina, or wheatgrass can turn your routine smoothie into a powerhouse of antioxidants and vitamins.
- **Teas and Beverages**: Dissolve herbal extracts like ginger, peppermint, or chamomile in hot water to create soothing teas. Liquid extracts can also be added to cold beverages for a nutritional boost.
- **Soups and Sauces**: Stir in a bit of turmeric or garlic powder to soups and sauces not only for the health benefits but also for added flavor complexity.
- **Baking**: Replace a portion of flour in recipes with herbal powders like flaxseed or hemp for an added nutritional punch in bread, muffins, and other baked goods.

Tips for Integrating Herbal Powders and Extracts into Your Daily Nutrition:

1. **Start Small**: If you're new to using herbal supplements, begin with small amounts to see how your body reacts.

2. **Quality Matters**: Invest in high-quality, organic products from reputable sources to ensure maximum purity and effectiveness.
3. **Consult Professionals**: Before incorporating any supplement into your routine, especially if you have existing health conditions, consult with a healthcare professional.

Herbal powders and extracts represent a convenient, versatile way to enhance your nutritional intake and support your overall health. With a little creativity, they can easily become a regular part of your diet, providing you with the myriad benefits that nature's pharmacy has to offer.

2.3 Herbs for Specific Health Conditions

Herbs have been revered throughout history for their medicinal properties, offering natural remedies to support health and well-being. In today's wellness landscape, the relevance of these potent plants continues to grow, with an increasing body of research supporting their therapeutic uses. This section delves into the specific health conditions that can benefit from herbal interventions, encompassing immune support, anti-inflammatory action, traditional remedies for common ailments, and mental health support.

Herbs to Boost Immunity and Fight Inflammation

The immune system is our body's defense mechanism against infections and diseases. Certain herbs have been identified to bolster this system, enhancing the body's ability to fight off pathogens. For example, Echinacea is widely recognized for its immune-boosting properties, often recommended at the onset of colds or flu. Similarly, Turmeric, with its active component curcumin, offers potent anti-inflammatory benefits, mitigating the effects of inflammatory conditions and promoting overall immune health.

- **Echinacea**: Known for enhancing the immune response, Echinacea can reduce the duration and severity of colds when taken at the first sign of symptoms.
- **Turmeric**: Beyond its culinary uses, turmeric is celebrated for its anti-inflammatory effects, beneficial for conditions from arthritis to cardiovascular health.

Herbal Remedies for Common Ailments

The natural pharmacy of herbs offers a plethora of remedies for everyday health complaints, from digestive issues to headaches and beyond. Ginger, with its warming and anti-nausea properties, is excellent for digestive discomfort, including motion sickness. Peppermint serves a dual purpose, easing indigestion and also offering relief from tension headaches when applied topically as an oil.

- **Ginger**: A staple in traditional medicine for its anti-nausea effects, making it a go-to remedy for stomach upset.
- **Peppermint**: Known for its soothing effect on the digestive system and its ability to alleviate headaches.

Using Herbs to Support Mental Health and Well-Being

Mental health, an integral component of overall well-being, can also benefit from herbal support. Herbs like St. John's Wort and Valerian have been researched for their impact on mood disorders and sleep disturbances, respectively. Lavender, through its calming scent, can reduce anxiety levels and improve sleep quality, making it a valuable ally in today's fast-paced world.

- **St. John's Wort**: Often used for mild to moderate depression, St. John's Wort is a well-known mood enhancer. However, it's important to note its potential interactions with prescription medications.
- **Valerian**: Used for its sedative qualities, Valerian can improve sleep quality without the grogginess associated with some sleep aids.
- **Lavender**: Renowned for its calming aroma, lavender oil can alleviate anxiety and improve sleep, making it a popular choice in aromatherapy.

The therapeutic potential of herbs offers a bridge to holistic health, emphasizing prevention, and natural care. Incorporating herbal remedies into your health regimen can provide a complementary approach to conventional medicine, affording gentle, yet effective, solutions to common health issues. It's essential, however, to approach herbal supplementation with an informed perspective, recognizing the importance of quality and appropriate dosing. Consulting with healthcare professionals, especially when managing specific health conditions or taking other medications, ensures a safe and synergistic approach to herbal medicine.

Embracing the wisdom of herbal traditions opens up a world of natural remedies, fostering a deeper connection with the healing power of nature. As we continue to explore and validate the benefits of these remarkable plants, the role of herbs in supporting health and well-being becomes ever more apparent, offering timeless solutions to modern-day health challenges.

Herbs to Boost Immunity and Fight Inflammation

Herbal remedies have been used for centuries to enhance the body's natural immune responses and fight inflammation, a root cause of many chronic diseases. Today, scientific research supports the use of various herbs for their health-promoting properties. Among these, echinacea, turmeric, and garlic stand out for their potent effects on our body's defense systems.

- **Echinacea**: Perhaps one of the most well-known herbs for boosting immunity, echinacea is often turned to at the first signs of a cold or flu. It works by increasing the production of white blood cells, which fight infections. A meta-analysis of studies has suggested that echinacea can reduce the chances of catching a cold by approximately 58% and shorten the duration of colds by almost 1.5 days. To incorporate echinacea into your regimen, consider taking supplements at the onset of cold symptoms or sipping echinacea tea as a preventive measure during cold and flu season.

- **Turmeric**: This bright yellow spice is not only a staple in culinary traditions around the world but also a powerhouse of medicinal benefits, primarily due to its active compound curcumin. Curcumin has been extensively studied for its potent anti-inflammatory properties and ability to boost antioxidant levels in the body. This makes turmeric an excellent supplement for reducing inflammation and pain associated with arthritis and other inflammatory conditions. Adding turmeric to your diet is simple; it can be sprinkled on meals, blended into smoothies, or taken as a supplement in capsule form.

- **Garlic**: Garlic's immune-boosting properties stem from its high concentration of sulfur-containing compounds, such as allicin. Studies have illustrated garlic's ability to enhance immune function by stimulating protective white blood cells like macrophages and lymphocytes. Additionally, garlic possesses antimicrobial and antiviral activities, making it effective against a broad spectrum of bacteria and viruses. Incorporating garlic into the diet is both easy and delicious. It can be added to a wide variety of dishes for flavor, or consumed raw or in supplement form for a more concentrated dose.

Incorporating these herbs into your daily routine can offer a simple yet powerful means to enhance your body's natural defenses against illness and inflammation. Whether through dietary adjustments or supplements, the inclusion of echinacea, turmeric, and garlic can contribute significantly to maintaining and improving overall health and well-being.

Herbal Remedies for Common Ailments

Herbal remedies have been used for centuries to treat a variety of common ailments, ranging from colds and headaches to digestive issues. These natural solutions offer a holistic approach to health, often with fewer side effects than conventional medications. Among the plethora of healing herbs, several stand out for their proven efficacy in treating these everyday health concerns.

Ginger: Known for its potent anti-inflammatory and antioxidant properties, ginger is a powerhouse when it comes to alleviating nausea and vomiting associated with motion sickness, pregnancy, and chemotherapy. Moreover, ginger can soothe an upset stomach, reduce menstrual pain, and relieve sore throats. For digestive health, ginger tea or fresh ginger root can be added to meals.

- **Peppermint**: A refreshing herb that is widely recognized for its ability to relieve digestive issues such as bloating, gas, and indigestion. Peppermint oil capsules are particularly effective in treating Irritable Bowel Syndrome (IBS). Additionally, inhaling peppermint essential oil can help reduce headaches and migraines.
- **Chamomile**: This gentle herb is best known for its calming and sedative qualities, making it a popular choice for treating insomnia and promoting better sleep. Chamomile tea can also help soothe stomach aches and menstrual cramps. Its anti-inflammatory and antioxidant effects make it beneficial for reducing cold symptoms and supporting overall immune health.

Incorporating these herbs into your daily routine can be simple. A cup of herbal tea, for example, can offer therapeutic benefits while providing hydration. For more targeted relief, herbal supplements in the form of capsules, tinctures, or essential oils may be appropriate. However, it's important to consult with a healthcare provider before beginning any herbal supplement regimen, especially for individuals with existing health conditions or those taking other medications, to avoid potential interactions.

Embracing herbal remedies as part of your healthcare routine can not only alleviate common ailments but also support a holistic approach to wellness. These natural solutions underscore the power of plants in promoting health and well-being, highlighting their relevance and sustainability as part of a balanced lifestyle.

Using Herbs to Support Mental Health and Well-Being

In today's fast-paced world, mental well-being often takes a backseat, leading to an increase in stress, anxiety, and other mental health issues. Fortunately, nature offers a bounty of herbs that have been used for centuries to foster mental health and emotional balance. Among these, St. John's Wort, valerian, and lavender stand out for their calming and mood-enhancing properties.

- **St. John's Wort (Hypericum perforatum)**: Renowned for its mood-stabilizing benefits, St. John's Wort has been a go-to herb for battling mild to moderate depression. The active compounds like hypericin and hyperforin contribute to its efficacy by modulating neurotransmitters in the brain, akin to many conventional antidepressants, but with fewer side effects. It's crucial, however, to consult with a healthcare provider before integrating it into your regimen, especially if you are taking other medications, to avoid potential interactions.

- **Valerian (Valeriana officinalis)**: Valerian root has been cherished for its sedative qualities that aid in alleviating anxiety and improving sleep quality. Its calming effect is attributed to valerenic acid that enhances the signaling of gamma-aminobutyric acid (GABA), a neurotransmitter responsible for regulating nerve impulses in your brain and nervous system. Valerian can be consumed as a tea or in capsule form. Its use is particularly beneficial in individuals grappling with insomnia or anxiety, fostering a sense of tranquility and promoting restful sleep.

- **Lavender (Lavandula angustifolia)**: Lavender is celebrated not only for its delightful fragrance but also for its profound calming and relaxing effects. Inhaling lavender essential oil or using it in aromatherapy sessions can significantly reduce stress levels, decrease anxiety, and improve sleep patterns. Lavender's soothing properties are primarily attributed to the compound linalool, which, when inhaled, can act directly on the brain to induce calmness and reduce agitation.

Incorporating these herbs into your daily life can vary from brewing herbal teas, using them in aromatherapy, to taking dietary supplements under the guidance of a healthcare professional. It is always prudent to start with lower doses to gauge your body's response and avoid potential side effects.

The journey towards mental well-being is multifaceted, involving a balanced diet, regular exercise, adequate sleep, and, when suitable, herbal support. By integrating these herbs into your wellness regimen, you harness the power of nature to nurture your mind, enhance emotional resilience, and foster overall well-being, all while steering through life's ups and downs with a more balanced outlook.

Chapter 3: Herbal Tea Recipes and Benefits

3.1 Introduction to Herbal Teas

Herbal teas have been cherished for centuries, transcending cultures and eras as a staple of wellness and culinary delight. They are more than just beverages; they are a blend of history, art, and healing. In this section, we delve into the rich tradition of herbal teas, unveil the secrets behind brewing the perfect cup, and explore their myriad health benefits. By understanding these elements, you can fully appreciate the timeless allure and modern relevance of herbal teas.

3.1.1 The History and Tradition of Herbal Teas

The journey of herbal teas stretches back to ancient civilizations. From the serene tea gardens of China to the aromatic kitchens of Medieval Europe, herbal teas have been integral to both cultural rituals and medicinal practices.

- ***Ancient China***: The origins of herbal teas can be traced to ancient China, where they were initially used for medicinal purposes. The legendary Emperor Shen Nong, often referred to as the "Divine Farmer," is credited with discovering the health benefits of herbs in 2737 BC. Shen Nong's meticulous documentation paved the way for the widespread use of herbal teas in traditional Chinese medicine.

- ***Ancient Egypt***: In Egypt, archaeological evidence reveals that herbal teas were used as early as 1550 BC. The Ebers Papyrus, one of the oldest medical texts, contains recipes for herbal infusions to treat various ailments. Chamomile, for instance, was revered for its calming properties.

- ***Grecian and Roman Empires:*** The Greeks and Romans also valued herbal teas, incorporating them into their daily lives. Hippocrates, the "Father of Medicine," documented the therapeutic uses of herbs such as mint and fennel.

- ***Middle Ages to Modern Times:*** During the Middle Ages, herbal teas became a cornerstone of European herbalism. Monastic gardens were teeming with medicinal herbs, which were used to create healing infusions. Today, the tradition continues, blending ancient wisdom with contemporary science to promote health and well-being.

3.1.2 The Art of Brewing the Perfect Cup

Brewing herbal teas is an art that requires attention to detail. The perfect cup brings out the full flavor and health benefits of the herbs, transforming a simple infusion into a delightful sensory experience.

Techniques for Brewing Herbal Teas

1. *Selecting Herbs:* Start by choosing high-quality herbs. Whether fresh or dried, ensure they are organically grown and free from contaminants.

2. *Water Quality*: Use filtered or spring water for the best results. Tap water can contain chemicals that may alter the flavor and efficacy of the tea.

3. *Water Temperature:* Different herbs require specific water temperatures to release their beneficial compounds. Generally, herbal teas are brewed with water just under boiling (around 190-200°F or 88-93°C).

4. *Steeping Time:* The steeping time can vary depending on the herb and desired strength of the tea. On average, steeping for 5-10 minutes is sufficient. However, some robust herbs may need up to 15 minutes to fully release their benefits.

5. *Covering the Tea:* Always cover the tea while it steeps. This practice traps the essential oils and volatile compounds, ensuring they do not evaporate.

6. *Straining and Serving:* After steeping, strain the herbs and pour the tea into a cup. Enjoy it plain, or add a touch of honey, lemon, or milk according to your preference.

3.1.3 Health Benefits of Herbal Teas

Herbal teas are celebrated not just for their exquisite flavors, but also for their impressive array of health benefits. Each herb brings its unique properties, offering a natural way to support various aspects of health.

Common Health Benefits

- *Digestive Health:* Many herbal teas, such as peppermint and ginger, are known for aiding digestion. They can help alleviate symptoms like bloating, nausea, and indigestion.

- *Relaxation and Stress Relief:* Teas like chamomile and lavender are renowned for their calming effects. They can promote relaxation and improve sleep quality, making them perfect for unwinding after a long day.

- *Immune Support:* Herbs like echinacea and elderberry are commonly used to boost the immune system. Regular consumption of these teas can help ward off colds and infections.

- *Anti-inflammatory Properties:* Herbal teas such as turmeric and ginger have natural anti-inflammatory effects. They can help reduce inflammation and pain, contributing to overall health.

- **Antioxidant Rich:** Many herbs, including rooibos and hibiscus, are packed with antioxidants. These compounds combat oxidative stress and can help protect against chronic diseases.

Specific Herbs and Their Benefits

- **Peppermint:** Known for its refreshing flavor, peppermint tea aids digestion and can relieve headaches and sinus congestion.
- **Chamomile:** A gentle, soothing tea, chamomile is excellent for relaxation and promoting restful sleep. It also has anti-inflammatory properties.
- **Ginger:** Spicy and invigorating, ginger tea is a powerful remedy for nausea and digestive issues. It also supports circulation and can help manage inflammation.
- **Rooibos:** This South African herb is caffeine-free and rich in antioxidants. It supports heart health and can improve skin conditions.
- **Hibiscus:** With its tart flavor, hibiscus tea is high in vitamin C and antioxidants. It supports immune health and can help manage blood pressure levels.
- **Echinacea:** Often used to prevent and treat the common cold, echinacea tea strengthens the immune system and has antimicrobial properties.

In conclusion, herbal teas are a captivating blend of tradition, art, and health. By embracing the rich history and honing the art of brewing, you can unlock the full potential of these remarkable infusions. Their health benefits are vast, making them a valuable addition to any wellness routine. As you explore the world of herbal teas, may you find both pleasure and health in every sip.

3.2 Herbal Tea Blends for Wellness

1) SOOTHING LAVENDER CHAMOMILE TEA

Ingredients:

- 1 Tbsp dried lavender buds
- 1 Tbsp dried chamomile flowers
- 2 cups boiling water
- Honey (optional)

Steps:

1. Add the dried lavender buds and chamomile flowers in a teapot.
2. Pour boiling water over the herbs.
3. Let steep for 6-8 min.
4. Divide the tea into cups.
5. Add honey to taste.

Usage Tips: This calming blend is perfect for winding down in the evening. Enjoy it before bed to promote relaxation and restful sleep.

2) MINT GINGER DIGESTIVE AID

Ingredients:

- 1 Tbsp dried peppermint leaves
- 1 Tbsp grated fresh ginger
- 2 Glasses of boiling water
- Lemon wedge

Steps:

1. Add the dried peppermint leaves and grated ginger in a teapot.
2. Pour boiling water over the herbs.
3. Let steep for 6-8 min.
4. Divide the tea into cups.
5. Add a squeeze of lemon.

Usage Tips: This refreshing blend aids digestion and can be enjoyed after meals to soothe the stomach.

3) REVITALIZING ROSEMARY LEMON BALM TEA

Ingredients:

- 1 Tbsp dried rosemary
- 1 Tbsp dried lemon balm
- 2 glasses boiling water
- Honey

Steps:

1. Add the dried rosemary and lemon balm in a teapot.
2. Pour boiling water over the herbs.
3. Let steep for 6-8 min.
4. Divide the tea into cups.
5. Add honey.

Usage Tips: This revitalizing blend is great for mental clarity and focus. Enjoy it in the afternoon to boost your concentration.

4) CALMING HOLY BASIL LICORICE ROOT TEA

Ingredients:

- 1 Tbsp dried holy basil leaves
- 1 Tbsp dried licorice root
- 2 glasses boiling water
- Honey

Steps:

1. Add the dried holy basil leaves and licorice root in a teapot.
2. Pour boiling water over the herbs.
3. Let steep for 6-8 min.
4. Divide the tea into cups.
5. Add honey.

Usage Tips: This soothing blend helps to reduce stress and anxiety. Enjoy it during stressful times to promote calmness

5) ENERGIZING GINSENG PEPPERMINT TEA

Ingredients:

- 1 Tbsp dried ginseng root
- 1 Tbsp dried peppermint leaves
- 2 glasses boiling water
- Honey

Steps:

1. Add the dried ginseng root and peppermint leaves in a teapot.
2. Pour boiling water over the herbs.
3. Let steep for 6-8 min.
4. Divide the tea into cups.
5. Add honey.

Usage Tips: This energizing blend provides a natural boost of energy. Enjoy it in the morning or early afternoon for a refreshing pick-me-up.

6) IMMUNE-BOOSTING ECHINACEA ELDERBERRY TEA

Ingredients:

- 1 Tbsp dried echinacea
- 1 Tbsp dried elderberries
- 2 glasses boiling water
- Honey

Steps:

1. Add the dried echinacea and elderberries in a teapot.
2. Pour boiling water over the herbs.
3. Let steep for 6-8 min.
4. Divide the tea into cups.
5. Add honey.

Usage Tips: This immune-boosting blend is great for preventing colds and flu. Enjoy it regularly during the cold season.

7) DETOXIFYING DANDELION NETTLE TEA

Ingredients:

- 1 Tbsp dried dandelion root
- 1 Tbsp dried nettle leaves
- 2 glasses boiling water
- Honey

Steps:

1. Add the dried dandelion root and nettle leaves in a teapot.
2. Pour boiling water over the herbs.
3. Let steep for 6-8 min.
4. Divide the tea into cups.
5. Add honey.

Usage Tips: This detoxifying blend supports liver function and overall detoxification. Enjoy it daily for a gentle cleanse.

8) ANTIOXIDANT-RICH HIBISCUS GREEN TEA

Ingredients:

- 1 Tbsp dried hibiscus flowers
- 1 Tbsp green tea leaves
- 2 glasses boiling water

- Honey

Steps:

1. Add the dried hibiscus flowers and green tea leaves in a teapot.
2. Pour boiling water over the herbs.
3. Let steep for 4-6 min.
4. Divide the tea into cups.
5. Add honey.

Usage Tips: This antioxidant-rich blend supports overall health and well-being. Enjoy it in the morning for a refreshing start to your day.

9) RELAXING VALERIAN LEMON BALM TEA

Ingredients:

- 1 Tbsp dried valerian root
- 1 Tbsp dried lemon balm
- 2 glasses boiling water
- Honey

Steps:

1. Add the dried valerian root and lemon balm in a teapot.
2. Pour boiling water over the herbs.
3. Let steep for 6-8 min.
4. Divide the tea into cups.
5. Add honey.

Usage Tips: This relaxing blend is perfect for promoting restful sleep. Enjoy it before bed to help unwind and relax.

10) CLEANSING FENNEL GINGER TEA

Ingredients:

- 1 Tbsp fennel seeds
- 1 Tbsp grated fresh ginger
- 2 glasses boiling water
- Honey

Steps:

1. Add the fennel seeds and grated ginger in a teapot.
2. Pour boiling water over the herbs.
3. Let steep for 6-8 min.
4. Divide the tea into cups.
5. Add honey.

Usage Tips: This cleansing blend aids digestion and supports detoxification. Enjoy it after meals to soothe the digestive system.

3.3 Herbal Teas for Everyday Enjoyment

11) LEMON VERBENA CITRUS TEA

Ingredients:

- 1 Tbsp dried lemon verbena
- 1 Tbsp dried orange peel
- 2 glasses boiling water
- Honey

Steps:

1 Add the dried lemon verbena and dried orange peel in a teapot.
2 Pour boiling water over the herbs.
3 Let steep for 6-8 min.
4 Divide the tea into cups.
5 Add honey.

Usage Tips: This refreshing tea has a bright citrus flavor. Enjoy it in the morning to start your day with a zesty boost.

12) PEPPERMINT LICORICE DELIGHT

Ingredients:

- 1 Tbsp dried peppermint leaves
- 1 Tbsp dried licorice root
- 2 glasses boiling water
- Honey

Steps:

1 Add the dried peppermint leaves and dried licorice root in a teapot.
2 Pour boiling water over the herbs.
3 Let steep for 6-8 min.
4 Divide the tea into cups.
5 Add honey.

Usage Tips: This soothing tea blend is perfect for an afternoon pick-me-up. The peppermint refreshes while the licorice root adds a natural sweetness.

13) CHAMOMILE ROSE BLISS

Ingredients:

- 1 Tbsp dried chamomile flowers
- 1 Tbsp dried rose petals
- 2 glasses boiling water
- Honey

Steps:

1 Add the dried chamomile flowers and dried rose petals in a teapot.
2 Pour boiling water over the herbs.
3 Let steep for 6-8 min.
4 Divide the tea into cups.
5 Add honey.

Usage Tips: This floral blend is calming and delightful. Enjoy it in the evening to unwind and relax.

14) LAVENDER EARL GREY

Ingredients:

- 1 Tbsp dried lavender buds
- 1 Tbsp Earl Grey tea leaves
- 2 glasses boiling water
- Honey or milk

Steps:

1 Add the dried lavender buds and Earl Grey tea leaves in a teapot.
2 Pour boiling water over the herbs.
3 Let steep for 4-6 min.
4 Divide the tea into cups.
5 Add honey or milk.

Usage Tips: This elegant blend combines the soothing properties of lavender with the bold flavor of Earl Grey. Enjoy it as an afternoon tea.

15) GINGER LEMONGRASS ZING

Ingredients:

- 1 Tbsp grated fresh ginger
- 1 Tbsp dried lemongrass
- 2 glasses boiling water
- Honey

Steps:

1 Add the grated fresh ginger and dried lemongrass in a teapot.
2 Pour boiling water over the herbs.
3 Let steep for 6-8 min.
4 Divide the tea into cups.
5 Add honey.

Usage Tips: This invigorating tea is perfect for boosting your energy levels. Enjoy it anytime you need a refreshing lift.

---

16)   BASIL MINT REFRESHER

Ingredients:

- 1 Tbsp dried basil leaves
- 1 Tbsp dried peppermint leaves
- 2 glasses boiling water
- Honey

Steps:

1. Add the dried basil leaves and dried peppermint leaves in a teapot.
2. Pour boiling water over the herbs.
3. Let steep for 6-8 min.
4. Divide the tea into cups.
5. Add honey.

Usage Tips: This refreshing blend is perfect for cooling down on a hot day. Serve it over ice for a delicious, iced tea.

---

17) SAGE THYME COMFORT

Ingredients:

- 1 Tbsp dried sage leaves
- 1 Tbsp dried thyme leaves
- 2 glasses boiling water
- Honey

Steps:

1. Add the dried sage leaves and dried thyme leaves in a teapot.
2. Pour boiling water over the herbs.
3. Let steep for 6-8 min.
4. Divide the tea into cups.
5. Add honey.

Usage Tips: This earthy blend is comforting and warming. Enjoy it in the evening for a cozy, relaxing experience.

---

18)   LEMON BALM HIBISCUS COOLER

Ingredients:

- 1 Tbsp dried lemon balm
- 1 Tbsp dried hibiscus flowers
- 2 glasses boiling water
- Honey

Steps:

1. Add the dried lemon balm and dried hibiscus flowers in a teapot.
2. Pour boiling water over the herbs.
3. Let steep for 6-8 min.
4. Divide the tea into cups.
5. Add honey.

Usage Tips: This tangy blend is perfect for a refreshing break. Enjoy it hot or iced, depending on your preference.

---

19)   ROSEMARY   MINT HARMONY

Ingredients:

- 1 Tbsp dried rosemary
- 1 dried peppermint leaves
- 2 glasses boiling water
- Honey

Steps:

1. Add the dried rosemary and dried peppermint leaves in a teapot.
2. Pour boiling water over the herbs.
3. Let steep for 6-8 min.
4. Divide the tea into cups.
5. Add honey.

Usage Tips: This refreshing and invigorating blend is great for mental clarity. Enjoy it in the afternoon to stay sharp and focused.

---

20)   ORANGE SPICE DELIGHT

Ingredients:

- 1 Tbsp dried orange peel
- 1 cinnamon stick
- 2 glasses boiling water
- Honey

Steps:

1. Add the dried orange peel and cinnamon stick in a teapot.
2. Pour boiling water over the herbs.
3. Let steep for 6-8 min.
4. Divide the tea into cups.
5. Add honey.

Usage Tips: This warm and spiced blend is perfect for cozy evenings. Enjoy it with a touch of honey for added sweetness

3.4 Herbal Teas for Specific Needs

3.4.1 Digestive Support Teas

21) MINT GINGER DIGESTIVE AID

Ingredients:

- 1 Tbsp dried peppermint leaves
- 1 Tbsp grated fresh ginger
- 2 glasses boiling water
- Honey

Steps:

1. Add the dried peppermint leaves and grated ginger in a teapot.
2. Pour boiling water over the herbs.
3. Let steep for 8-9 min.
4. Divide the tea into cups.
5. Add honey.

Usage Tips: This refreshing blend aids digestion and can be enjoyed after meals to soothe the stomach.

22) STOMACH SOOTHING FENNEL PEPPERMINT TEA

Ingredients:

- 1 Tbsp fennel seeds
- 1 Tbsp dried peppermint leaves
- 2 glasses boiling water
- Honey

Steps:

1. Add the fennel seeds and dried peppermint leaves in a teapot.
2. Pour boiling water over the herbs.
3. Let steep for 8-9 min.
4. Divide the tea into cups.
5. Add honey.

Usage Tips: This blend is excellent for soothing an upset stomach. Drink it after meals to aid digestion and reduce bloating.

23) CLEANSING FENNEL GINGER TEA

Ingredients:

- 1 Tbsp fennel seeds
- 1 Tbsp grated fresh ginger
- 2 glasses boiling water
- Honey

Steps:

1. Add the fennel seeds and grated fresh ginger in a teapot.
2. Pour boiling water over the herbs.
3. Let steep for 8-9 min.
4. Divide the tea into cups.
5. Add honey.

Usage Tips: This cleansing blend aids digestion and supports detoxification. Enjoy it after meals to soothe the digestive system.

3.4.2 Sleep-Enhancing Teas

24) RELAXING VALERIAN LEMON BALM TEA

Ingredients:

- 1 Tbsp dried valerian root
- 1 Tbsp dried lemon balm
- 2 glasses boiling water
- Honey

Steps:

1. Add the dried valerian root and lemon balm in a teapot.
2. Pour boiling water over the herbs.
3. Let steep for 8-9 min.
4. Divide the tea into cups.

5. Add honey.

Usage Tips: This relaxing blend is perfect for promoting restful sleep. Enjoy it before bed to help unwind and relax.

25) CALMING SKULLCAP VALERIAN TEA

Ingredients:

- 1 Tbsp dried skullcap
- 1 Tbsp dried valerian root
- 2 glasses boiling water
- Honey

Steps:

1. Add the dried skullcap and dried valerian root in a teapot.
2. Pour boiling water over the herbs.
3. Let steep for 8-9 min.
4. Divide the tea into cups.
5. Add honey.

Usage Tips: This calming blend helps reduce anxiety and stress. Drink it in the evening to unwind and relax.

26) SLEEP AID CHAMOMILE HOPS TEA

Ingredients:

- 1 Tbsp dried chamomile flowers
- 1 Tbsp dried hops flowers
- 2 glasses boiling water
- Honey

Steps:

1. Add the dried chamomile flowers and dried hops flowers in a teapot.
2. Pour boiling water over the herbs.
3. Let steep for 8-9 min.
4. Divide the tea into cups.
5. Add honey.

Usage Tips: This sleep aid blend promotes restful sleep. Drink it before bed to help unwind and prepare for a good night's rest.

3.4.3 Detoxifying Teas

27) DETOXIFYING DANDELION NETTLE TEA

Ingredients:

- 1 Tbsp dried dandelion root
- 1 Tbsp dried nettle leaves
- 2 glasses boiling water
- Honey

Steps:

1. Add the dried dandelion root and nettle leaves in a teapot.
2. Pour boiling water over the herbs.
3. Let steep for 8-9 min.
4. Divide the tea into cups.
5. Add honey.

Usage Tips: This detoxifying blend supports liver function and overall detoxification. Enjoy it daily for a gentle cleanse.

28) DETOXIFYING BURDOCK ROOT DANDELION TEA

Ingredients:

- 1 Tbsp dried burdock root
- 1 Tbsp dried dandelion root
- 2 glasses boiling water
- Honey

Steps:

1. Add the dried burdock root and dried dandelion root in a teapot.
2. Pour boiling water over the herbs.
3. Let steep for 8-9 min.
4. Divide the tea into cups.
5. Add honey.

Usage Tips: This detoxifying blend supports liver function and overall detoxification. Enjoy it daily for a gentle cleanse.

29) CLEANSING NETTLE DANDELION TEA

Ingredients:

- 1 Tbsp dried nettle leaves
- 1 Tbsp dried dandelion leaves
- 2 glasses boiling water
- Honey

Steps:

1. Add the dried nettle leaves and dried dandelion leaves in a teapot.

3.4.4 Energy-Boosting Teas

30) ENERGIZING GINSENG PEPPERMINT TEA

Ingredients:

- 1 Tbsp dried ginseng root
- 1 Tbsp dried peppermint leaves
- 2 glasses boiling water
- Honey

Steps:

1. Add the dried ginseng root and peppermint leaves in a teapot.
2. Pour boiling water over the herbs.
3. Let steep for 8-9min.
4. Divide the tea into cups.
6. Add honey.

Usage Tips: This energizing blend provides a natural boost of energy. Enjoy it in the morning or early afternoon for a refreshing pick-me-up.

31) FOCUS AND CLARITY GOTU KOLA TEA

Ingredients:

- 1 Tbsp dried gotu kola
- 1 Tbsp dried rosemary
- 2 glasses boiling water
- Honey

Steps:

1. Add the dried gotu kola and dried rosemary in a teapot.

2. Pour boiling water over the herbs.
3. Let steep for 8-9 min.
4. Divide the tea into cups.
5. Add honey.

Usage Tips: This cleansing blend supports kidney function and detoxification. Drink it regularly to help cleanse the body.

2. Pour boiling water over the herbs.
3. Let steep for 8-9 min.
4. Divide the tea into cups.
5. Add honey.

Usage Tips: This blend enhances focus and mental clarity. Drink it in the morning or afternoon to boost cognitive function.

32) GINGER LEMONGRASS ZING

Ingredients:

- 1 Tbsp grated fresh ginger
- 1 Tbsp dried lemongrass
- 2 glasses boiling water
- Honey

Steps:

1. Add the grated fresh ginger and dried lemongrass in a teapot.
2. Pour boiling water over the herbs.
3. Let steep for 8-9 min.
4. Divide the tea into cups.
5. Add honey.

Usage Tips: This invigorating tea is perfect for boosting your energy levels. Enjoy it anytime you need a refreshing lift.

33) CALMING HOLY BASIL LICORICE ROOT TEA

Ingredients:

- 1 Tbsp dried holy basil leaves
- 1 Tbsp dried licorice root
- 2 glasses boiling water
- Honey

Steps:

1. Add the dried holy basil leaves and licorice root in a teapot.
2. Pour boiling water over the herbs.
3. Let steep for 8-9 min.
4. Divide the tea into cups.
5. Add honey.

Usage Tips: This soothing blend helps to reduce stress and anxiety. Enjoy it during stressful times to promote calmness.

34) ANTI-ANXIETY LEMON BALM CATNIP TEA

Ingredients:

- 1 Tbsp dried lemon balm
- 1 Tbsp dried catnip
- 2 glasses boiling water
- Honey

Steps:

1. Add the dried lemon balm and dried catnip in a teapot.
2. Pour boiling water over the herbs.
3. Let steep for 8-9 min.
4. Divide the tea into cups.
5. Add honey.

Usage Tips: This anti-anxiety blend is calming and soothing. Drink it in the evening to help relax and reduce stress.

35) CALMING LAVENDER LEMON BALM TEA

Ingredients:

- 1 Tbsp dried lavender buds
- 1 Tbsp dried lemon balm
- 2 glasses boiling water
- Honey

Steps:

1. Add the dried lavender buds and dried lemon balm in a teapot.
2. Pour boiling water over the herbs.
3. Let steep for 8-9 min.
4. Divide the tea into cups.
5. Add honey.

Usage Tips: This calming blend helps reduce stress and anxiety. Enjoy it in the evening to help relax and unwind.

Chapter 4: Recipes for Meals, Beverages, and Desserts

Welcome to a culinary journey where herbs take center stage, transforming everyday meals, beverages, and desserts into extraordinary delights. In this chapter, we explore the versatile role of herbs in culinary arts, providing insights into their flavor-enhancing properties, nutritional benefits, and how they can elevate your cooking. From hearty breakfasts to savory dinners, refreshing beverages to indulgent desserts, and tantalizing appetizers to sweet treats, each recipe showcases the unique charm of herbs. Discover tips for using fresh and dried herbs, learn basic techniques for herbal infusions, and embrace the art of cooking with these natural wonders.

4.1 Introduction to Wholesome Herbal Cooking

Discover the vibrant world of herbal culinary delights, where fresh and dried herbs bring new dimensions of flavor, aroma, and health benefits to your cooking. In this section, we explore the transformative role of herbs in the kitchen, offering practical tips for incorporating them into your meals. Learn basic techniques for creating herbal infusions and master the art of enhancing dishes with nature's finest ingredients.

4.1.1 The Role of Herbs in Culinary Arts

Enhancing and Balancing Flavors

Herbs are essential for enhancing and balancing flavors in culinary arts. Fresh herbs like basil, cilantro, and parsley add a burst of freshness and color to salads, soups, and sauces. Dried herbs, such as oregano, thyme, and rosemary, are ideal for slow-cooked dishes, infusing them with deep, earthy flavors. By understanding each herb's distinct characteristics, cooks can create harmonious flavor profiles that elevate simple ingredients into gourmet dishes.

Natural Preservation and Nutritional Value

Herbs serve as natural preservatives and are recognized for their antimicrobial properties. Herbs like rosemary, thyme, and sage can help extend the shelf life of foods, particularly meats and dairy products. This enhances food safety and reduces waste, aligning with sustainable cooking practices. Additionally, herbs contribute to the nutritional value of meals. For instance, parsley is rich in vitamins C and K, while basil contains compounds supporting heart health and reducing inflammation. Incorporating various herbs into daily meals boosts essential nutrient intake.

Therapeutic Properties and Health Benefits

Herbs are known for their therapeutic properties, supporting overall well-being. Traditional medicine systems like Ayurveda and Traditional Chinese Medicine have long used herbs for their healing properties. Culinary herbs such as ginger, turmeric, and garlic are noted for their anti-inflammatory, digestive, and immune-boosting benefits. Integrating these herbs into everyday cooking allows for the enjoyment of their health-promoting effects naturally and deliciously.

Creativity, Artistry, and Cultural Significance

Herbs add creativity and artistry to cooking. Their vibrant colors, textures, and shapes can transform the visual appeal of dishes, making meals more enticing. Garnishing with fresh herbs like cilantro, dill, or chives enhances flavor and adds a decorative touch, elevating the dining experience. Beyond the kitchen, herbs hold cultural and historical significance. Many herbs are integral to the culinary traditions of various cultures worldwide. For example, basil is central to Italian cuisine, cilantro is a staple in Mexican dishes, and lemongrass is essential in Thai cooking. Understanding the cultural context of herbs deepens appreciation for global cuisines and inspires culinary exploration.

4.1.2 Tips for Cooking with Fresh and Dried Herbs

Cooking with herbs can transform ordinary dishes into extraordinary culinary delights. Understanding the nuances between fresh and dried herbs and knowing how to use them effectively can make all the difference in your cooking.

Understanding Fresh vs. Dried Herbs

Fresh and dried herbs have distinct flavors and uses. Fresh herbs are vibrant and delicate, best added at the end of cooking or as a garnish. Dried herbs have concentrated flavors and are ideal for slow-cooked dishes, providing depth and complexity. Knowing when and how to use each type can enhance your dishes significantly.

Top 10 Tips for Using Herbs in Cooking

1. ***Add fresh herbs at the end:*** Preserve their flavor and color.

2. ***Use dried herbs early:*** Allow them to infuse and release flavors.

3. ***Double the amount of fresh herbs if substituting for dried:*** Fresh herbs have a milder flavor.

4. ***Store fresh herbs properly:*** Keep them in the fridge, wrapped in a damp paper towel.

5. ***Crush dried herbs before use***: Release their essential oils and maximize flavor.

6. ***Combine herbs thoughtfully:*** Pair complementary herbs for balanced flavors.

7. ***Experiment with herb blends:*** Create custom blends for unique flavor profiles.

8. ***Use herb stems:*** They are flavorful and can be added to stocks and broths.

9. ***Dry your own herbs:*** Preserve fresh herbs by drying them for later use.

10. ***Taste as you go:*** Adjust the amount of herbs to suit your taste preference.

Enhancing Culinary Creativity with Herbs

Herbs are a fantastic way to unleash culinary creativity. Experimenting with different combinations and techniques can lead to discovering new flavors and dishes. For instance, making herb-infused oils and vinegars can add a gourmet touch to salads and marinades. Herbs can also be blended into butters, salts, and sugars, providing a unique twist to your culinary creations. Embrace the versatility of herbs and enjoy the endless possibilities they offer in cooking.

4.1.3 Basic Techniques for Herbal Infusions in Cooking

Herbal infusions are a fantastic way to impart the rich flavors and aromas of herbs into various dishes. Understanding the basic techniques for herbal infusions can enhance your culinary creations, making them more flavorful and aromatic. Here are three essential techniques for using herbal infusions in cooking:

Infused Oils

Infused oils are a versatile and flavorful addition to many dishes. To create an herb-infused oil, follow these steps:

1. Choose a neutral oil such as olive, grapeseed, or sunflower oil.

2. Heat the oil gently over low heat until warm, but not boiling.

3. Add your chosen fresh or dried herbs (e.g., rosemary, thyme, basil, garlic).

4. Let the mixture steep over low heat for 20-30 minutes, ensuring the herbs do not burn.

5. Strain the oil through a fine-mesh sieve or cheesecloth to remove the herbs.

6. Store the infused oil in a clean, airtight container in the refrigerator for up to two weeks.

Usage tips: Use herb-infused oils for drizzling over salads, roasting vegetables, marinating meats, or enhancing the flavor of pasta dishes.

Herbal Vinegars

Herbal vinegars are simple to make and can add a burst of flavor to dressings, marinades, and sauces. Here's how to make herb-infused vinegar:

1. Choose a base vinegar such as white wine, apple cider, or rice vinegar.

2. Fill a clean glass jar with your chosen fresh herbs (e.g., tarragon, dill, chives).

3. Pour the vinegar over the herbs, ensuring they are fully submerged.

4. Seal the jar tightly and let it sit in a cool, dark place for 2-4 weeks to allow the flavors to meld.

5. Strain the vinegar through a fine-mesh sieve or cheesecloth to remove the herbs.

6. Transfer the infused vinegar to a clean, airtight bottle for storage.

Usage tips: Use herb-infused vinegars in salad dressings, marinades, or as a flavorful addition to sauces and dips.

Herb-Infused Butters

Herb-infused butters are perfect for adding a burst of flavor to breads, vegetables, and meats. To make herb-infused butter, follow these steps:

1. Soften unsalted butter at room temperature.

2. Finely chop your chosen fresh herbs (e.g., parsley, chives, thyme, sage).

3. In a bowl, mix the softened butter with the chopped herbs until well combined.

4. Transfer the herb butter to a sheet of parchment paper or plastic wrap.

5. Shape the butter into a log and wrap tightly.

6. Refrigerate until firm, then slice as needed.

Usage tips: Use herb-infused butters for spreading on bread, melting over grilled meats, or tossing with cooked vegetables and pasta.

These basic techniques for herbal infusions can elevate your culinary creations, bringing fresh and vibrant flavors to your dishes. Experiment with different herbs and combinations to discover your favorite flavor profiles.

4.2 Herbal Breakfast Recipes

36) ROSEMARY AND TOMATO FRITTATA

Ingredients:

- 6 large eggs
- 1/4 cup milk
- 1/2 cup cherry tomatoes, halved
- 2 tablespoons fresh rosemary, chopped
- 1/4 cup grated Parmesan cheese
- Salt and pepper to taste
- 1 tablespoon olive oil

Steps:

1. Preheat the oven to 375°F (190°C).
2. In a bowl, whisk together the eggs, milk, salt, and pepper.
3. Heat the olive oil in a skillet over medium heat.
4. Add the cherry tomatoes and cook for 2-3 minutes.
5. Pour the egg mixture into the skillet and sprinkle with rosemary and Parmesan cheese.
6. Cook for 5 minutes until the edges start to set.
7. Transfer the skillet to the oven and bake for 10-12 minutes until fully set.
8. Cut into wedges and serve.

Usage Tips: This frittata is a savory and herbaceous breakfast option. Serve it with a side of fresh greens or toast.

37) MINT AND BERRY OVERNIGHT OATS

Ingredients:

- 1 cup rolled oats
- 1 cup almond milk
- 1/2 cup Greek yogurt
- 1/2 cup mixed berries
- 1 tablespoon fresh mint, chopped
- 1 tablespoon honey
- 1 teaspoon chia seeds

Steps:

1. In a mason jar or bowl, combine the oats, almond milk, Greek yogurt, honey, and chia seeds.
2. Stir in the mixed berries and chopped mint.
3. Cover and refrigerate overnight.
4. Stir before serving and add more berries or mint if desired.

Usage Tips: This refreshing and nutritious breakfast can be prepared the night before for a quick and easy start to your day.

38) LEMON THYME PANCAKES

Ingredients:

- 1 cup all-purpose flour
- 1 tablespoon sugar
- 1 teaspoon baking powder
- 1/2 teaspoon baking soda
- 1/4 teaspoon salt
- 1 cup buttermilk
- 1 large egg
- 2 tablespoons melted butter
- 1 tablespoon fresh thyme leaves
- 1 tablespoon lemon zest

Steps:

1. In a bowl, mix the flour, sugar, baking powder, baking soda, and salt.
2. In another bowl, whisk together the buttermilk, egg, and melted butter.
3. Combine the wet and dry ingredients, then fold in the thyme leaves and lemon zest.
4. Heat a non-stick skillet over medium heat and grease with butter or oil.
5. Pour 1/4 cup of batter onto the skillet and cook until bubbles form on the surface.
6. Flip and cook until golden brown.
7. Repeat with the remaining batter.

Usage Tips: Serve these fragrant pancakes with a drizzle of maple syrup and a sprinkle of fresh thyme leaves.

39) CILANTRO AND AVOCADO BREAKFAST BURRITO

Ingredients:

- 4 large eggs
- 1/4 cup milk
- 1 avocado, sliced
- 1/4 cup fresh cilantro, chopped
- 1/4 cup shredded cheese
- Salt and pepper to taste
- 2 large flour tortillas
- 1 tablespoon olive oil

Steps:

1. In a bowl, whisk together the eggs, milk, salt, and pepper.
2. Heat the olive oil in a non-stick skillet over medium heat.
3. Pour the egg mixture into the skillet and scramble until fully cooked.
4. Place the scrambled eggs in the center of each tortilla.
5. Top with avocado slices, cilantro, and shredded cheese.
6. Roll up the tortillas to form burritos.
7. Serve immediately.

Usage Tips: These breakfast burritos are filling and flavorful. Add a splash of hot sauce for an extra kick.

40) LAVENDER HONEY BREAKFAST BISCUITS

Ingredients:

- 2 cups all-purpose flour
- 1 tablespoon baking powder
- 1/2 teaspoon salt
- 1/2 cup cold butter, cubed
- 1 tablespoon dried lavender buds
- 3/4 cup milk
- 2 tablespoons honey

Steps:

1. Preheat the oven to 425°F (220°C).
2. In a large bowl, mix the flour, baking powder, and salt.
3. Cut in the butter until the mixture resembles coarse crumbs.
4. Stir in the dried lavender buds.

5. Add the milk and honey, mixing until just combined.
6. Turn the dough out onto a floured surface and knead gently.
7. Roll out to 1/2-inch thickness and cut into biscuits.
8. Place the biscuits on a baking sheet and bake for 12-15 minutes until golden brown.

Usage Tips: Serve these fragrant biscuits with butter and a drizzle of honey for a delightful breakfast treat.

41) OREGANO AND MUSHROOM BREAKFAST QUICHE

Ingredients:

- 1 pre-made pie crust
- 1 cup sliced mushrooms
- 1/2 cup grated cheese
- 1/4 cup fresh oregano leaves, chopped
- 4 large eggs
- 1 cup milk
- Salt and pepper to taste
- 1 tablespoon olive oil

Steps:

1. Preheat the oven to 375°F (190°C).
2. Heat the olive oil in a skillet over medium heat.
3. Add the mushrooms and cook until soft, about 5 minutes.
4. Place the pie crust in a pie dish and sprinkle with the cooked mushrooms and grated cheese.
5. In a bowl, whisk together the eggs, milk, oregano, salt, and pepper.
6. Pour the egg mixture over the mushrooms and cheese.
7. Bake for 35-40 minutes until the quiche is set and golden brown.
8. Let cool slightly before serving.

Usage Tips: This savory quiche is perfect for a weekend breakfast or brunch. Serve with a side salad for a complete meal.

42) THYME AND APPLE BREAKFAST MUFFINS

Ingredients:

- 1 1/2 cups all-purpose flour
- 1/2 cup sugar
- 1 teaspoon baking powder
- 1/2 teaspoon baking soda
- 1/4 teaspoon salt
- 1/2 teaspoon ground cinnamon
- 1/4 teaspoon ground nutmeg
- 1/2 cup milk
- 1/4 cup vegetable oil
- 1 large egg
- 1 apple, peeled and diced
- 1 tablespoon fresh thyme leaves

Steps:

1. Preheat the oven to 350°F (175°C).
2. In a large bowl, mix the flour, sugar, baking powder, baking soda, salt, cinnamon, and nutmeg.
3. In another bowl, whisk together the milk, vegetable oil, and egg.
4. Combine the wet and dry ingredients, then fold in the diced apple and thyme leaves.
5. Spoon the batter into a greased muffin tin, filling each cup about 2/3 full.
6. Bake for 20-25 minutes until a toothpick inserted into the center comes out clean.
7. Cool in the tin for 5 minutes, then transfer to a wire rack to cool completely.

Usage Tips: These muffins are moist and flavorful, with a hint of thyme that complements the sweetness of the apples. Enjoy them warm or at room temperature.

43) PARSLEY AND FETA SCRAMBLED EGGS

Ingredients:

- 4 large eggs
- 1/4 cup milk
- 1/4 cup crumbled feta cheese
- 2 tablespoons fresh parsley, chopped
- Salt and pepper to taste
- 1 tablespoon butter

Steps:

1. In a bowl, whisk together the eggs, milk, salt, and pepper.
2. Heat the butter in a non-stick skillet over medium heat.
3. Pour the egg mixture into the skillet and cook, stirring gently.
4. When the eggs are almost set, sprinkle in the feta cheese and parsley.
5. Continue cooking until the eggs are fully set.
6. Serve hot.

Usage Tips: These scrambled eggs are creamy and flavorful. Serve with whole-grain toast for a complete breakfast.

44) SAGE AND SAUSAGE BREAKFAST CASSEROLE

Ingredients:

- 1 pound breakfast sausage
- 1/2 cup chopped onion
- 1/2 cup chopped red bell pepper
- 1/4 cup fresh sage leaves, chopped
- 6 large eggs
- 1 cup milk
- 1 cup shredded cheese
- 4 cups cubed bread
- Salt and pepper to taste

Steps:

1. Preheat the oven to 350°F (175°C).
2. In a skillet, cook the sausage over medium heat until browned. Drain excess fat.
3. Add the onion and red bell pepper to the skillet and cook until soft.
4. In a large bowl, whisk together the eggs, milk, sage, salt, and pepper.
5. Add the cooked sausage mixture, shredded cheese, and cubed bread to the bowl and mix well.
6. Pour the mixture into a greased baking dish.
7. Bake for 30-35 minutes until the casserole is set and golden brown.
8. Let cool slightly before serving.

Usage Tips: This hearty breakfast casserole can be prepared the night before and baked in the morning for a convenient and delicious start to the day.

45) BASIL AND SPINACH BREAKFAST SMOOTHIE

Ingredients:

- 1 cup spinach leaves
- 1/2 cup fresh basil leaves
- 1 banana
- 1/2 cup Greek yogurt
- 1 cup almond milk
- 1 tablespoon honey

Steps:

1. Combine all ingredients in a blender.
2. Blend until smooth and creamy.
3. Pour into a glass and serve immediately.

Usage Tips: This green smoothie is packed with nutrients and offers a refreshing start to your day. Adjust the sweetness by adding more or less honey.

4.3 Herbal Lunch Recipes

46) LEMON BASIL CHICKEN SALAD

Ingredients:

- 2 cups cooked chicken breast, shredded
- 1/4 cup mayonnaise
- 2 tablespoons Greek yogurt
- 1 tablespoon fresh lemon juice
- 1 tablespoon fresh basil leaves, chopped
- 1/4 cup celery, diced
- Salt and pepper to taste

Steps:

1. In a large bowl, combine the mayonnaise, Greek yogurt, lemon juice, salt, and pepper.
2. Add the shredded chicken, basil leaves, and diced celery to the bowl.
3. Mix well until all ingredients are evenly coated.
4. Refrigerate for at least 30 minutes before serving.

Usage Tips: This refreshing chicken salad is perfect for a light lunch. Serve it on a bed of mixed greens or in a sandwich.

47) ROSEMARY GARLIC GRILLED VEGGIE WRAP

Ingredients:

- 1 zucchini, sliced
- 1 red bell pepper, sliced
- 1 yellow bell pepper, sliced
- 1 red onion, sliced
- 2 tablespoons olive oil
- 1 tablespoon fresh rosemary, chopped
- 2 cloves garlic, minced
- Salt and pepper to taste
- 4 large whole wheat tortillas
- 1/2 cup hummus

Steps:

1. Preheat the grill to medium-high heat.
2. In a large bowl, toss the zucchini, bell peppers, and onion with olive oil, rosemary, garlic, salt, and pepper.
3. Grill the vegetables for 5-7 minutes, turning occasionally, until tender and slightly charred.
4. Spread a thin layer of hummus on each tortilla.
5. Divide the grilled vegetables among the tortillas and wrap tightly.
6. Serve immediately.

Usage Tips: These grilled veggie wraps are packed with flavor and perfect for a quick lunch. Add a sprinkle of feta cheese for extra richness.

48) MINTY QUINOA TABBOULEH

Ingredients:

- 1 cup quinoa, rinsed
- 2 cups water

- 1 cup fresh parsley, chopped
- 1/2 cup fresh mint, chopped
- 2 tomatoes, diced
- 1 cucumber, diced
- 1/4 cup olive oil
- 1/4 cup fresh lemon juice
- Salt and pepper to taste

Steps:

1. In a medium pot, bring the water to a boil. Add the quinoa, reduce heat, and simmer for 15 minutes until water is absorbed.
2. Fluff the quinoa with a fork and let it cool to room temperature.
3. In a large bowl, combine the cooled quinoa, parsley, mint, tomatoes, and cucumber.
4. In a small bowl, whisk together the olive oil, lemon juice, salt, and pepper.
5. Pour the dressing over the quinoa mixture and toss to combine.
6. Refrigerate for at least 30 minutes before serving.

Usage Tips: This minty quinoa tabbouleh is a refreshing and healthy lunch option. Serve it as a side dish or add grilled chicken for a complete meal.

49) CILANTRO LIME SHRIMP TACOS

Ingredients:

- 1 pound shrimp, peeled and deveined
- 1 tablespoon olive oil
- 2 cloves garlic, minced
- 1/4 cup fresh cilantro, chopped
- 1 tablespoon fresh lime juice
- 8 small corn tortillas
- 1 avocado, sliced
- 1/4 cup red onion, thinly sliced
- Salt and pepper to taste

Steps:

1. In a large skillet, heat the olive oil over medium-high heat.
2. Add the garlic and cook for 1 minute until fragrant.
3. Add the shrimp and cook for 3-4 minutes until pink and opaque.

4. Remove the skillet from heat and stir in the cilantro and lime juice.
5. Season with salt and pepper to taste.
6. Warm the tortillas in a dry skillet or microwave.
7. Divide the shrimp among the tortillas and top with avocado slices and red onion.
8. Serve immediately.

Usage Tips: These cilantro lime shrimp tacos are light and flavorful. Serve with a side of black beans and rice for a satisfying lunch.

50) BASIL PESTO PASTA SALAD

Ingredients:

- 8 ounces rotini pasta
- 1/2 cup basil pesto
- 1 cup cherry tomatoes, halved
- 1/2 cup mozzarella balls, halved
- 1/4 cup black olives, sliced
- 1/4 cup red onion, thinly sliced
- Salt and pepper to taste

Steps:

1. Cook the pasta according to package instructions. Drain and rinse with cold water to cool.
2. In a large bowl, combine the cooked pasta, basil pesto, cherry tomatoes, mozzarella balls, black olives, and red onion.
3. Toss to combine and season with salt and pepper to taste.
4. Refrigerate for at least 30 minutes before serving.

Usage Tips: This basil pesto pasta salad is a great make-ahead lunch. It's perfect for picnics or as a side dish for grilled meats.

51) THYME AND LEMON ROASTED CHICKEN

Ingredients:

- 4 chicken thighs, bone-in and skin-on
- 2 tablespoons olive oil
- 1 tablespoon fresh thyme leaves
- 1 lemon, sliced
- 4 cloves garlic, minced

- Salt and pepper to taste

Steps:

1. Preheat the oven to 400°F (200°C).
2. In a large bowl, toss the chicken thighs with olive oil, thyme leaves, garlic, salt, and pepper.
3. Place the chicken thighs in a baking dish and top with lemon slices.
4. Roast in the oven for 35-40 minutes until the chicken is cooked through and the skin is crispy.
5. Serve hot.

Usage Tips: This thyme and lemon roasted chicken is flavorful and easy to prepare. Serve with a side of roasted vegetables or a simple green salad.

52) DILL AND CUCUMBER YOGURT DIP

Ingredients:

- 1 cup Greek yogurt
- 1 cucumber, grated and excess water squeezed out
- 2 tablespoons fresh dill, chopped
- 1 clove garlic, minced
- 1 tablespoon fresh lemon juice
- Salt and pepper to taste

Steps:

1. In a medium bowl, combine the Greek yogurt, grated cucumber, dill, garlic, lemon juice, salt, and pepper.
2. Mix well until all ingredients are evenly incorporated.
3. Refrigerate for at least 30 minutes before serving.

Usage Tips: This dill and cucumber yogurt dip is refreshing and versatile. Serve it with fresh vegetables, pita bread, or as a topping for grilled meats.

53) SAGE AND SWEET POTATO SOUP

Ingredients:

- 2 large sweet potatoes, peeled and diced
- 1 onion, chopped
- 2 cloves garlic, minced
- 1 tablespoon fresh sage, chopped

- 4 cups vegetable broth
- 1/2 cup coconut milk
- Salt and pepper to taste
- 2 tablespoons olive oil

Steps:

1. In a large pot, heat the olive oil over medium heat.
2. Add the onion and garlic and cook for 5 minutes until soft.
3. Add the sweet potatoes and cook for another 5 minutes.
4. Pour in the vegetable broth and bring to a boil.
5. Reduce heat and simmer for 20 minutes until the sweet potatoes are tender.
6. Remove from heat and stir in the sage and coconut milk.
7. Use an immersion blender to puree the soup until smooth.
8. Season with salt and pepper to taste.

Usage Tips: This sage and sweet potato soup is creamy and comforting. Serve with crusty bread for a complete lunch.

54) PARSLEY AND LEMON CHICKPEA SALAD

Ingredients:

- 1 can chickpeas, drained and rinsed
- 1/4 cup fresh parsley, chopped
- 1/4 cup red onion, diced
- 1/4 cup cherry tomatoes, halved
- 1 tablespoon olive oil
- 1 tablespoon fresh lemon juice
- Salt and pepper to taste

Steps:

1. In a large bowl, combine the chickpeas, parsley, red onion, and cherry tomatoes.
2. In a small bowl, whisk together the olive oil, lemon juice, salt, and pepper.
3. Pour the dressing over the chickpea mixture and toss to combine.
4. Refrigerate for at least 30 minutes before serving.

Usage Tips: This parsley and lemon chickpea salad is light and refreshing. Serve it on its own or as a side dish with grilled chicken or fish.

55) HERB-CRUSTED SALMON

Ingredients:

- 4 salmon fillets
- 1/4 cup fresh dill, chopped
- 1/4 cup fresh parsley, chopped
- 2 tablespoons fresh thyme leaves
- 2 cloves garlic, minced
- 2 tablespoons olive oil
- Salt and pepper to taste

Steps:

1. Preheat the oven to 400°F (200°C).
2. In a small bowl, combine the dill, parsley, thyme, garlic, olive oil, salt, and pepper.
3. Place the salmon fillets on a baking sheet lined with parchment paper.
4. Spread the herb mixture evenly over the top of each fillet.
5. Bake for 15-20 minutes until the salmon is cooked through and flakes easily with a fork.
6. Serve hot.

Usage Tips: This herb-crusted salmon is flavorful and healthy. Serve with a side of steamed vegetables or a fresh salad.

56) ROSEMARY AND TOMATO FRITTATA

Ingredients:

- 6 large eggs
- 1/4 cup milk
- 1/2 cup cherry tomatoes, halved
- 2 tablespoons fresh rosemary, chopped
- 1/4 cup grated Parmesan cheese
- Salt and pepper to taste
- 1 tablespoon olive oil

Steps:

1. Preheat the oven to 375°F (190°C).
2. In a bowl, whisk together the eggs, milk, salt, and pepper.
3. Heat the olive oil in a skillet over medium heat.
4. Add the cherry tomatoes and cook for 2-3 minutes.
5. Pour the egg mixture into the skillet and sprinkle with rosemary and Parmesan cheese.

6. Cook for 5 minutes until the edges start to set.
7. Transfer the skillet to the oven and bake for 10-12 minutes until fully set.
8. Cut into wedges and serve.

Usage Tips: This frittata is a savory and herbaceous breakfast option. Serve it with a side of fresh greens or toast.

57) LEMON THYME PANCAKES

Ingredients:

- 1 cup all-purpose flour
- 1 tablespoon sugar
- 1 teaspoon baking powder
- 1/2 teaspoon baking soda
- 1/4 teaspoon salt
- 1 cup buttermilk
- 1 large egg
- 2 tablespoons melted butter
- 1 tablespoon fresh thyme leaves
- 1 tablespoon lemon zest

Steps:

1. In a bowl, mix the flour, sugar, baking powder, baking soda, and salt.
2. In another bowl, whisk together the buttermilk, egg, and melted butter.
3. Combine the wet and dry ingredients, then fold in the thyme leaves and lemon zest.
4. Heat a non-stick skillet over medium heat and grease with butter or oil.
5. Pour 1/4 cup of batter onto the skillet and cook until bubbles form on the surface.
6. Flip and cook until golden brown.
7. Repeat with the remaining batter.

Usage Tips: Serve these fragrant pancakes with a drizzle of maple syrup and a sprinkle of fresh thyme leaves.

58) PARSLEY AND FETA SCRAMBLED EGGS

Ingredients:

- 4 large eggs
- 1/4 cup milk
- 1/4 cup crumbled feta cheese

- 2 tablespoons fresh parsley, chopped
- Salt and pepper to taste
- 1 tablespoon butter

Steps:

1. In a bowl, whisk together the eggs, milk, salt, and pepper.
2. Heat the butter in a non-stick skillet over medium heat.
3. Pour the egg mixture into the skillet and cook, stirring gently.
4. When the eggs are almost set, sprinkle in the feta cheese and parsley.
5. Continue cooking until the eggs are fully set.
6. Serve hot.

Usage Tips: These scrambled eggs are creamy and flavorful. Serve with whole-grain toast for a complete breakfast.

59) CILANTRO AND AVOCADO BREAKFAST BURRITO

Ingredients:

- 4 large eggs
- 1/4 cup milk
- 1 avocado, sliced
- 1/4 cup fresh cilantro, chopped
- 1/4 cup shredded cheese
- Salt and pepper to taste
- 2 large flour tortillas
- 1 tablespoon olive oil

Steps:

1. In a bowl, whisk together the eggs, milk, salt, and pepper.
2. Heat the olive oil in a non-stick skillet over medium heat.
3. Pour the egg mixture into the skillet and scramble until fully cooked.
4. Place the scrambled eggs in the center of each tortilla.
5. Top with avocado slices, cilantro, and shredded cheese.
6. Roll up the tortillas to form burritos.
7. Serve immediately.

Usage Tips: These breakfast burritos are filling and flavorful. Add a splash of hot sauce for an extra kick.

60) LAVENDER HONEY BREAKFAST BISCUITS

Ingredients:

- 2 cups all-purpose flour
- 1 tablespoon baking powder
- 1/2 teaspoon salt
- 1/2 cup cold butter, cubed
- 1 tablespoon dried lavender buds
- 3/4 cup milk
- 2 tablespoons honey

Steps:

1. Preheat the oven to 425°F (220°C).
2. In a large bowl, mix the flour, baking powder, and salt.
3. Cut in the butter until the mixture resembles coarse crumbs.
4. Stir in the dried lavender buds.
5. Add the milk and honey, mixing until just combined.
6. Turn the dough out onto a floured surface and knead gently.
7. Roll out to 1/2-inch thickness and cut into biscuits.
8. Place the biscuits on a baking sheet and bake for 12-15 minutes until golden brown.

Usage Tips: Serve these fragrant biscuits with butter and a drizzle of honey for a delightful breakfast treat.

61) OREGANO AND MUSHROOM BREAKFAST QUICHE

Ingredients:

- 1 pre-made pie crust
- 1 cup sliced mushrooms
- 1/2 cup grated cheese
- 1/4 cup fresh oregano leaves, chopped
- 4 large eggs
- 1 cup milk
- Salt and pepper to taste
- 1 tablespoon olive oil

Steps:

1. Preheat the oven to 375°F (190°C).
2. Heat the olive oil in a skillet over medium heat.

3. Add the mushrooms and cook until soft, about 5 minutes.
4. Place the pie crust in a pie dish and sprinkle with the cooked mushrooms and grated cheese.
5. In a bowl, whisk together the eggs, milk, oregano, salt, and pepper.
6. Pour the egg mixture over the mushrooms and cheese.
7. Bake for 35-40 minutes until the quiche is set and golden brown.
8. Let cool slightly before serving.

Usage Tips: This savory quiche is perfect for a weekend breakfast or brunch. Serve with a side salad for a complete meal.

62) THYME AND APPLE BREAKFAST MUFFINS

Ingredients:

- 1 1/2 cups all-purpose flour
- 1/2 cup sugar
- 1 teaspoon baking powder
- 1/2 teaspoon baking soda
- 1/4 teaspoon salt
- 1/2 teaspoon ground cinnamon
- 1/4 teaspoon ground nutmeg
- 1/2 cup milk
- 1/4 cup vegetable oil
- 1 large egg
- 1 apple, peeled and diced
- 1 tablespoon fresh thyme leaves

Steps:

1. Preheat the oven to 350°F (175°C).
2. In a large bowl, mix the flour, sugar, baking powder, baking soda, salt, cinnamon, and nutmeg.
3. In another bowl, whisk together the milk, vegetable oil, and egg.
4. Combine the wet and dry ingredients, then fold in the diced apple and thyme leaves.
5. Spoon the batter into a greased muffin tin, filling each cup about 2/3 full.
6. Bake for 20-25 minutes until a toothpick inserted into the center comes out clean.
7. Cool in the tin for 5 minutes, then transfer to a wire rack to cool completely.

Usage Tips: These muffins are moist and flavorful, with a hint of thyme that complements the sweetness of the apples. Enjoy them warm or at room temperature.

63) MINT AND BERRY OVERNIGHT OATS

Ingredients:

- 1 cup rolled oats
- 1 cup almond milk
- 1/2 cup Greek yogurt
- 1/2 cup mixed berries
- 1 tablespoon fresh mint, chopped
- 1 tablespoon honey
- 1 teaspoon chia seeds

Steps:

1. In a mason jar or bowl, combine the oats, almond milk, Greek yogurt, honey, and chia seeds.
2. Stir in the mixed berries and chopped mint.
3. Cover and refrigerate overnight.
4. Stir before serving and add more berries or mint if desired.

Usage Tips: This refreshing and nutritious breakfast can be prepared the night before for a quick and easy start to your day.

64) SAGE AND SAUSAGE BREAKFAST CASSEROLE

Ingredients:

- 1 pound breakfast sausage
- 1/2 cup chopped onion
- 1/2 cup chopped red bell pepper
- 1/4 cup fresh sage leaves, chopped
- 6 large eggs
- 1 cup milk
- 1 cup shredded cheese
- 4 cups cubed bread
- Salt and pepper to taste

Steps:

1. Preheat the oven to 350°F (175°C).
2. In a skillet, cook the sausage over medium heat until browned. Drain excess fat.

3. Add the onion and red bell pepper to the skillet and cook until soft.
4. In a large bowl, whisk together the eggs, milk, sage, salt, and pepper.
5. Add the cooked sausage mixture, shredded cheese, and cubed bread to the bowl and mix well.
6. Pour the mixture into a greased baking dish.
7. Bake for 30-35 minutes until the casserole is set and golden brown.
8. Let cool slightly before serving.

Usage Tips: This hearty breakfast casserole can be prepared the night before and baked in the morning for a convenient and delicious start to the day.

65) BASIL AND SPINACH BREAKFAST SMOOTHIE

Ingredients:

- 1 cup spinach leaves
- 1/2 cup fresh basil leaves
- 1 banana
- 1/2 cup Greek yogurt
- 1 cup almond milk
- 1 tablespoon honey

Steps:

1. Combine all ingredients in a blender.
2. Blend until smooth and creamy.
3. Pour into a glass and serve immediately.

Usage Tips: This green smoothie is packed with nutrients and offers a refreshing start to your day. Adjust the sweetness by adding more or less honey.

4.3 Herbal Dinner Recipes

66) LEMON BASIL CHICKEN SALAD

Ingredients:

- 2 cups cooked chicken breast, shredded
- 1/4 cup mayonnaise
- 2 tablespoons Greek yogurt
- 1 tablespoon fresh lemon juice
- 1 tablespoon fresh basil leaves, chopped
- 1/4 cup celery, diced
- Salt and pepper to taste

Steps:

1. In a large bowl, combine the mayonnaise, Greek yogurt, lemon juice, salt, and pepper.
2. Add the shredded chicken, basil leaves, and diced celery to the bowl.
3. Mix well until all ingredients are evenly coated.
4. Refrigerate for at least 30 minutes before serving.

Usage Tips: This refreshing chicken salad is perfect for a light lunch. Serve it on a bed of mixed greens or in a sandwich.

67) THYME AND LEMON ROASTED CHICKEN

Ingredients:

- 4 chicken thighs, bone-in and skin-on

- 2 tablespoons olive oil
- 1 tablespoon fresh thyme leaves
- 1 lemon, sliced
- 4 cloves garlic, minced
- Salt and pepper to taste

Steps:

1. Preheat the oven to 400°F (200°C).
2. In a large bowl, toss the chicken thighs with olive oil, thyme leaves, garlic, salt, and pepper.
3. Place the chicken thighs in a baking dish and top with lemon slices.
4. Roast in the oven for 35-40 minutes until the chicken is cooked through and the skin is crispy.
5. Serve hot.

Usage Tips: This thyme and lemon roasted chicken is flavorful and easy to prepare. Serve with a side of roasted vegetables or a simple green salad.

68) ROSEMARY GARLIC GRILLED VEGGIE WRAP

Ingredients:

- 1 zucchini, sliced
- 1 red bell pepper, sliced
- 1 yellow bell pepper, sliced
- 1 red onion, sliced
- 2 tablespoons olive oil
- 1 tablespoon fresh rosemary, chopped
- 2 cloves garlic, minced
- Salt and pepper to taste
- 4 large whole wheat tortillas
- 1/2 cup hummus

Steps:

1. Preheat the grill to medium-high heat.
2. In a large bowl, toss the zucchini, bell peppers, and onion with olive oil, rosemary, garlic, salt, and pepper.
3. Grill the vegetables for 5-7 minutes, turning occasionally, until tender and slightly charred.
4. Spread a thin layer of hummus on each tortilla.
5. Divide the grilled vegetables among the tortillas and wrap tightly.
6. Serve immediately.

Usage Tips: These grilled veggie wraps are packed with flavor and perfect for a quick lunch. Add a sprinkle of feta cheese for extra richness.

69) MINTY QUINOA TABBOULEH

Ingredients:

- 1 cup quinoa, rinsed
- 2 cups water
- 1 cup fresh parsley, chopped
- 1/2 cup fresh mint, chopped
- 2 tomatoes, diced
- 1 cucumber, diced
- 1/4 cup olive oil
- 1/4 cup fresh lemon juice
- Salt and pepper to taste

Steps:

1. In a medium pot, bring the water to a boil. Add the quinoa, reduce heat, and simmer for 15 minutes until water is absorbed.
2. Fluff the quinoa with a fork and let it cool to room temperature.
3. In a large bowl, combine the cooled quinoa, parsley, mint, tomatoes, and cucumber.
4. In a small bowl, whisk together the olive oil, lemon juice, salt, and pepper.
5. Pour the dressing over the quinoa mixture and toss to combine.
6. Refrigerate for at least 30 minutes before serving.

Usage Tips: This minty quinoa tabbouleh is a refreshing and healthy lunch option. Serve it as a side dish or add grilled chicken for a complete meal.

70) CILANTRO LIME SHRIMP TACOS

Ingredients:

- 1 pound shrimp, peeled and deveined
- 1 tablespoon olive oil
- 2 cloves garlic, minced
- 1/4 cup fresh cilantro, chopped
- 1 tablespoon fresh lime juice
- 8 small corn tortillas

- 1 avocado, sliced
- 1/4 cup red onion, thinly sliced
- Salt and pepper to taste

Steps:

1. In a large skillet, heat the olive oil over medium-high heat.
2. Add the garlic and cook for 1 minute until fragrant.
3. Add the shrimp and cook for 3-4 minutes until pink and opaque.
4. Remove the skillet from heat and stir in the cilantro and lime juice.
5. Season with salt and pepper to taste.
6. Warm the tortillas in a dry skillet or microwave.
7. Divide the shrimp among the tortillas and top with avocado slices and red onion.
8. Serve immediately.

Usage Tips: These cilantro lime shrimp tacos are light and flavorful. Serve with a side of black beans and rice for a satisfying lunch.

71) BASIL PESTO PASTA SALAD

Ingredients:

- 8 ounces rotini pasta
- 1/2 cup basil pesto
- 1 cup cherry tomatoes, halved
- 1/2 cup mozzarella balls, halved
- 1/4 cup black olives, sliced
- 1/4 cup red onion, thinly sliced
- Salt and pepper to taste

Steps:

1. Cook the pasta according to package instructions. Drain and rinse with cold water to cool.
2. In a large bowl, combine the cooked pasta, basil pesto, cherry tomatoes, mozzarella balls, black olives, and red onion.
3. Toss to combine and season with salt and pepper to taste.
4. Refrigerate for at least 30 minutes before serving.

Usage Tips: This basil pesto pasta salad is a great make-ahead lunch. It's perfect for picnics or as a side dish for grilled meats.

72) DILL AND CUCUMBER YOGURT DIP

Ingredients:

- 1 cup Greek yogurt
- 1 cucumber, grated and excess water squeezed out
- 2 tablespoons fresh dill, chopped
- 1 clove garlic, minced
- 1 tablespoon fresh lemon juice
- Salt and pepper to taste

Steps:

1. In a medium bowl, combine the Greek yogurt, grated cucumber, dill, garlic, lemon juice, salt, and pepper.
2. Mix well until all ingredients are evenly incorporated.
3. Refrigerate for at least 30 minutes before serving.

Usage Tips: This dill and cucumber yogurt dip is refreshing and versatile. Serve it with fresh vegetables, pita bread, or as a topping for grilled meats.

73) SAGE AND SWEET POTATO SOUP

Ingredients:

- 2 large sweet potatoes, peeled and diced
- 1 onion, chopped
- 2 cloves garlic, minced
- 1 tablespoon fresh sage, chopped
- 4 cups vegetable broth
- 1/2 cup coconut milk
- Salt and pepper to taste
- 2 tablespoons olive oil

Steps:

1. In a large pot, heat the olive oil over medium heat.
2. Add the onion and garlic and cook for 5 minutes until soft.
3. Add the sweet potatoes and cook for another 5 minutes.
4. Pour in the vegetable broth and bring to a boil.
5. Reduce heat and simmer for 20 minutes until the sweet potatoes are tender.

6. Remove from heat and stir in the sage and coconut milk.
7. Use an immersion blender to puree the soup until smooth.
8. Season with salt and pepper to taste.

Usage Tips: This sage and sweet potato soup is creamy and comforting. Serve with crusty bread for a complete lunch.

74) PARSLEY AND LEMON CHICKPEA SALAD

Ingredients:

- 1 can chickpeas, drained and rinsed
- 1/4 cup fresh parsley, chopped
- 1/4 cup red onion, diced
- 1/4 cup cherry tomatoes, halved
- 1 tablespoon olive oil
- 1 tablespoon fresh lemon juice
- Salt and pepper to taste

Steps:

1. In a large bowl, combine the chickpeas, parsley, red onion, and cherry tomatoes.
2. In a small bowl, whisk together the olive oil, lemon juice, salt, and pepper.
3. Pour the dressing over the chickpea mixture and toss to combine.
4. Refrigerate for at least 30 minutes before serving.

76) THYME AND LEMON ROAST CHICKEN

Ingredients:

- 1 whole chicken
- 1/4 cup olive oil
- 4 cloves garlic, minced
- 2 tablespoons fresh thyme leaves
- 1 lemon, sliced
- Salt and pepper to taste

Steps:

1. Preheat the oven to 375°F (190°C).
2. In a small bowl, mix the olive oil, garlic, thyme, salt, and pepper.
3. Rub the mixture all over the chicken, including under the skin.

Usage Tips: This parsley and lemon chickpea salad is light and refreshing. Serve it on its own or as a side dish with grilled chicken or fish.

75) HERB-CRUSTED SALMON

Ingredients:

- 4 salmon fillets
- 1/4 cup fresh dill, chopped
- 1/4 cup fresh parsley, chopped
- 2 tablespoons fresh thyme leaves
- 2 cloves garlic, minced
- 2 tablespoons olive oil
- Salt and pepper to taste

Steps:

1. Preheat the oven to 400°F (200°C).
2. In a small bowl, combine the dill, parsley, thyme, garlic, olive oil, salt, and pepper.
3. Place the salmon fillets on a baking sheet lined with parchment paper.
4. Spread the herb mixture evenly over the top of each fillet.
5. Bake for 15-20 minutes until the salmon is cooked through and flakes easily with a fork.
6. Serve hot.

Usage Tips: This herb-crusted salmon is flavorful and healthy. Serve with a side of steamed vegetables or a fresh salad.

4. Place the lemon slices inside the chicken cavity and around the chicken in the roasting pan.
5. Roast the chicken for 1 hour and 30 minutes, or until the internal temperature reaches 165°F (75°C).
6. Let the chicken rest for 10 minutes before carving.

Usage Tips: This thyme and lemon roast chicken is flavorful and tender. Serve with roasted vegetables and potatoes for a complete dinner.

77)   ROSEMARY GARLIC LAMB CHOPS

Ingredients:

- 8 lamb chops
- 3 tablespoons olive oil
- 4 cloves garlic, minced
- 2 tablespoons fresh rosemary, chopped
- Salt and pepper to taste

Steps:

1. In a large bowl, combine the olive oil, garlic, rosemary, salt, and pepper.
2. Add the lamb chops and coat them well with the marinade.
3. Cover and refrigerate for at least 2 hours.
4. Preheat the grill to medium-high heat.
5. Grill the lamb chops for 4-5 minutes per side, or until desired doneness.
6. Let rest for a few minutes before serving.

Usage Tips: These rosemary garlic lamb chops are perfect for a special dinner. Serve with a side of mashed potatoes and green beans.

78)   BASIL PESTO PASTA WITH GRILLED SHRIMP

Ingredients:

- 8 ounces pasta
- 1 pound shrimp, peeled and deveined
- 1/4 cup basil pesto
- 1/4 cup grated Parmesan cheese
- 2 tablespoons olive oil
- Salt and pepper to taste

Steps:

1. Cook the pasta according to package instructions. Drain and set aside.
2. In a large bowl, toss the shrimp with olive oil, salt, and pepper.
3. Preheat a grill or grill pan to medium-high heat.
4. Grill the shrimp for 2-3 minutes per side, until pink and opaque.
5. In a large bowl, toss the cooked pasta with basil pesto and Parmesan cheese.
6. Top with grilled shrimp and serve immediately.

Usage Tips: This basil pesto pasta with grilled shrimp is fresh and delicious. Add a squeeze of lemon juice for extra flavor.

79)   OREGANO AND LEMON BAKED COD

Ingredients:

- 4 cod fillets
- 1/4 cup olive oil
- 2 cloves garlic, minced
- 2 tablespoons fresh oregano, chopped
- 1 lemon, sliced
- Salt and pepper to taste

Steps:

1. Preheat the oven to 375°F (190°C).
2. In a small bowl, mix the olive oil, garlic, oregano, salt, and pepper.
3. Place the cod fillets in a baking dish and brush with the olive oil mixture.
4. Top with lemon slices.
5. Bake for 20-25 minutes, or until the fish flakes easily with a fork.
6. Serve hot.

Usage Tips: This oregano and lemon baked cod is light and flavorful. Serve with a side of rice and steamed vegetables.

80)   MINT AND CILANTRO GRILLED LAMB KEBABS

Ingredients:

- 1 pound ground lamb
- 1/4 cup fresh mint, chopped
- 1/4 cup fresh cilantro, chopped
- 2 cloves garlic, minced
- 1 tablespoon ground cumin
- Salt and pepper to taste
- Skewers

Steps:

1. In a large bowl, combine the ground lamb, mint, cilantro, garlic, cumin, salt, and pepper.
2. Form the mixture into small patties and thread onto skewers.
3. Preheat a grill or grill pan to medium-high heat.

4. Grill the kebabs for 4-5 minutes per side, or until cooked through.
5. Serve hot.

Usage Tips: These mint and cilantro grilled lamb kebabs are full of flavor. Serve with a side of yogurt sauce and pita bread.

81) SAGE AND BROWN BUTTER GNOCCHI

Ingredients:

- 1 pound gnocchi
- 1/4 cup unsalted butter
- 2 tablespoons fresh sage, chopped
- 1/4 cup grated Parmesan cheese
- Salt and pepper to taste

Steps:

1. Cook the gnocchi according to package instructions. Drain and set aside.
2. In a large skillet, melt the butter over medium heat until it turns golden brown and smells nutty.
3. Add the sage and cook for 1 minute.
4. Add the cooked gnocchi to the skillet and toss to coat with the brown butter.
5. Season with salt and pepper.
6. Serve topped with grated Parmesan cheese.

Usage Tips: This sage and brown butter gnocchi is rich and delicious. Pair it with a simple green salad for a balanced dinner.

82) TARRAGON CHICKEN ALFREDO

Ingredients:

- 2 boneless, skinless chicken breasts
- 8 ounces fettuccine pasta
- 1 cup heavy cream
- 1/2 cup grated Parmesan cheese
- 2 tablespoons fresh tarragon, chopped
- 2 tablespoons butter
- Salt and pepper to taste

Steps:

1. Cook the pasta according to package instructions. Drain and set aside.

2. Season the chicken breasts with salt and pepper.
3. In a large skillet, melt the butter over medium heat.
4. Add the chicken breasts and cook for 6-7 minutes per side, or until cooked through.
5. Remove the chicken from the skillet and let rest for a few minutes before slicing.
6. In the same skillet, add the heavy cream and bring to a simmer.
7. Stir in the grated Parmesan cheese and tarragon.
8. Add the cooked pasta and sliced chicken to the skillet and toss to combine.
9. Serve hot.

Usage Tips: This tarragon chicken Alfredo is creamy and flavorful. Serve with garlic bread and a side of steamed vegetables.

83) DILL AND LEMON ROASTED SALMON

Ingredients:

- 4 salmon fillets
- 1/4 cup olive oil
- 2 tablespoons fresh dill, chopped
- 1 lemon, sliced
- Salt and pepper to taste

Steps:

1. Preheat the oven to 375°F (190°C).
2. In a small bowl, mix the olive oil, dill, salt, and pepper.
3. Place the salmon fillets in a baking dish and brush with the olive oil mixture.
4. Top with lemon slices.
5. Bake for 15-20 minutes, or until the salmon is cooked through and flakes easily with a fork.
6. Serve hot.

Usage Tips: This dill and lemon roasted salmon is light and healthy. Serve with quinoa and roasted asparagus.

84) BASIL AND TOMATO STUFFED PEPPERS

Ingredients:

- 4 large bell peppers, tops cut off and seeds removed
- 1 cup cooked quinoa
- 1 cup cherry tomatoes, halved
- 1/2 cup mozzarella cheese, shredded
- 1/4 cup fresh basil, chopped
- 2 cloves garlic, minced
- Salt and pepper to taste

Steps:

1. Preheat the oven to 375°F (190°C).
2. In a large bowl, combine the cooked quinoa, cherry tomatoes, mozzarella cheese, basil, garlic, salt, and pepper.
3. Stuff the bell peppers with the quinoa mixture and place them in a baking dish.
4. Bake for 30-35 minutes, or until the peppers are tender and the cheese is melted.
5. Serve hot.

Usage Tips: These basil and tomato stuffed peppers are colorful and nutritious. Serve with a side salad for a complete meal.

85) CILANTRO LIME CHICKEN SKEWERS

Ingredients:

- 1 pound chicken breast, cut into cubes
- 1/4 cup olive oil
- 1/4 cup fresh cilantro, chopped
- 2 tablespoons fresh lime juice
- 2 cloves garlic, minced
- Salt and pepper to taste
- Skewers

Steps:

1. In a large bowl, combine the olive oil, cilantro, lime juice, garlic, salt, and pepper.
2. Add the chicken cubes and toss to coat.
3. Cover and refrigerate for at least 30 minutes.
4. Preheat a grill or grill pan to medium-high heat.
5. Thread the chicken onto skewers.
6. Grill the skewers for 4-5 minutes per side, or until the chicken is cooked through.
7. Serve hot.

Usage Tips: These cilantro lime chicken skewers are zesty and flavorful. Serve with a side of rice and grilled vegetables

4.5 Herbal Snacks and Appetizers

86) ROSEMARY PARMESAN POPCORN

Ingredients:

- 1/4 cup popcorn kernels
- 2 tablespoons olive oil
- 1 tablespoon fresh rosemary, chopped
- 1/4 cup grated Parmesan cheese
- Salt to taste

Steps:

1. Heat the olive oil in a large pot over medium heat.
2. Add the popcorn kernels and cover the pot with a lid.
3. Cook, shaking the pot occasionally, until the popping slows down.

4. Remove from heat and transfer the popcorn to a large bowl.
5. Sprinkle with chopped rosemary, grated Parmesan cheese, and salt.
6. Toss to combine and serve.

Usage Tips: This rosemary Parmesan popcorn is a savory snack perfect for movie nights. Adjust the amount of rosemary and Parmesan to taste.

87) MINT AND FETA STUFFED MINI PEPPERS

Ingredients:

- 12 mini bell peppers
- 1 cup feta cheese, crumbled
- 2 tablespoons fresh mint, chopped
- 1 tablespoon olive oil

- Salt and pepper to taste

Steps:

1. Preheat the oven to 375°F (190°C).
2. Cut the tops off the mini bell peppers and remove the seeds.
3. In a bowl, mix the feta cheese, mint, olive oil, salt, and pepper.
4. Stuff the mini bell peppers with the feta mixture.
5. Place the stuffed peppers on a baking sheet and bake for 15 minutes.
6. Serve warm.

Usage Tips: These mint and feta stuffed mini peppers are a flavorful appetizer. Serve them as a starter at your next dinner party.

88) BASIL AND TOMATO BRUSCHETTA

Ingredients:

- 1 baguette, sliced
- 1 cup cherry tomatoes, diced
- 1/4 cup fresh basil, chopped
- 2 cloves garlic, minced
- 2 tablespoons olive oil
- Salt and pepper to taste

Steps:

1. Preheat the oven to 400°F (200°C).
2. Place the baguette slices on a baking sheet and drizzle with olive oil.
3. Toast in the oven for 8-10 minutes until golden brown.
4. In a bowl, combine the cherry tomatoes, basil, garlic, salt, and pepper.
5. Top each baguette slice with the tomato mixture.
6. Serve immediately.

Usage Tips: This basil and tomato bruschetta is a classic appetizer. For added flavor, rub the toasted baguette slices with a clove of garlic before topping with the tomato mixture.

89) DILL AND CUCUMBER CANAPÉS

Ingredients:

- 1 cucumber, sliced into rounds
- 1/2 cup cream cheese, softened
- 2 tablespoons fresh dill, chopped
- 1 tablespoon lemon juice
- Salt and pepper to taste

Steps:

1. In a bowl, mix the cream cheese, dill, lemon juice, salt, and pepper until well combined.
2. Spread a small amount of the cream cheese mixture onto each cucumber round.
3. Arrange on a serving platter and garnish with additional dill if desired.
4. Serve chilled.

Usage Tips: These dill and cucumber canapés are light and refreshing. They make a great snack or appetizer for summer gatherings.

90) THYME AND LEMON GOAT CHEESE CROSTINI

Ingredients:

- 1 baguette, sliced
- 1/2 cup goat cheese
- 1 tablespoon fresh thyme leaves
- 1 tablespoon lemon zest
- 2 tablespoons olive oil
- Salt and pepper to taste

Steps:

1. Preheat the oven to 400°F (200°C).
2. Place the baguette slices on a baking sheet and drizzle with olive oil.
3. Toast in the oven for 8-10 minutes until golden brown.
4. In a bowl, mix the goat cheese, thyme, lemon zest, salt, and pepper.
5. Spread the goat cheese mixture onto each baguette slice.
6. Serve immediately.

Usage Tips: These thyme and lemon goat cheese crostini are elegant and flavorful. Serve them as an appetizer at your next gathering.

91) BASIL AND MOZZARELLA STUFFED MUSHROOMS

Ingredients:

- 12 large mushrooms, stems removed
- 1/2 cup mozzarella cheese, shredded
- 1/4 cup fresh basil, chopped
- 2 cloves garlic, minced
- 2 tablespoons olive oil
- Salt and pepper to taste

Steps:

1. Preheat the oven to 375°F (190°C).
2. In a bowl, mix the mozzarella cheese, basil, garlic, salt, and pepper.
3. Stuff each mushroom with the cheese mixture.
4. Place the stuffed mushrooms on a baking sheet and drizzle with olive oil.
5. Bake for 15-20 minutes until the mushrooms are tender and the cheese is melted.
6. Serve warm.

Usage Tips: These basil and mozzarella stuffed mushrooms are a delicious appetizer. Serve them warm for the best flavor.

92) ROSEMARY AND SEA SALT CRACKERS

Ingredients:

- 1 cup all-purpose flour
- 1 tablespoon fresh rosemary, chopped
- 1/2 teaspoon sea salt
- 1/4 cup olive oil
- 1/4 cup water

Steps:

1. Preheat the oven to 400°F (200°C).
2. In a bowl, combine the flour, rosemary, and sea salt.
3. Add the olive oil and water, and mix until a dough forms.
4. Roll out the dough on a floured surface to about 1/8-inch thickness.
5. 5 Cut into desired shapes and place on a baking sheet.
6. Bake for 10-12 minutes until golden brown.
7. Let cool before serving.

Usage Tips: These rosemary and sea salt crackers are perfect for serving with cheese or dips. Store them in an airtight container to keep them fresh.

93) MINT AND PEA HUMMUS

Ingredients:

- 1 cup frozen peas, thawed
- 1 can chickpeas, drained and rinsed
- 2 tablespoons fresh mint, chopped
- 1/4 cup tahini
- 2 tablespoons olive oil
- 1 tablespoon lemon juice
- 2 cloves garlic, minced
- Salt and pepper to taste

Steps:

1. In a food processor, combine the peas, chickpeas, mint, tahini, olive oil, lemon juice, garlic, salt, and pepper.
2. Blend until smooth, adding a little water if needed to reach the desired consistency.
3. Transfer to a serving bowl and drizzle with additional olive oil if desired.
4. Serve with pita bread or fresh vegetables.

Usage Tips: This mint and pea hummus is a fresh take on a classic dip. Serve it as a healthy snack or appetizer.

94) SAGE AND CHEDDAR CHEESE STRAWS

Ingredients:

- 1 sheet puff pastry, thawed
- 1/2 cup grated cheddar cheese
- 1 tablespoon fresh sage, chopped
- 1 egg, beaten
- Salt and pepper to taste

Steps:

1. Preheat the oven to 400°F (200°C).
2. On a floured surface, roll out the puff pastry to a 1/8-inch thickness.
3. Brush with beaten egg and sprinkle with cheddar cheese, sage, salt, and pepper.
4. Cut into 1/2-inch wide strips and twist each strip several times.

5. Place on a baking sheet lined with parchment paper.
6. Bake for 12-15 minutes until golden brown.
7. Let cool before serving.

Usage Tips: These sage and cheddar cheese straws are perfect for snacking. Serve them as a party appetizer or with soup.

95)   LEMON THYME CHICKEN SKEWERS

Ingredients:

- 1 pound chicken breast, cut into cubes
- 2 tablespoons olive oil
- 1 tablespoon fresh thyme leaves
- 1 tablespoon lemon zest
- 1 tablespoon lemon juice
- Salt and pepper to taste
- Skewers

Steps:

1. In a bowl, combine the olive oil, thyme, lemon zest, lemon juice, salt, and pepper.
2. Add the chicken cubes and toss to coat.
3. Cover and refrigerate for at least 30 minutes.
4. Preheat a grill or grill pan to medium-high heat.
5. Thread the chicken onto skewers.
6. Grill the skewers for 4-5 minutes per side, or until the chicken is cooked through.
7. Serve hot.

Usage Tips: These lemon thyme chicken skewers are a light and flavorful appetizer. Serve with a side of tzatziki sauce for dipping.

4.6 Herbal Desserts and Sweet Treats

96)   LAVENDER HONEY ICE CREAM

Ingredients:

- 2 cups heavy cream
- 1 cup whole milk
- 3/4 cup honey
- 2 tablespoons dried lavender buds
- 5 large egg yolks
- 1 teaspoon vanilla extract

Steps:

1. In a saucepan, combine the heavy cream, whole milk, honey, and dried lavender buds.
2. Heat over medium heat until the mixture begins to simmer. Remove from heat and let steep for 30 minutes.
3. Strain the mixture to remove the lavender buds.
4. In a bowl, whisk the egg yolks.
5. Slowly add the warm cream mixture to the egg yolks, whisking constantly.
6. Return the mixture to the saucepan and cook over low heat, stirring constantly, until it thickens and coats the back of a spoon.
7. Remove from heat and stir in the vanilla extract.
8. Chill the mixture in the refrigerator for at least 4 hours or overnight.
9. Churn in an ice cream maker according to the manufacturer's instructions.
10.   Transfer to a container and freeze until firm.

Usage Tips: This lavender honey ice cream is fragrant and creamy. Serve it with a drizzle of honey or fresh lavender sprigs.

97)   MINT CHOCOLATE CHIP BROWNIES

Ingredients:

- 1 cup unsalted butter, melted
- 2 cups sugar
- 4 large eggs

- 1 teaspoon vanilla extract
- 1/2 cup fresh mint leaves, finely chopped
- 1 cup all-purpose flour
- 1 cup cocoa powder
- 1 teaspoon salt
- 1 cup chocolate chips

Steps:

1. Preheat the oven to 350°F (175°C).
2. In a large bowl, mix the melted butter and sugar until well combined.
3. Add the eggs, one at a time, mixing well after each addition.
4. Stir in the vanilla extract and chopped mint leaves.
5. In a separate bowl, whisk together the flour, cocoa powder, and salt.
6. Gradually add the dry ingredients to the wet ingredients, mixing until just combined.
7. Fold in the chocolate chips.
8. Pour the batter into a greased 9x13-inch baking pan.
9. Bake for 25-30 minutes, or until a toothpick inserted into the center comes out with a few moist crumbs.
10.   Cool completely before cutting into squares.

Usage Tips: These mint chocolate chip brownies are rich and fudgy with a hint of fresh mint. Serve them with a scoop of vanilla ice cream for an extra treat.

98) LEMON VERBENA POUND CAKE

Ingredients:

- 1 cup unsalted butter, softened
- 1 1/2 cups granulated sugar
- 4 large eggs
- 2 tablespoons fresh lemon verbena leaves, finely chopped
- 1 teaspoon lemon zest
- 1 teaspoon vanilla extract
- 2 cups all-purpose flour
- 1/2 teaspoon baking powder
- 1/4 teaspoon salt
- 1/2 cup whole milk

Steps:

1. Preheat the oven to 350°F (175°C).
2. In a large bowl, cream the butter and granulated sugar until light and fluffy.
3. Add the eggs, one at a time, mixing well after each addition.
4. Stir in the lemon verbena leaves, lemon zest, and vanilla extract.
5. In a separate bowl, whisk together the flour, baking powder, and salt.
6. Gradually add the dry ingredients to the wet ingredients, alternating with the milk, beginning and ending with the dry ingredients.
7. Pour the batter into a greased loaf pan.
8. Bake for 50-60 minutes, or until a toothpick inserted into the center comes out clean.
9. Cool in the pan for 10 minutes, then transfer to a wire rack to cool completely.

Usage Tips: This lemon verbena pound cake is moist and fragrant. Serve it with a dusting of powdered sugar or a glaze made from lemon juice and powdered sugar.

99) LAVENDER LEMON BARS

Ingredients:

- 1 cup all-purpose flour
- 1/2 cup powdered sugar
- 1/2 cup unsalted butter, softened
- 2 tablespoons dried lavender buds
- 1 cup granulated sugar
- 2 tablespoons all-purpose flour
- 1/2 teaspoon baking powder
- 3 large eggs
- 1/3 cup fresh lemon juice
- 1 tablespoon lemon zest

Steps:

1. Preheat the oven to 350°F (175°C).
2. In a bowl, mix 1 cup flour, powdered sugar, and butter until crumbly. Press into the bottom of a greased 9x9-inch baking pan.
3. Bake for 15-20 minutes, or until lightly golden.
4. In another bowl, combine granulated sugar, 2 tablespoons flour, baking powder, eggs, lemon juice, lemon zest,

and lavender buds. Mix until well blended.

5. Pour over the baked crust.
6. Bake for an additional 20-25 minutes, or until the filling is set.
7. Cool completely before cutting into bars.

Usage Tips: These lavender lemon bars are tangy and aromatic. Store them in the refrigerator to keep them fresh and serve chilled.

---

100) THYME AND HONEY PANNA COTTA

Ingredients:

- 2 cups heavy cream
- 1/2 cup whole milk
- 1/4 cup honey
- 2 teaspoons fresh thyme leaves
- 1 packet gelatin (2 1/2 teaspoons)
- 2 tablespoons cold water
- 1 teaspoon vanilla extract

Steps:

1. In a saucepan, combine the heavy cream, whole milk, honey, and thyme leaves. Heat over medium heat until it begins to simmer.
2. Remove from heat and let steep for 15 minutes.
3. Strain the mixture to remove the thyme leaves.
4. In a small bowl, sprinkle the gelatin over the cold water and let sit for 5 minutes.
5. Reheat the cream mixture until warm, then stir in the gelatin until fully dissolved.
6. Stir in the vanilla extract.
7. Pour the mixture into ramekins and refrigerate for at least 4 hours, or until set.

Usage Tips: This thyme and honey panna cotta is creamy and subtly herbal. Serve it with fresh berries or a drizzle of honey.

---

101) ROSE PETAL JAM THUMBPRINT COOKIES

Ingredients:

- 1 cup unsalted butter, softened
- 1/2 cup granulated sugar
- 1 large egg yolk
- 1 teaspoon vanilla extract
- 2 cups all-purpose flour
- 1/4 teaspoon salt
- 1/2 cup rose petal jam

Steps:

1. Preheat the oven to 350°F (175°C).
2. In a large bowl, cream the butter and granulated sugar until light and fluffy.
3. Add the egg yolk and vanilla extract, mixing well.
4. Gradually add the flour and salt, mixing until just combined.
5. Roll the dough into 1-inch balls and place on a baking sheet lined with parchment paper.
6. Press your thumb into the center of each ball to create an indentation.
7. Fill each indentation with a small amount of rose petal jam.
8. Bake for 12-15 minutes, or until the edges are lightly golden.
9. Cool on a wire rack before serving.

Usage Tips: These rose petal jam thumbprint cookies are delicate and floral. Serve them with tea for a perfect afternoon treat.

---

102) ROSEMARY LEMON SHORTBREAD COOKIES

Ingredients:

- 1 cup unsalted butter, softened
- 1/2 cup powdered sugar
- 2 cups all-purpose flour
- 1 tablespoon fresh rosemary, finely chopped
- 1 tablespoon lemon zest
- 1/2 teaspoon salt

Steps:

1. Preheat the oven to 350°F (175°C).
2. In a large bowl, cream the butter and powdered sugar until light and fluffy.

3. Add the flour, rosemary, lemon zest, and salt. Mix until combined.
4. Roll the dough into a log and wrap in plastic wrap. Chill in the refrigerator for at least 1 hour.
5. Slice the dough into 1/4-inch thick rounds and place on a baking sheet lined with parchment paper.
6. Bake for 12-15 minutes until the edges are lightly golden.
7. Cool on a wire rack before serving.

Usage Tips: These rosemary lemon shortbread cookies are perfect for tea time. Store them in an airtight container to keep them fresh.

103)   BASIL STRAWBERRY SORBET

Ingredients:

- 2 cups fresh strawberries, hulled
- 1/2 cup water
- 1/2 cup sugar
- 1/4 cup fresh basil leaves
- 1 tablespoon lemon juice

Steps:

1. In a small saucepan, combine the water and sugar. Heat over medium heat until the sugar dissolves. Remove from heat and let cool.
2. In a blender, combine the strawberries, basil leaves, lemon juice, and cooled sugar syrup. Blend until smooth.
3. Strain the mixture through a fine-mesh sieve to remove any seeds.
4. Chill the mixture in the refrigerator for at least 1 hour.
5. Churn in an ice cream maker according to the manufacturer's instructions.
6. Transfer to a container and freeze until firm.

Usage Tips: This basil strawberry sorbet is refreshing and light. Serve it as a palate cleanser or a light dessert on a hot day.

104)   CHAMOMILE AND HONEY POACHED PEARS

Ingredients:

- 4 ripe pears, peeled and cored
- 2 cups water
- 1 cup honey
- 1 cup chamomile tea (brewed from 2 chamomile tea bags)
- 1 cinnamon stick
- 1 teaspoon vanilla extract

Steps:

1. In a large saucepan, combine the water, honey, chamomile tea, cinnamon stick, and vanilla extract.
2. Bring to a simmer over medium heat.
3. Add the pears and reduce the heat to low.
4. Simmer the pears for 20-25 minutes, or until tender.
5. Remove the pears from the liquid and set aside.
6. Continue to simmer the liquid until it reduces by half and becomes syrupy.
7. Serve the pears drizzled with the chamomile-honey syrup.

Usage Tips: These chamomile and honey poached pears are a light and elegant dessert. Serve them warm or chilled, with a scoop of vanilla ice cream.

105) CARDAMOM AND ORANGE RICE PUDDING

Ingredients:

- 1 cup Arborio rice
- 4 cups whole milk
- 1/2 cup granulated sugar
- 1 teaspoon ground cardamom
- 1 tablespoon orange zest
- 1 teaspoon vanilla extract
- 1/4 cup raisins (optional)

Steps:

1. In a large saucepan, combine the rice, milk, sugar, cardamom, and orange zest.
2. Bring to a simmer over medium heat, stirring frequently.
3. Reduce the heat to low and cook, stirring occasionally, until the rice is tender and the mixture is creamy, about 25-30 minutes.
4. Stir in the vanilla extract and raisins (if using).
5. Remove from heat and let cool slightly before serving.

Usage Tips: This cardamom and orange rice pudding is creamy and aromatic. Serve it warm or chilled, with a sprinkle of ground cardamom or additional orange zest.

4.7 Herbal Beverages Beyond Tea

106) ROSEMARY LEMONADE

Ingredients:

- 1 cup fresh lemon juice
- 1/2 cup honey
- 4 cups water
- 2 sprigs fresh rosemary
- Ice cubes
- Lemon slices for garnish

Steps:

1. In a small saucepan, combine the honey and 1 cup of water. Heat over medium heat, stirring until the honey is dissolved. Remove from heat and add the rosemary sprigs. Let steep for 30 minutes.
2. Remove the rosemary sprigs and let the syrup cool to room temperature.
3. In a pitcher, combine the lemon juice, rosemary syrup, and the remaining 3 cups of water.
4. Stir well and refrigerate until chilled.
5. Serve over ice and garnish with lemon slices.

Usage Tips: This rosemary lemonade is refreshing and aromatic. Perfect for hot summer days or as a unique drink at gatherings.

107) LAVENDER BLUEBERRY SMOOTHIE

Ingredients:

- 1 cup fresh or frozen blueberries
- 1 banana
- 1/2 cup Greek yogurt
- 1/2 cup almond milk
- 1 teaspoon dried lavender buds
- 1 tablespoon honey

Steps:

1. In a blender, combine the blueberries, banana, Greek yogurt, almond milk, lavender buds, and honey.
2. Blend until smooth.
3. Pour into a glass and serve immediately.

Usage Tips: This lavender blueberry smoothie is a calming and nutritious start to your day. Adjust the sweetness with more or less honey as desired.

108) LEMON VERBENA POUND CAKE

Ingredients:

- 1 cup unsalted butter, softened
- 1 1/2 cups granulated sugar

- 4 large eggs
- 2 tablespoons fresh lemon verbena leaves, finely chopped
- 1 teaspoon lemon zest
- 1 teaspoon vanilla extract
- 2 cups all-purpose flour
- 1/2 teaspoon baking powder
- 1/4 teaspoon salt
- 1/2 cup whole milk

Steps:

1. Preheat the oven to 350°F (175°C).
2. In a large bowl, cream the butter and granulated sugar until light and fluffy.
3. Add the eggs, one at a time, mixing well after each addition.
4. Stir in the lemon verbena leaves, lemon zest, and vanilla extract.
5. In a separate bowl, whisk together the flour, baking powder, and salt.
6. Gradually add the dry ingredients to the wet ingredients, alternating with the milk, beginning and ending with the dry ingredients.
7. Pour the batter into a greased loaf pan.
8. Bake for 50-60 minutes, or until a toothpick inserted into the center comes out clean.
9. Cool in the pan for 10 minutes, then transfer to a wire rack to cool completely.

Usage Tips: This lemon verbena pound cake is moist and fragrant. Serve it with a dusting of powdered sugar or a glaze made from lemon juice and powdered sugar.

109) GINGER TURMERIC TONIC

Ingredients:

- 2 cups water
- 1 tablespoon fresh ginger, grated
- 1 tablespoon fresh turmeric, grated
- 1 tablespoon honey
- Juice of 1 lemon

Steps:

1. In a saucepan, bring the water to a boil.
2. Add the grated ginger and turmeric. Reduce heat and simmer for 10 minutes.

3. Remove from heat and strain the liquid into a mug.
4. Stir in the honey and lemon juice.
5. Serve warm or chilled.

Usage Tips: This ginger turmeric tonic is soothing and anti-inflammatory. Drink it warm in the morning for a health boost or chilled for a refreshing beverage.

110) BASIL LIME COOLER

Ingredients:

- 1/2 cup fresh lime juice
- 1/4 cup sugar
- 4 cups sparkling water
- 1/4 cup fresh basil leaves
- Ice cubes
- Lime slices for garnish

Steps:

1. In a small saucepan, combine the sugar and 1/2 cup of water. Heat over medium heat, stirring until the sugar is dissolved. Remove from heat and add the basil leaves. Let steep for 15 minutes.
2. Remove the basil leaves and let the syrup cool to room temperature.
3. In a pitcher, combine the lime juice, basil syrup, and sparkling water.
4. Stir well and refrigerate until chilled.
5. Serve over ice and garnish with lime slices.

Usage Tips: This basil lime cooler is light and zesty. It's a great non-alcoholic option for parties and gatherings.

111) THYME LEMON FIZZ

Ingredients:

- 1/2 cup fresh lemon juice
- 1/4 cup thyme syrup (see steps)
- 4 cups sparkling water
- Ice cubes
- Lemon slices and thyme sprigs for garnish

Steps:

1. To make the thyme syrup, combine 1/4 cup sugar, 1/4 cup water, and 2 sprigs of fresh thyme in a small saucepan. Heat

over medium heat until the sugar is dissolved. Remove from heat and let steep for 15 minutes. Strain to remove the thyme sprigs.

2. In a pitcher, combine the lemon juice, thyme syrup, and sparkling water.
3. Stir well and refrigerate until chilled.
4. Serve over ice and garnish with lemon slices and thyme sprigs.

Usage Tips: This thyme lemon fizz is refreshing and aromatic. Serve it at brunch or as a non-alcoholic option at parties.

112) CHAMOMILE ORANGE SPRITZER

Ingredients:

- 1 cup chamomile tea, brewed and cooled
- 1 cup fresh orange juice
- 1 cup sparkling water
- 1 tablespoon honey
- Ice cubes
- Orange slices for garnish

Steps:

1. In a pitcher, combine the chamomile tea, orange juice, and honey. Stir well until the honey is dissolved.
2. Add the sparkling water and stir gently.
3. Serve over ice and garnish with orange slices.

Usage Tips: This chamomile orange spritzer is calming and revitalizing. Enjoy it as a mid-afternoon refreshment.

113) MINT AND CUCUMBER INFUSED WATER

Ingredients:

- 1 cucumber, thinly sliced
- 1/4 cup fresh mint leaves
- 8 cups water
- Ice cubes

Steps:

1. In a large pitcher, combine the cucumber slices, mint leaves, and water.
2. Stir well and refrigerate for at least 2 hours to allow the flavors to infuse.

3. Serve over ice.

Usage Tips: This mint and cucumber infused water is refreshing and hydrating. Perfect for staying cool and hydrated throughout the day.

114) ROSE PETAL MILK

Ingredients:

- 2 cups whole milk
- 1/4 cup dried rose petals
- 1 tablespoon honey
- 1/2 teaspoon vanilla extract

Steps:

1. In a saucepan, heat the milk over medium heat until it begins to simmer.
2. Remove from heat and add the dried rose petals. Let steep for 15 minutes.
3. Strain the milk to remove the rose petals.
4. Stir in the honey and vanilla extract.
5. Serve warm.

Usage Tips: This rose petal milk is fragrant and soothing. Enjoy it as a relaxing bedtime drink.

115) BASIL PINEAPPLE SMOOTHIE

Ingredients:

- 1 cup fresh pineapple chunks
- 1/2 cup coconut milk
- 1/2 cup Greek yogurt
- 1/4 cup fresh basil leaves
- 1 tablespoon honey
- 1 cup ice cubes

Steps:

1. In a blender, combine the pineapple, coconut milk, Greek yogurt, basil leaves, honey, and ice cubes.
2. Blend until smooth.
3. Pour into a glass and serve immediately.

Usage Tips: This basil pineapple smoothie is tropical and refreshing. It's perfect for a healthy breakfast or a post-workout snack.

116)   MINT AND CUCUMBER INFUSED WATER

Ingredients:

- 1 cucumber, thinly sliced
- 1/4 cup fresh mint leaves
- 8 cups water
- Ice cubes

Steps:

1. In a large pitcher, combine the cucumber slices, mint leaves, and water.
2. Stir well and refrigerate for at least 2 hours to allow the flavors to infuse.
3. Serve over ice.

Usage Tips: This mint and cucumber infused water is refreshing and hydrating. Perfect for staying cool and hydrated throughout the day

117)   CILANTRO LIME AGUA FRESCA

Ingredients:

- 1 cup fresh lime juice
- 1/2 cup cilantro leaves
- 4 cups water
- 1/4 cup sugar
- Ice cubes
- Lime slices for garnish

Steps:

1. In a blender, combine the lime juice, cilantro leaves, water, and sugar. Blend until smooth.
2. Strain the mixture through a fine-mesh sieve to remove the solids.
3. Pour into a pitcher and refrigerate until chilled.
4. Serve over ice and garnish with lime slices.

Usage Tips: This cilantro lime agua fresca is refreshing and slightly tangy. Serve it as a cooling drink on a hot day.

The Power of Feedback
A Challenge for You!

Hey, you!

Yes, if you've made it this far, something must have resonated with you.

So, here's a challenge: grab your device and leave a review on Amazon.

It doesn't matter if it's long or short, if it changed your life or just made you think.

Every word counts, and your opinion could be the spark that ignites another reader's curiosity.

Do you accept the challenge?

Leaving feedback is simple, and I treasure each piece of insight. Just go to the ORDERS section of your Amazon account and click on the "Write a product review" button, or SCAN THIS QR CODE to go directly to the review section.

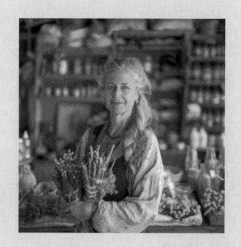

Thank you for accepting the challenge!

Serena Moss

BOOK 4: HERBAL BEAUTY AND PERSONAL CARE

Chapter 1: DIY Skincare, Haircare, and Body Care Products

1.1 Herbs for Radiant Skin.

1. BRIGHTENING BASIL AND CUCUMBER MASK

Ingredients:

- 1/2 cucumber, peeled and diced
- 1 tbsp fresh basil leaves, chopped
- 1 tbsp plain yogurt
- 1 tsp honey

Steps:

1 Put all ingredients in a blender.
2 Blend until the mixture is smooth.
3 Apply the mask to your face and leave it on for 15-20 minutes.
4 Rinse off with warm water.

Usage Tips: Use this mask once a week to brighten and refresh your skin.

2. ROSEWATER AND WITCH HAZEL TONER

Ingredients:

- 1/2 cup rosewater
- 1/2 cup witch hazel
- 4 drops lavender essential oil

Steps:

1 Mix rosewater and witch hazel in a spray bottle.
2 Add lavender essential oil and mix well.
3 Spritz onto your face after cleansing.

Usage Tips: Store the toner in the refrigerator for a refreshing and soothing effect.

3. GREEN TEA ANTIOXIDANT FACIAL STEAM

Ingredients:

- 1 tbsp dried green tea leaves
- 1 tbsp dried chamomile flowers
- 1 quart boiling water

Steps:

1 Combine green tea leaves and chamomile flowers in a large bowl.
2 Pour boiling water into the bowl.
3 Lean over the bowl with a towel draped over your head to trap the steam.
4 Steam your face for 12-14 min.

Usage Tips: Follow up with a moisturizer to lock in the benefits of the steam.

---

4. CALENDULA HEALING SALVE

Ingredients:

- 1/3 cup dried calendula flowers
- 1/2 cup olive oil
- 1/3 cup beeswax pellets

Steps:

1. Heat olive oil with calendula flowers on low for approximately 90 minutes to infuse.
2. Strain the infused oil and transfer it to a clean pot.
3. Add beeswax pellets and heat until they melt.
4. Pour the blend into small jars and allow it to cool and solidify.

Usage Tips: Apply the salve to cuts, scrapes, and dry skin for healing and soothing effects.

---

5. LAVENDER HONEY BRIGHTENING SCRUB

Ingredients:

- 1/3 cup sugar
- 1 tbsp honey
- 1 tbsp dried lavender flowers
- 2 tbsp coconut oil

Steps:

1. Mix all ingredients in a bowl until well combined.
2. Gently apply the scrub to your face using circular motions.
3. Rinse off with warm water.

Usage Tips: Use this scrub once or twice a week to exfoliate and brighten your skin.

---

6. HERBAL ANTI-AGING FACE SERUM

Ingredients:

- 1 tbsp rosehip oil
- 1 tbsp jojoba oil
- 4 drops frankincense essential oil
- 4 drops lavender essential oil

Steps:

1. Transfer all ingredients in a small bottle.
2. Mix well.
3. Apply a few drops to your face and neck after cleansing.

Usage Tips: Use this serum nightly to nourish and rejuvenate your skin.

---

7. CHAMOMILE SOOTHING MIST

Ingredients:

- 1/2 cup chamomile tea (cooled)
- 1/2 cup distilled water
- 1 tsp aloe vera gel

Steps:

1. Combine chamomile tea, distilled water, and aloe vera gel in a spray bottle.
2. Mix well.
3. Spritz onto your face as needed for soothing and hydration.

Usage Tips: Keep the mist in the refrigerator for an extra cooling effect.

---

8. NETTLE PURIFYING CLAY MASK

Ingredients:

- 1 tbsp bentonite clay
- 1 tbsp dried nettle leaf powder
- 2 tbsp water
- 1 tsp apple cider vinegar

Steps:

1. Combine bentonite clay and nettle leaf powder in a bowl.
2. Add water and apple cider vinegar and mix until a smooth paste forms.
3. Apply the mask to your face and let it sit for 12-14 min.
4. Rinse off with warm water.

Usage Tips: Use it once a week to purify and detoxify your skin.

---

9. SAFFRON GLOW ELIXIR

Ingredients:

- 1/3 cup almond oil

- 8 strands of saffron
- 4 drops rose essential oil

Steps:

1. Slightly heat the almond oil and add saffron strands.
2. Allow the saffron to infuse in the oil for 24 hours.
3. Mix in rose essential oil thoroughly.
4. Apply a few drops to your face and neck.

Usage Tips: Use this elixir daily to enhance your skin's natural glow.

10.   EVENING PRIMROSE SKIN REPAIR OIL

Ingredients:

- 2 tbsp evening primrose oil
- 2 tbsp jojoba oil
- 5 drops lavender essential oil

Steps:

1. Transfer all ingredients in a small bottle.
2. Mix well.
3. Apply a few drops to your face and neck before bed.

Usage Tips: Use this oil nightly to repair and nourish your skin while you sleep.

11. ALOE VERA RESILIENCE GEL

Ingredients:

- 1/3 cup fresh aloe vera gel
- 1 tsp vitamin E oil
- 5 drops tea tree essential oil

Steps:

1. Mix all ingredients in a bowl until well combined.
2. Transfer the mixture to a jar or bottle.
3. Apply a thin layer to your face and neck.

Usage Tips: Use this gel daily to soothe and protect your skin.

1.2 Natural Hair Care with Herbs and Oils #1

12. ROSEMARY AND MINT SCALP TREATMENT

Ingredients:

- 1/3 cup olive oil
- 1 tbsp dried rosemary
- 1 tbsp dried mint

Steps:

1. Warm the olive oil slightly and add dried rosemary and mint.
2. Let the herbs infuse in the oil for 1 hour.
3. Strain the oil and pour it into a bottle.
4. Massage a small amount into your scalp and leave it on for 30 minutes.
5. Rinse thoroughly.

Usage Tips: Use this treatment once a week to stimulate hair growth and refresh your scalp.

13. HERBAL HAIR RINSE FOR SHINE

Ingredients:

- 1/3 cup dried chamomile
- 1/3 cup dried rosemary
- 2 cups boiling water

Steps:

1. Put dried chamomile and rosemary in a bowl.
2. Pour boiling water into the bowl.
3. Let it steep for 30 minutes.
4. Strain the liquid and let it cool.
5. Use as a final rinse after shampooing.

Usage Tips: Rinse your hair with this mixture after washing to add shine and softness.

14. COCONUT AND HIBISCUS CURL ENHANCER

Ingredients:

- 1/3 cup coconut oil
- 2 tbsp hibiscus powder
- 1 tbsp aloe vera gel

Steps:

1. Melt the coconut oil and combine with hibiscus powder and aloe vera gel.
2. Mix well until smooth.
3. Apply to damp hair and style as usual.

Usage Tips: Use this enhancer to define curls and reduce frizz.

15. NOURISHING FENUGREEK SEED HAIR PACK

Ingredients:

- 2 tbsp fenugreek seeds
- 1/3 cup yogurt

Steps:

1. Soak fenugreek seeds in water overnight.
2. Blend soaked seeds into a paste.
3. Mix the fenugreek paste with yogurt.
4. Apply to your hair and scalp and leave for half an hour.
5. Rinse thoroughly.

Usage Tips: Use this hair pack weekly to nourish and strengthen your hair.

16. SAGE AND NETTLE HAIR GROWTH SERUM

Ingredients:

- 1/3 cup sage leaves
- 1/3 cup nettle leaves
- 1 cup water
- 1/3 cup castor oil

Steps:

1. Boil sage and nettle leaves in water for 8-9 min.
2. Strain the mixture and let it cool.
3. Mix the herbal water with castor oil.
4. Massage into your scalp and leave overnight.
5. Wash out in the morning.

Usage Tips: Apply this serum twice a week to promote hair growth.

17. LAVENDER AND JOJOBA HAIR OIL

Ingredients:

- 1/3 cup jojoba oil
- 12 drops lavender essential oil

Steps:

1. transfer jojoba oil and lavender essential oil in a bottle.
2. Mix well.
3. Apply a few drops to your hair and scalp.

Usage Tips: Use this hair oil daily to add moisture and shine.

18. CHAMOMILE LIGHTENING SPRAY

Ingredients:

- 1/2 cup chamomile tea (strongly brewed and cooled)
- 1/3 cup lemon juice
- 1 tbsp honey

Steps:

1. Combine chamomile tea, lemon juice, and honey in a spray bottle.
2. Mix well.
3. Spritz onto your hair and leave for 1-2 hours in the sun.
4. Rinse thoroughly.

Usage Tips: Use this spray regularly to naturally lighten your hair.

19. BURDOCK ROOT HAIR THICKENER

Ingredients:

- 1/3 cup dried burdock root
- 1 cup water
- 1/3 cup castor oil

Steps:

1. Boil dried burdock root in water for 8-9 min.
2. Strain the mixture and let it cool.

3 Mix the burdock root water with castor oil.
4 Massage into your scalp and leave overnight.
5 Wash out in the morning.

Usage Tips: Use this treatment twice a week to thicken your hair.

20. TEA TREE SCALP SOOTHER

Ingredients:

- 1/3 cup coconut oil
- 12 drops tea tree essential oil

Steps:

1 Melt the coconut oil and combine with tea tree essential oil.
2 Mix well and transfer to a bottle.
3 Massage a small amount into your scalp.

Usage Tips: Apply this soothing oil to relieve scalp irritation and dandruff.

21. HORSETAIL STRENGTHENING SPRAY

Ingredients:

- 1/3 cup dried horsetail
- 1 cup water
- 1 tbsp apple cider vinegar

Steps:

1 Simmer dried horsetail in water for 8-9 minutes.
2 Strain the liquid and allow it to cool.
3 Mix in apple cider vinegar thoroughly.
4 Transfer the mixture to a spray bottle and apply to your hair.

Usage Tips: Spray this mixture onto your hair after washing to strengthen and add shine.

22. HERBAL HAIR PROTECTION LOTION

Ingredients:

- 1/3 cup shea butter
- 1/3 cup coconut oil
- 1 tbsp dried rosemary
- 1 tbsp dried lavender

Steps:

1 Using a double boiler, melt the shea butter and coconut oil together.
2 Stir in the dried rosemary and lavender.
3 Allow the herbs to infuse for 30 minutes, then strain the mixture to remove the herbs.
4 Transfer the infused oil into a jar and let it cool.

Usage Tips: Apply this lotion to your hair before styling to protect it from heat and environmental damage.

1.3 Natural Hair Care with Herbs and Oils #2

23. ZINC AND HERB SUNSCREEN CREAM

Ingredients:

- 1/3 cup coconut oil
- 1/3 cup shea butter
- 1/3 cup beeswax pellets
- 2 tbsp zinc oxide
- 1 tbsp aloe vera gel
- 8 drops lavender essential oil

Steps:

1 Using a double boiler, melt coconut oil, shea butter, and beeswax pellets together.
2 Remove from heat and mix in zinc oxide, aloe vera gel, and lavender essential oil.
3 Transfer the blend into a jar and allow it to cool completely.

Usage Tips: Apply this sunscreen cream before sun exposure to protect your skin from UV rays.

24. PROTECTIVE HERBAL LIP BALM

Ingredients:

- 2 tbsp beeswax pellets
- 2 tbsp coconut oil
- 2 tbsp shea butter
- 4 drops peppermint essential oil

Steps:

1. Melt beeswax pellets, coconut oil, and shea butter together in a double boiler.
2. Once melted, remove from heat and stir in peppermint essential oil.
3. Pour the mixture into lip balm tubes and let them cool down.

Usage Tips: Apply this lip balm regularly to keep your lips hydrated and protected.

25. SKIN BARRIER BOOSTING BALM

Ingredients:

- 1/3 cup shea butter
- 1/3 cup coconut oil
- 1 tbsp beeswax pellets
- 4 drops lavender essential oil
- 4 drops tea tree essential oil

Steps:

1. In a double boiler, melt together shea butter, coconut oil, and beeswax pellets.
2. Once melted, remove from heat and mix in lavender and tea tree essential oils.
3. Transfer the blend into a jar and allow it to cool.

Usage Tips: Apply this balm to areas prone to dryness and irritation to boost your skin's natural barrier.

26. ELDERBERRY SKIN DEFENSE SERUM

Ingredients:

- 1/3 cup elderberry juice
- 1/3 cup aloe vera gel
- 1 tbsp vitamin E oil
- 5 drops tea tree essential oil

Steps:

1. Mix all ingredients in a small bottle.
2. Shake to mix.
3. Apply a few drops to your face and neck.

Usage Tips: Use this serum daily to protect your skin from environmental damage.

27. HERBAL ANTI-RASH CREAM

Ingredients:

- 1/3 cup calendula oil
- 1/3 cup coconut oil
- 1/3 cup shea butter
- 1 tbsp beeswax pellets
- 4 drops chamomile essential oil

Steps:

1. Melt calendula oil, coconut oil, shea butter, and beeswax pellets together in a double boiler.
2. Remove from heat and stir in chamomile essential oil.
3. Transfer the mixture into a jar and let it cool.

Usage Tips: Apply this cream to rashes and irritated skin to soothe and heal.

28. PROTECTIVE OATMEAL AND LAVENDER BATH SOAK

Ingredients:

- 1 cup oatmeal
- 1/3 cup dried lavender flowers
- 1/3 cup baking soda

Steps:

1. Combine oatmeal, dried lavender flowers, and baking soda in a bowl and blend.
2. Transfer to a jar or airtight container.
3. Add 1/2 cup of the mixture to a warm bath and soak for 20 minutes.

Usage Tips: Use this bath soak to soothe and protect your skin, especially during dry seasons.

29. MARSHMALLOW AND COCOA BUTTER HAND CREAM

Ingredients:

- 1/3 cup marshmallow root
- 1/3 cup cocoa butter
- 1/3 cup coconut oil
- 1 tbsp vitamin E oil

Steps:

1. Infuse marshmallow root in coconut oil by heating on low for 1 hour.
2. Strain the mixture and return to a clean pot.
3. Add cocoa butter and heat until melted.
4. Remove from heat and stir in vitamin E oil.
5. Transfer the mixture into a jar and let it cool.

Usage Tips: Use this hand cream daily to moisturize and soothe dry hands.

30. NATURAL BUG REPELLENT WITH ESSENTIAL OILS

Ingredients:

- 1/3 cup witch hazel
- 1/3 cup distilled water
- 8 drops citronella essential oil
- 8 drops eucalyptus essential oil
- 8 drops lavender essential oil

Steps:

1. Combine all ingredients in a spray bottle.
2. Mix well.
3. Spray onto skin and clothing before going outside.

Usage Tips: Reapply as needed to keep bugs away naturally.

31. THYME AND CLOVER LEAF ANTI-POLLUTION SPRAY

Ingredients:

- 1 cup distilled water
- 1/3 cup witch hazel
- 1 tbsp dried thyme
- 1 tbsp dried clover leaves

Steps:

1. Combine dried thyme and clover leaves in a bowl.
2. Pour boiling water into the bowl and let steep for 30 minutes.
3. Strain the mixture and let it cool.
4. Add witch hazel and mix well.
5. Transfer to a spray bottle.

Usage Tips: Spray this mixture onto your face before going out to protect your skin from pollution.

32. ANTIOXIDANT BERRY AND HERB LOTION

Ingredients:

- 1/3 cup almond oil
- 1/3 cup shea butter
- 1/3 cup beeswax pellets
- 1/3 cup mixed berries (strawberries, blueberries, raspberries)
- 2 tbsp dried rosemary

Steps:

1. In a double boiler, melt together almond oil, shea butter, and beeswax pellets.
2. Puree the mixed berries and dried rosemary in a blender.
3. Combine the melted oils with the berry puree and mix until well blended.
4. Pour the lotion into a jar and let it set and cool.

Usage Tips: Use this antioxidant-rich lotion daily to nourish and protect your skin.

33. GOLDENROD AND MYRRH HEALING SLVE

Ingredients:

- 1/3 cup dried goldenrod
- 1/3 cup olive oil
- 1/3 cup beeswax pellets
- 4 drops myrrh essential oil

Steps:

1. Gently heat dried goldenrod in olive oil on low for one hour.
2. Strain the infusion and pour it back into a clean pot.
3. Add beeswax pellets and heat until fully melted.

4 Remove from heat and stir in myrrh essential oil.
5 Pour the mixture into a jar and let it set and cool.

Usage Tips: Use this salve to heal cuts, scrapes, and minor skin irritations.

1.4 Herbs for Hair Health

34. GINGER ROOT HAIR REVITALIZER

Ingredients:

- 1/3 cup fresh ginger root, grated
- 1/3 cup coconut oil
- 1 tbsp honey

Steps:

1 Combine grated ginger root, coconut oil, and honey in a small pot.
2 Heat gently for 8-9 min.
3 Strain the mixture and pour into a bottle.
4 Massage a small amount into your scalp and leave for 30 minutes.
5 Rinse thoroughly.

Usage Tips: Use this revitalizer once a week to stimulate hair growth and add shine.

35. PEPPERMINT AND EUCALYPTUS SCALP AWAKENING

Ingredients:

- 1/3 cup olive oil
- 12 drops peppermint essential oil
- 12 drops eucalyptus essential oil

Steps:

1 Mix olive oil, peppermint essential oil, and eucalyptus essential oil in a bottle.
2 Mix well.
3 Massage a small amount into your scalp.

Usage Tips: Apply this oil blend to awaken and invigorate your scalp.

36. LEMONGRASS HAIR DEODORIZER

Ingredients:

- 1 cup distilled water
- 1/3 cup witch hazel
- 12 drops lemongrass essential oil

Steps:

1 Combine distilled water, witch hazel, and lemongrass essential oil in a spray bottle.
2 Mix well.
3 Spritz onto your hair as needed.

Usage Tips: Use this deodorizer to freshen your hair between washes.

37. FLAXSEED AND ROSEMARY HAIR GEL

Ingredients:

- 1/3 cup flaxseeds
- 2 cups water
- 1 tbsp dried rosemary

Steps:

1 Mix flaxseeds and water in a saucepan.
2 Bring to a boil, then simmer for 8-9 minutes.
3 Strain the mixture and allow it to cool.
4 Stir in dried rosemary thoroughly.
5 Pour into a jar.

Usage Tips: Use this gel to style your hair naturally.

38. PUMPKIN SEED HAIR STRENGTHENING MASK

Ingredients:

- 1/3 cup pumpkin seed oil
- 1/3 cup coconut oil

- 1 tbsp honey

Steps:

1. Melt coconut oil and combine with pumpkin seed oil and honey.
2. Mix well until smooth.
3. Apply to damp hair and leave for 30 minutes.
4. Rinse thoroughly.

Usage Tips: Use this mask once a week to strengthen and nourish your hair.

39. LICORICE ROOT SCALP TREATMENT

Ingredients:

- 1/3 cup dried licorice root
- 1 cup water
- 1 tbsp olive oil

Steps:

1. Boil dried licorice root in water for 8-9 minutes.
2. Strain and let the mixture cool.
3. Combine the herbal infusion with olive oil.Massage into your scalp and leave it on for 30 minutes.
4. Rinse thoroughly.

Usage Tips: Apply this treatment once a week to soothe and condition your scalp.

40. CILANTRO HAIR DETOXIFIER

Ingredients:

- 1/3 cup fresh cilantro, chopped
- 1 cup water
- 1 tbsp apple cider vinegar

Steps:

1. Put fresh cilantro and water in a blender.
2. Mix until the mixture is smooth.
3. Strain and add apple cider vinegar.
4. Mix well and pour into a spray bottle.

Usage Tips: Spray this detox solution onto your hair and scalp, leave it on for 15 minutes, then rinse thoroughly.

41. YARROW ANTI-BREAKAGE FORMULA

Ingredients:

- 1/3 cup dried yarrow
- 1 cup water
- 2 tbsp coconut oil

Steps:

1. Simmer dried yarrow in water for 8-9 minutes.
2. Strain the mixture and allow it to cool.
3. Mix the cooled herbal infusion with coconut oil.
4. Apply to your hair and leave it on for 30 minutes.
5. Rinse thoroughly.

Usage Tips: Use this formula once a week to strengthen your hair and prevent breakage.

42. PARSLEY SCALP RENEWAL TONIC

Ingredients:

- 1/3 cup fresh parsley, chopped
- 1 cup water
- 1 tbsp apple cider vinegar

Steps:

1. Combine fresh parsley and water in a blender.
2. Blend until smooth.
3. Strain the mixture and add apple cider vinegar.
4. Mix well and transfer to a spray bottle.

Usage Tips: Spritz this tonic onto your scalp, let it sit for 15 minutes, and then rinse thoroughly.

43. HERBAL CONDITIONING HAIR WRAP

Ingredients:

- 1/3 cup dried chamomile
- 1/3 cup dried lavender
- 1 cup water
- 2 tbsp olive oil

Steps:

1. Simmer dried chamomile and lavender in water for 8-9 minutes.
2. Strain and let the herbal infusion cool.

3 Combine the cooled herbal water with olive oil.
4 Apply to your hair and cover with a shower cap.
5 Leave it on for 30 minutes, then rinse thoroughly.

Usage Tips: Use this conditioning wrap once a week to add moisture and shine to your hair.

---

44. HERBAL DANDRUFF CONTROL SHAMPOO

Ingredients:

- 1/3 cup liquid castile soap
- 1/3 cup distilled water
- 1 tbsp dried rosemary
- 1 tbsp dried thyme
- 12 drops tea tree essential oil

Steps:

1 Mix liquid castile soap and distilled water in a bottle.
2 Add dried rosemary and thyme to the bottle.
3 Allow the mixture to infuse for 24 hours.
4 Strain the liquid and add tea tree essential oil.
5 Shake well before each use.

Usage Tips: Use this shampoo regularly to control dandruff and soothe your scalp.

1.5 Preparing the Home with Natural Scents

---

45. RELAXING LAVENDER ROOM SPRAY

Ingredients:

- 1 cup distilled water
- 1/3 cup witch hazel
- 12 drops lavender essential oil

Steps:

1 Combine distilled water, witch hazel, and lavender essential oil in a spray bottle.
2 Stir well to mix.
3 Spray around your home to create a relaxing atmosphere.

Usage Tips: Use this spray in the evening to promote a calm and peaceful environment.

---

46. CITRUS AND MINT MOOD ENHANCER

Ingredients:

- 1 cup distilled water
- 1/3 cup witch hazel
- 12 drops orange essential oil
- 12 drops peppermint essential oil

Steps:

1 Combine distilled water, witch hazel, orange essential oil, and peppermint essential oil in a spray bottle.
2 Shake well to blend.
3 Spray around your home to elevate your mood.

Usage Tips: Use this spray in the morning to invigorate and uplift your spirits.

---

47. JASMINE AND VANILLA HOME PERFUME

Ingredients:

- 1 cup distilled water
- 1/3 cup witch hazel
- 8 drops jasmine essential oil
- 8 drops vanilla essential oil

Steps:

1 Mix distilled water, witch hazel, jasmine essential oil, and vanilla essential oil in a spray bottle.
2 Shake thoroughly to combine.
3 Spray around your home for a luxurious fragrance.

Usage Tips: Use this home perfume in living areas and bedrooms for a soothing and romantic scent.

48. PINE AND CEDARWOOD WINTER AIR FRESHENER

Ingredients:

- 1 cup distilled water
- 1/3 cup witch hazel
- 12 drops pine essential oil
- 12 drops cedarwood essential oil

Steps:

1 Transfer distilled water, witch hazel, pine essential oil, and cedarwood essential oil in a spray bottle.
2 Mix well.
3 Spray around your home to create a cozy winter atmosphere.

Usage Tips: Use this air freshener during the winter months to bring a fresh, woodsy scent indoors.

49. SWEET ORANGE AND CLOVE SIMMER POT

Ingredients:

- 1 orange, sliced
- 1 tbsp whole cloves
- 2 cinnamon sticks
- 4 cups water

Steps:

1 Transfer all ingredients in a pot.
2 Bring to a simmer on the stove.
3 Let simmer, adding water as needed.

Usage Tips: Simmer this mixture on the stove to fill your home with a warm, inviting aroma.

50. HERBAL POTPOURRI MIX

Ingredients:

- 1 cup dried rose petals
- 1 cup dried lavender flowers
- 1 cup dried orange peel
- 1 tbsp ground cinnamon
- 12 drops rose essential oil

Steps:

1 Transfer all dried ingredients in a bowl and mix.

2 Add rose essential oil and stir to combine.
3 Place the potpourri in a decorative bowl or sachet.

Usage Tips: Use the potpourri in various rooms to naturally scent your home.

51. SANDALWOOD AND BERGAMOT OIL DIFFUSER BLEND

Ingredients:

- 12 drops sandalwood essential oil
- 12 drops bergamot essential oil
- 1/3 cup distilled water

Steps:

1 Combine all ingredients in an oil diffuser.
2 Mix well and start the diffuser.

Usage Tips: Use this blend in an oil diffuser to create a calming and uplifting environment.

52. DIY HERBAL INCENSE CONES

Ingredients:

- 1/3 cup dried lavender flowers
- 1/3 cup dried rosemary
- 1/3 cup dried sage
- 1/3 cup water
- 2 tbsp gum arabic

Steps:

1 Grind dried lavender flowers, rosemary, and sage into a fine powder.
2 Mix the herb powder with water and gum arabic to form a thick paste.
3 Shape the paste into small cones and let them dry completely.

Usage Tips: Light these incense cones to create a calming and fragrant atmosphere in your home.

53. SOOTHING HERBAL WAX MELTS

Ingredients:

- 1/2 cup soy wax
- 1/34 cup dried lavender flowers
- 12 drops lavender essential oil

Steps:

1 Melt the soy wax in a double boiler.
2 Stir in dried lavender flowers and lavender essential oil.
3 Transfer the mixture into silicone molds and let it cool completely.

Usage Tips: Place the wax melts in a warmer to release a soothing lavender scent in your home.

---

54.   EUCALYPTUS SHOWER BOMBS

Ingredients:

- 1 cup baking soda
- 1/3 cup citric acid
- 12 drops eucalyptus essential oil
- Water (as needed)

Steps:

1 Combine baking soda and citric acid in a bowl.
2 Add eucalyptus essential oil and shale.
3 Spritz with water and mix until the mixture holds its shape.
4 Press the mixture into molds and let them dry completely.

Usage Tips: Place a shower bomb on the floor of your shower to release a refreshing eucalyptus scent.

---

55.   PEPPERMINT AND SAGE HOME DISINFECTANT SPRAY

Ingredients:

- 1 cup distilled water
- 1/3 cup witch hazel
- 12 drops peppermint essential oil
- 8 drops sage essential oil

Steps:

1 Combine distilled water, witch hazel, peppermint essential oil, and sage essential oil in a spray bottle.
2 Mix well.
3 Spray onto surfaces and wipe clean.

Usage Tips: Use this disinfectant spray to naturally clean and freshen your home.

Chapter 2: Body Care and Aromatherapy

2.1 Herbal Infusions for Vitality

56. ENERGIZING GINSENG AND GINKGO TEA

Ingredients:

- 1 tsp dried ginseng root
- 1 tsp dried ginkgo leaves
- 1 cup boiling water
- Honey to taste

Steps:

1 Add ginseng root and ginkgo leaves to a teapot.
2 Pour hot water into the teapot.
3 Steep for 8-9 minutes.
4 Strain the tea into a cup.
5 Sweeten with honey to taste.

Usage Tips: Enjoy this tea in the morning to boost energy and improve mental clarity.

57. VITALITY BOOSTING ROOIBOS TONIC

Ingredients:

- 1 tsp rooibos tea
- 1/2 tsp dried ginger root
- 1 cup boiling water
- Lemon slice for garnish

Steps:

1 Put rooibos tea and dried ginger root in your teapot.
2 Pour hot water into the teapot.
3 Steep for 8-9 minutes.
4 Strain the infusion into a cup.
5 Garnish with a lemon slice.

Usage Tips: Enjoy this tonic in the afternoon to sustain energy levels throughout the day.

58. GREEN TEA AND HIBISCUS REFRESHER

Ingredients:

- 1 tsp green tea leaves
- 1 tsp dried hibiscus flowers
- 1 cup boiling water
- Honey to taste

Steps:

1 Add green tea leaves and dried hibiscus flowers to a teapot.
2 Pour hot water into the teapot.
3 Steep for 5-7 minutes.
4 Strain the tea into a cup.
5 Add honey to taste.

Usage Tips: This refreshing tea is perfect for a mid-morning pick-me-up.

59. INVIGORATING PEPPERMINT AND LICORICE BREW

Ingredients:

- 1 tsp dried peppermint leaves
- 1/2 tsp dried licorice root
- 1 cup boiling water
- Honey to taste

Steps:

1 Place dried peppermint leaves and licorice root in your teapot.
2 Pour hot water into the teapot.
3 Steep for 8-9 minutes.
4 Strain the liquid into a cup.
5 Add honey to taste.

Usage Tips: Enjoy this brew in the afternoon to invigorate and soothe digestion.

60. DETOXIFYING DANDELION AND BURDOCK DRINK

Ingredients:

- 1 tsp dried dandelion root
- 1 tsp dried burdock root
- 1 cup boiling water
- Lemon slice for garnish

Steps:

1. Combine dandelion root and burdock root in your teapot.
2. Pour hot water into the teapot.
3. Steep for 8-9 minutes.
4. Strain the tea into a cup.
5. Garnish with a lemon slice.

Usage Tips: Drink this detoxifying blend daily to support liver and kidney health.

61. MORNING KICKSTART TURMERIC AND LEMON INFUSION

Ingredients:

- 1/2 tsp turmeric powder
- 1 cup boiling water
- Juice of 1 lemon
- Honey to taste

Steps:

1. Place turmeric powder in a cup.
2. Put boiling water over the turmeric.
3. Stir in lemon juice and honey.
4. Mix well and serve.

Usage Tips: Start your day with this infusion to boost metabolism and reduce inflammation.

62. CARDAMOM AND BLACK PEPPER WARMER

Ingredients:

- 1 tsp crushed cardamom pods
- 1/4 tsp black peppercorns
- 1 cup boiling water
- Honey to taste

Steps:

1. Add crushed cardamom pods and black peppercorns to a teapot.
2. Pour hot water over the spices.

3. Steep for 8-9 minutes.
4. Strain the liquid into a cup.
5. Add honey to taste.

Usage Tips: Enjoy this warm, spicy drink in the evening to improve digestion and circulation.

63. HERBAL MATE ENERGY ELIXIR

Ingredients:

- 1 tsp yerba mate
- 1/2 tsp dried peppermint leaves
- 1 cup boiling water
- Honey to taste

Steps:

1. Place yerba mate and dried peppermint leaves in your teapot.
2. Pour hot water into the teapot.
3. Let it steep for 8-9 minutes.
4. Strain the tea into a cup.
5. Add honey to taste.

Usage Tips: Drink this elixir in the morning for a natural energy boost and enhanced focus.

64. SCHISANDRA BERRY VITALITY SHOT

Ingredients:

- 1 tsp dried schisandra berries
- 1 cup boiling water
- Honey to taste

Steps:

1. Add dried schisandra berries to a teapot.
2. Pour hot water over the berries.
3. Let it steep for 8-9 minutes.
4. Strain the liquid into a cup.
5. Sweeten with honey if desired.

Usage Tips: Enjoy this vitality boost daily to support energy levels and adaptogenic health.

65. ADAPTOGENIC ASHWAGANDHA AND HOLY BASIL TEA

Ingredients:

- 1 tsp dried ashwagandha root
- 1 tsp dried holy basil leaves

- 1 cup boiling water
- Honey to taste

Steps:

1 Combine ashwagandha root and holy basil leaves in your teapot.
2 Pour hot water into the teapot.
3 Steep for 8-9 minutes.
4 Strain the tea into a cup.
5 Add honey to taste.

Usage Tips: Drink this adaptogenic tea in the evening to reduce stress and promote relaxation.

66. REFRESHING CITRUS AND MINT ICED INFUSION

Ingredients:

- 1 tsp dried mint leaves
- 1 cup boiling water
- Juice of 1 orange
- Ice

Steps:

1 Place dried mint leaves in your teapot.
2 Pour hot water over the mint.
3 Steep for 8-9 minutes, then strain.
4 Stir in orange juice and pour over ice.

Usage Tips: This refreshing iced infusion is perfect for a hot summer day to stay cool and hydrated.

2.2 Natural Baths for Relaxation and Wellness

67. SOOTHING LAVENDER AND EPSOM SALT BATH

Ingredients:

- 1 cup Epsom salts
- 1/2 cup baking soda
- 12 drops lavender essential oil

Steps:

1 In a bowl, combine Epsom salts, baking soda, and lavender essential oil.
2 Mix thoroughly and transfer to a jar.
3 Add 1/2 cup of the blend to warm bathwater.

Usage Tips: Soak in this bath for 20 minutes to soothe sore muscles and promote relaxation.

68. DETOXIFYING SEAWEED SOAK

Ingredients:

- 1 cup dried seaweed
- 1 cup Epsom salts
- 1/2 cup baking soda

Steps:

1 In a bowl, mix dried seaweed, Epsom salts, and baking soda.
2 Stir well and transfer to a jar.
3 Add 1/2 cup of the mixture to warm bathwater.

Usage Tips: Use this soak to detoxify the body and replenish minerals.

69. MOISTURIZING OATMEAL AND HONEY BATH

Ingredients:

- 1 cup finely ground oatmeal
- 1/2 cup honey
- 1/3 cup coconut oil

Steps:

1 Combine finely ground oatmeal, honey, and coconut oil in a bowl.
2 Stir until well mixed and transfer to a jar.
3 Add 1/2 cup of the mixture to warm bathwater.

Usage Tips: Soak in this bath to moisturize and soothe dry, irritated skin.

70. RELAXING CHAMOMILE AND MILK BATH

Ingredients:

- 1/2 cup dried chamomile flowers
- 1 cup powdered milk
- 1/3 cup baking soda

Steps:

1 Mix dried chamomile flowers, powdered milk, and baking soda in a bowl.
2 Stir well and transfer to a jar.
3 Add 1/2 cup of the blend to warm bathwater.

Usage Tips: This bath is perfect for relaxing and softening the skin before bedtime.

71. ENERGIZING CITRUS AND ROSEMARY BATH SALTS

Ingredients:

- 1 cup Epsom salts
- 1/3 cup sea salt
- 12 drops rosemary essential oil
- 12 drops orange essential oil

Steps:

1 Combine Epsom salts, sea salt, rosemary essential oil, and orange essential oil in a bowl.
2 Mix thoroughly and transfer to a jar.
3 Add 1/2 cup of the mixture to warm bathwater.

Usage Tips: Use this bath to energize and invigorate your body and mind.

72. CALMING JASMINE AND COCONUT MILK BATH

Ingredients:

- 1/2 cup dried jasmine flowers
- 1 cup powdered coconut milk
- 1/3 cup baking soda

Steps:

1 Mix dried jasmine flowers, powdered coconut milk, and baking soda in a bowl.
2 Stir well and transfer to a jar.
3 Add 1/2 cup of the blend to warm bathwater.

Usage Tips: Soak in this luxurious bath to calm your senses and hydrate your skin.

73. REJUVENATING GREEN TEA BATH

Ingredients:

- 1/2 cup dried green tea leaves
- 1 cup Epsom salts
- 1/3 cup baking soda

Steps:

1 Combine dried green tea leaves, Epsom salts, and baking soda in a bowl.
2 Mix well and transfer to a jar.
3 Add 1/2 cup of the mixture to warm bathwater.

Usage Tips: This bath rejuvenates your skin and provides powerful antioxidants.

74. SOOTHING MUSCLE RELIEF BATH WITH EUCALYPTUS

Ingredients:

- 1 cup Epsom salts
- 1/2 cup sea salt
- 12 drops eucalyptus essential oil

Steps:

1 Combine Epsom salts, sea salt, and eucalyptus essential oil in a bowl.
2 Stir and transfer to a jar.
3 Add 1/2 cup of the mixture to warm bathwater.

Usage Tips: Use this bath to soothe sore muscles and relieve tension after a long day.

75. SLEEP PROMOTING VALERIAN AND HOPS BATH

Ingredients:

- 1/3 cup dried valerian root
- 1/3 cup dried hops
- 1 cup Epsom salts
- 1/3 cup baking soda

Steps:

1 Combine dried valerian root, dried hops, Epsom salts, and baking soda in a bowl.

2 Mix well and transfer to a jar.
3 Add 1/2 cup of the mixture to warm bathwater.

Usage Tips: This bath promotes restful sleep and helps you unwind before bed.

76. INVIGORATING GINGER AND EUCALYPTUS STEAM BATH

Ingredients:

- 1/2 cup dried ginger root
- 12 drops eucalyptus essential oil
- 1 cup Epsom salts
- 1/3 cup baking soda

Steps:

1 Combine dried ginger root, eucalyptus essential oil, Epsom salts, and baking soda in a bowl.
2 Mix well and transfer to a jar.
3 Add 1/2 cup of the mixture to warm bathwater.

Usage Tips: Use this bath to invigorate your senses and open your airways.

77. BALANCING ROSE PETAL AND SALT BATH

Ingredients:

- 1/3 cup dried rose petals
- 1 cup Epsom salts
- 1/3 cup sea salt
- 1/3 cup baking soda

Steps:

1 Combine dried rose petals, Epsom salts, sea salt, and baking soda in a bowl.
2 Stir and transfer to a jar.
3 Add 1/2 cup of the mixture to warm bathwater.

Usage Tips: This bath helps balance your mood and provides a calming, aromatic experience.

2.3 Massages with Essential Oils

78. STRESS RELIEF LAVENDER MASSAGE OIL

Ingredients:

- 1/3 cup sweet almond oil
- 12 drops lavender essential oil

Steps:

1 Mix sweet almond oil and lavender essential oil in a small bottle.
2 Mix well.
3 Apply a small amount to the skin and massage gently.

Usage Tips: Use this massage oil to relieve stress and promote relaxation.

79. REVITALIZING ORANGE AND PEPPERMINT MASSAGE BLEND

Ingredients:

- 1/3 cup coconut oil
- 5 drops orange essential oil
- 5 drops peppermint essential oil

Steps:

1 Mix coconut oil, orange essential oil, and peppermint essential oil in a small bottle.
2 Stir to mix.
3 Apply a small amount to the skin and massage gently.

Usage Tips: This blend is perfect for a refreshing and revitalizing massage.

80. RELAXING CHAMOMILE AND ALMOND OIL MIX

Ingredients:

- 1/3 cup sweet almond oil
- 12 drops chamomile essential oil

Steps:

1 Combine sweet almond oil and chamomile essential oil in a small bottle.
2 Stir to mix.
3 Apply a small amount to the skin and massage gently.

Usage Tips: Use this mix to relax muscles and soothe the skin.

81. DEEP TISSUE EUCALYPTUS AND WINTERGREEN OIL

Ingredients:

- 1/3 cup jojoba oil
- 5 drops eucalyptus essential oil
- 5 drops wintergreen essential oil

Steps:

1 Mix jojoba oil, eucalyptus essential oil, and wintergreen essential oil in a small bottle.
2 Stir to mix.
3 Apply a small amount to the skin and massage deeply.

Usage Tips: Use this oil for deep tissue massage to relieve muscle tension and pain.

82. ENERGIZING GINGER AND BLACK PEPPER BODY RUB

Ingredients:

- 1/3 cup coconut oil
- 5 drops ginger essential oil
- 5 drops black pepper essential oil

Steps:

1 Mix coconut oil, ginger essential oil, and black pepper essential oil in a small bottle.

2 Stir to mix.
3 Apply a small amount to the skin and massage vigorously.

Usage Tips: This body rub is ideal for energizing the body and warming up muscles.

83. DETOX MASSAGE OIL WITH GRAPEFRUIT AND JUNIPER

Ingredients:

- 1/3 cup jojoba oil
- 5 drops grapefruit essential oil
- 5 drops juniper essential oil

Steps:

1 Mix jojoba oil, grapefruit essential oil, and juniper essential oil in a small bottle.
2 Stir to mix.
3 Apply a small amount to the skin and massage in circular motions.

Usage Tips: Use this detox massage oil to promote lymphatic drainage and detoxification.

84. MUSCLE SOOTHING ARNICA AND ROSEMARY OIL

Ingredients:

- 1/3 cup sweet almond oil
- 12 drops arnica oil
- 6 drops rosemary essential oil

Steps:

1 Mix sweet almond oil, arnica oil, and rosemary essential oil in a small bottle.
2 Stir to mix.
3 Apply a small amount to the skin and massage gently.

Usage Tips: This oil is perfect for soothing sore muscles and reducing inflammation.

85. CALMING YLANG-YLANG AND CEDARWOOD ESSENCE

Ingredients:

- 1/3 cup coconut oil
- 5 drops ylang-ylang essential oil
- 5 drops cedarwood essential oil

Steps:

1 Mix coconut oil, ylang-ylang essential oil, and cedarwood essential oil in a small bottle.
2 Stir to mix.
3 Apply a small amount to the skin and massage gently.

Usage Tips: Use this essence to calm the mind and relax the body.

86. ROMANTIC ROSE AND SANDALWOOD MASSAGE OIL

Ingredients:

- 1/3 cup jojoba oil
- 8 drops rose essential oil
- 6 drops sandalwood essential oil

Steps:

1 Mix jojoba oil, rose essential oil, and sandalwood essential oil in a small bottle.
2 Stir to mix.
3 Apply a small amount to the skin and massage gently.

Usage Tips: This massage oil is ideal for creating a romantic and soothing atmosphere.

87. IMMUNE BOOSTING THYME AND LEMON MASSAGE OIL

Ingredients:

- 1/3 cup sweet almond oil
- 5 drops thyme essential oil
- 5 drops lemon essential oil

Steps:

1 Mix sweet almond oil, thyme essential oil, and lemon essential oil in a small bottle.
2 Stir to mix.
3 Apply a small amount to the skin and massage gently.

Usage Tips: Use this oil during cold and flu season to boost immunity and promote well-being.

88. COOLING PEPPERMINT AND ALOE VERA GEL FOR FOOT MASSAGE

Ingredients:

- 1/3 cup aloe vera gel
- 2 drops peppermint essential oil

Steps:

1 Combine aloe vera gel and peppermint essential oil in a small bottle.
2 Mix well.
3 Apply a small amount to the feet and massage gently.

Usage Tips: This gel is perfect for cooling and soothing tired feet after a long day.

2.4 Aromatic Waters for Body and Spirit

89. REFRESHING ROSEWATER FACIAL MIST

Ingredients:

- 1/3 cup distilled water
- 1/3 cup rosewater
- 14 drops rose essential oil

Steps:

1 Combine distilled water, rosewater, and rose essential oil in a spray bottle.
2 Stir well to mix.
3 Spray onto your face as needed.

Usage Tips: Use this facial mist to refresh and hydrate your skin throughout the day.

90. SOOTHING LAVENDER AND CHAMOMILE SPRAY

Ingredients:

- 1/2 cup distilled water
- 1/3 cup witch hazel
- 12 drops lavender essential oil
- 12 drops chamomile essential oil

Steps:

1 Combine distilled water, witch hazel, lavender essential oil, and chamomile essential oil in a spray bottle.
2 Mix well.
3 Spray onto your body or pillow as needed.

Usage Tips: This spray is perfect for promoting relaxation and restful sleep.

91. PURIFYING PEPPERMINT AND TEA TREE FOOT SPRAY

Ingredients:

- 1/2 cup distilled water
- 1/3 cup witch hazel
- 12 drops peppermint essential oil
- 12 drops tea tree essential oil

Steps:

1 Combine distilled water, witch hazel, peppermint essential oil, and tea tree essential oil in a spray bottle.
2 Stir well to mix.
3 Spray onto your feet as needed.

Usage Tips: This foot spray is perfect for keeping feet fresh and purifying them naturally.

92. ENERGIZING CITRUS BODY SPLASH

Ingredients:

- 1/2 cup distilled water
- 1/3 cup witch hazel
- 12 drops orange essential oil
- 12 drops grapefruit essential oil

Steps:

1 Combine distilled water, witch hazel, orange essential oil, and grapefruit essential oil in a spray bottle.
2 Mix well.
3 Spray onto your body as needed.

Usage Tips: Use this body splash to energize and uplift your spirits throughout the day.

93. BALANCING SAGE AND ROSEMARY HAIR MIST

Ingredients:

- 1/2 cup distilled water
- 1/3 cup witch hazel
- 12 drops sage essential oil
- 12 drops rosemary essential oil

Steps:

1 Combine distilled water, witch hazel, sage essential oil, and rosemary essential oil in a spray bottle.
2 Mix well.
3 Spray onto your hair as needed.

Usage Tips: This hair mist is perfect for balancing the scalp and adding shine to your hair.

94.   RELAXING VETIVER AND BERGAMOT SKIN TONIC

Ingredients:

- 1/2 cup distilled water
- 1/3 cup witch hazel
- 12 drops vetiver essential oil
- 12 drops bergamot essential oil

Steps:

1. Combine distilled water, witch hazel, vetiver essential oil, and bergamot essential oil in a spray bottle.
2. Stir well to mix.
3. Spray onto your skin as needed.

Usage Tips: Use this skin tonic to relax and rejuvenate your skin.

95.   INVIGORATING GINGER AND BASIL SCALP REFRESH

Ingredients:

- 1/2 cup distilled water
- 1/3 cup witch hazel
- 12 drops ginger essential oil
- 12 drops basil essential oil

Steps:

1. Mix distilled water, witch hazel, ginger essential oil, and basil essential oil in a spray bottle.
2. Stir well to mix.
3. Spray onto your scalp as needed.

Usage Tips: Use this scalp refresh to invigorate and stimulate your scalp.

96.   CALMING NEROLI AND ORANGE BLOSSOM FACE TONIC

Ingredients:

- 1/2 cup distilled water
- 1/3 cup witch hazel
- 12 drops neroli essential oil
- 12 drops orange blossom essential oil

Steps:

1. Combine distilled water, witch hazel, neroli essential oil, and orange blossom essential oil in a spray bottle.
2. Stir well to mix.

3. Spray onto your face as needed.

Usage Tips: This face tonic is perfect for calming and hydrating the skin.

97.   REVITALIZING MINT AND CUCUMBER COOLING SPRAY

Ingredients:

- 1/2 cup distilled water
- 1/3 cup witch hazel
- 12 drops peppermint essential oil
- 1/3 cup cucumber juice

Steps:

1. Combine distilled water, witch hazel, peppermint essential oil, and cucumber juice in a spray bottle.
2. Stir well to mix.
3. Spray onto your skin as needed.

Usage Tips: This cooling spray is perfect for hot days and refreshing your skin.

98.   DETOXIFYING LEMON AND THYME BODY MIST

Ingredients:

- 1/2 cup distilled water
- 1/3 cup witch hazel
- 12 drops lemon essential oil
- 12 drops thyme essential oil

Steps:

1. Combine distilled water, witch hazel, lemon essential oil, and thyme essential oil in a spray bottle.
2. Stir well to mix.
3. Spray onto your body as needed.

Usage Tips: This body mist is perfect for detoxifying and refreshing your skin.

99.   UPLIFTING JASMINE AND GREEN TEA AROMA SPRAY

Ingredients:

- 1/2 cup distilled water
- 1/3 cup witch hazel
- 12 drops jasmine essential oil

- 1/3 cup green tea

Steps:

1 Combine distilled water, witch hazel, jasmine essential oil, and green tea in a spray bottle.
2 Stir well to mix.
3 Spray around your home as needed.

Usage Tips: This aroma spray is perfect for uplifting and refreshing your home environment.

2.5 Evening Herbal Comfort Rituals

100.   CALMING CHAMOMILE NIGHT TEA

Ingredients:

- 1 tsp dried chamomile flowers
- 1 cup boiling water
- Honey to taste

Steps:

1 Put dried chamomile flowers in a cup.
2 Pour boiling water over the flowers.
3 Let steep for 8-9 min.
4 Strain into a cup and add honey to taste.

Usage Tips: Drink this tea before bedtime to promote relaxation and restful sleep.

101.   RELAXING VALERIAN ROOT SLEEP TINCTURE

Ingredients:

- 1/3 cup dried valerian root
- 1 cup vodka or glycerin (for alcohol-free version)

Steps:

1 Place dried valerian root in a jar.
2 Pour vodka or glycerin over the root, ensuring it is fully submerged.
3 Seal the jar and let it sit for about 30 days, shaking occasionally.
4 Strain the tincture into a dropper bottle.

Usage Tips: Take a few drops of this tincture before bedtime to promote restful sleep.

102.   SOOTHING LAVENDER PILLOW SPRAY

Ingredients:

- 1/2 cup distilled water
- 1/3 cup witch hazel
- 12 drops lavender essential oil

Steps:

1 Combine distilled water, witch hazel, and lavender essential oil in a spray bottle.
2 Stir well to mix.
3 Spray onto your pillow before bedtime.

Usage Tips: Use this spray to create a calming atmosphere and promote restful sleep.

103.   NIGHTLY NOURISHING MOON MILK

Ingredients:

- 1 cup milk (dairy or non-dairy)
- 1 tsp honey
- 1/2 tsp ashwagandha powder
- 1/3 tsp cinnamon
- 1/3 tsp nutmeg

Steps:

1 Heat the milk in a small pot until warm.
2 Stir in honey, ashwagandha powder, cinnamon, and nutmeg.
3 Mix well and serve warm.

Usage Tips: Drink this moon milk before bed to nourish your body and promote deep sleep.

104. GENTLE EVENING YOGA HERBAL INCENSE

Ingredients:

- 1/3 cup dried sage
- 1/3 cup dried lavender flowers
- 1/3 cup dried rosemary
- 1/3 cup dried rose petals

Steps:

1 Mix all dried herbs in a bowl and mix well.
2 Place a small amount on a heat-resistant dish or incense burner.
3 Light the herbs and let the smoke fill your space.

Usage Tips: Burn this incense during evening yoga or meditation to create a peaceful environment.

105. RELAXING MAGNESIUM AND HERB BATH SOAK

Ingredients:

- 1 cup Epsom salts
- 1/2 cup baking soda
- 1/3 cup dried lavender flowers
- 12 drops lavender essential oil

Steps:

1 Combine Epsom salts, baking soda, dried lavender flowers, and lavender essential oil in a bowl.
2 Stir well and transfer to a jar.
3 Add 1/2 cup of the mixture to warm bathwater.

Usage Tips: Soak in this bath for 20 minutes to relax muscles and calm the mind before bed.

106. SLEEP-PROMOTING HOPS AND MUGWORT SACHET

Ingredients:

- 1/3 cup dried hops
- 1/3 cup dried mugwort
- Small fabric sachets

Steps:

1 Combine dried hops and mugwort in a bowl and mix well.

2 Fill small fabric sachets with the herb blend.
3 Tie or sew the sachets closed.

Usage Tips: Place these sachets under your pillow to promote restful sleep.

107. WARM GOLDEN MILK WITH TURMERIC AND CARDAMOM

Ingredients:

- 1 cup milk (dairy or non-dairy)
- 1/2 tsp turmeric powder
- 1/4 tsp ground cardamom
- 1 tsp honey

Steps:

1 Heat the milk in a small pot until warm.
2 Stir in turmeric powder, ground cardamom, and honey.
3 Mix well and serve warm.

Usage Tips: Drink this golden milk in the evening to reduce inflammation and promote relaxation.

108. SOOTHING EVENING FOOT SOAK WITH LAVENDER AND EPSOM SALT

Ingredients:

- 1 cup Epsom salts
- 1/3 cup baking soda
- 12 drops lavender essential oil

Steps:

1 Mix Epsom salts, baking soda, and lavender essential oil in a bowl.
2 Stir and transfer to a jar.
3 Add 1/2 cup of the mixture to warm foot bathwater.

Usage Tips: Soak your feet in this soothing bath to relax and relieve foot tension before bed.

109. CALMING BEDTIME HERBAL CAPSULES

Ingredients:

- 1/3 cup dried chamomile flowers
- 1/3 cup dried valerian root

- Empty gelatin or vegetarian capsules

Steps:

1. Grind dried chamomile flowers and valerian root into a fine powder using a coffee grinder.
2. Fill the empty capsules with the powdered herbs using a capsule machine or by hand.
3. Store the filled capsules in an airtight container.

Usage Tips: Take one capsule 30 minutes before bedtime to promote relaxation and restful sleep.

---

110. NIGHTTIME SKIN REPLENISHING HERBAL SERUM

Ingredients:

- 1/3 cup jojoba oil
- 12 drops lavender essential oil
- 6 drops frankincense essential oil

Steps:

1. Combine jojoba oil, lavender essential oil, and frankincense essential oil in a small bottle.
2. Stir well to mix.
3. Apply a few drops to your face before bed.

Usage Tips: Use this serum nightly to replenish and nourish your skin while you sleep.

2.6 Morning Revitalizing Herbal Routines

111. MORNING WAKE-UP PEPPERMINT AND LEMON WATER

Ingredients:

- 1 cup warm water
- 1/2 tsp peppermint extract
- 1/2 lemon (juice)

Steps:

1. Combine warm water, peppermint extract, and lemon juice in a cup.
2. Stir well and serve.

Usage Tips: Drink this refreshing water first thing in the morning to wake up your senses and start your day.

---

112. ENERGIZING GINSENG AND ORANGE SMOOTHIE

Ingredients:

- 1 banana
- 1 orange, peeled
- 1 cup almond milk
- 1 tsp ginseng powder
- 1 tbsp honey

Steps:

1. Transfer all ingredients in a blender.
2. Mix until smooth.
3. Pour into a glass and serve immediately.

Usage Tips: Enjoy this smoothie in the morning for a natural energy boost and enhanced focus.

---

113. REFRESHING HERBAL FACE TONER WITH GREEN TEA

Ingredients:

- 1 cup brewed green tea, cooled
- 1/3 cup witch hazel
- 12 drops tea tree essential oil

Steps:

1. Combine brewed green tea, witch hazel, and tea tree essential oil in a spray bottle.
2. Stir well to mix.
3. Spray onto your face after cleansing.

Usage Tips: Use this toner to refresh and tighten your skin in the morning.

114. MORNING METABOLISM BOOST TEA

Ingredients:

- 1 tsp dried green tea leaves
- 1/2 tsp dried ginger root
- 1 cup boiling water
- Honey to taste

Steps:

1 Transfer dried green tea leaves and ginger root in your teapot.
2 Pour boiling water into the teapot.
3 Let steep for 8-9 min.
4 Strain into a cup and add honey to taste.

Usage Tips: Drink this tea in the morning to boost your metabolism and start your day right.

115. DETOXIFYING HERBAL GREEN JUICE

Ingredients:

- 1 cucumber
- 1 handful spinach
- 1 apple
- 1 lemon, juiced
- 1 tsp spirulina powder

Steps:

1 Transfer all ingredients in a juicer.
2 Juice until smooth.
3 Pour into a glass and serve immediately.

Usage Tips: Drink this green juice in the morning to detoxify your body and boost your energy.

116. SUNRISE STRETCHING AROMATIC OIL BLEND

Ingredients:

- 1/3 cup sweet almond oil
- 6 drops orange essential oil
- 6 drops peppermint essential oil

Steps:

1 Transfer sweet almond oil, orange essential oil, and peppermint essential oil in a small bottle.
2 Stir well to mix.
3 Apply a small amount to your wrists and inhale deeply.

Usage Tips: Use this aromatic blend during morning stretches to invigorate and uplift your senses.

117. AWAKENING HERBAL BREATH FRESHENER SPRAY

Ingredients:

- 1/2 cup distilled water
- 1/3 cup witch hazel
- 12 drops peppermint essential oil

Steps:

1 Transfer distilled water, witch hazel, and peppermint essential oil in a spray bottle.
2 Stir well to mix.
3 Spray into your mouth as needed.

Usage Tips: Use this spray in the morning to freshen your breath and awaken your senses.

118. REVITALIZING ROSEMARY AND MINT SHAMPOO

Ingredients:

- 1/3 cup liquid castile soap
- 1/3 cup distilled water
- 12 drops rosemary essential oil
- 12 drops peppermint essential oil

Steps:

1 Combine liquid castile soap, distilled water, rosemary essential oil, and peppermint essential oil in a bottle.
2 Stir well to mix.
3 Apply to wet hair, lather, and rinse thoroughly.

Usage Tips: Use this shampoo to cleanse and invigorate your scalp in the morning.

119. BRIGHTENING COFFEE AND CINNAMON BODY SCRUB

Ingredients:

- 1/2 cup coffee grounds
- 1/3 cup coconut oil
- 1/3 cup brown sugar
- 1 tsp ground cinnamon

Steps:

1 Combine coffee grounds, coconut oil, brown sugar, and ground cinnamon in a bowl.
2 Stir and transfer to a jar.
3 Apply to damp skin in circular motions, then rinse off.

Usage Tips: Utilize this scrub in the morning shower to exfoliate and brighten your skin.

120. INVIGORATING EUCALYPTUS SHOWER STEAMERS

Ingredients:

- 1 cup baking soda
- 1/3 cup citric acid
- 12 drops eucalyptus essential oil
- Water (as needed)

Steps:

1 Combine baking soda and citric acid in a bowl.
2 Add eucalyptus essential oil and stir well.
3 Spritz with water and mix until the mixture holds its shape.
4 Press the mixture into molds and let them dry completely.

Usage Tips: Place a shower steamer on the floor of your shower to release invigorating eucalyptus steam.

121. STIMULATING SCALP MASSAGE OIL WITH ROSEMARY AND CEDARWOOD

Ingredients:

- 1/3 cup jojoba oil
- 12 drops rosemary essential oil
- 6 drops cedarwood essential oil

Steps:

1 Transfer jojoba oil, rosemary essential oil, and cedarwood essential oil in a small bottle.
2 Stir well to mix.
3 Apply a small amount to your scalp and massage gently.

Usage Tips: Use this oil for a stimulating scalp massage to promote hair growth and relaxation.

Chapter 3: Benefits of Herbs in Beauty Routines

3.1 General Benefits of Herbal Beauty Treatments

Herbal beauty treatments have been used for centuries across various cultures to maintain and enhance skin and hair health. Unlike many conventional beauty products that are laden with synthetic chemicals, herbal treatments utilize natural plant extracts known for their therapeutic properties. The benefits of these treatments are manifold and can significantly improve the overall health and appearance of the skin and hair.

One of the primary advantages of herbal beauty treatments is their holistic approach to skincare and haircare. These treatments often address the root cause of issues rather than just masking symptoms. For instance, herbs like chamomile and calendula have anti-inflammatory properties that can soothe irritated skin and promote healing from within. Similarly, herbs like rosemary and nettle can strengthen hair from the roots, promoting healthier growth and reducing breakage.

Moreover, herbal beauty treatments are packed with natural antioxidants, vitamins, and minerals that provide essential nutrients to the skin and hair. Antioxidants found in herbs like green tea and rosehip help combat free radicals, which are responsible for premature aging. This results in a more youthful and radiant appearance over time.

Another significant benefit of herbal beauty treatments is their compatibility with various skin types. Whether you have oily, dry, sensitive, or combination skin, there are specific herbs that can cater to your unique needs. This versatility makes herbal treatments suitable for a wide range of individuals, minimizing the risk of adverse reactions that are often associated with chemical-laden products.

Furthermore, the use of herbs in beauty routines promotes sustainability and environmental consciousness. Herbs are renewable resources, and their cultivation typically has a lower environmental impact compared to the production of synthetic ingredients. By opting for herbal beauty treatments, you contribute to a more sustainable and eco-friendly beauty regimen.

In summary, herbal beauty treatments offer a natural, effective, and sustainable alternative to conventional beauty products. They provide a holistic approach to skincare and haircare, delivering long-term benefits and promoting overall wellness. Through the utilization of herbs, individuals can achieve healthier, more radiant skin and hair while supporting environmental sustainability.

3.1.1 The Science Behind Herbal Efficacy

The effectiveness of herbal beauty treatments is rooted in the rich array of bioactive compounds found in plants. These compounds include antioxidants, vitamins, minerals, and essential oils, all of which play crucial roles in maintaining and enhancing skin and hair health. Understanding the science behind herbal efficacy can help demystify why these natural ingredients are so beneficial.

Bioactive Compounds and Their Roles

Herbs are rich in bioactive compounds that interact with the body at a cellular level. For example, antioxidants such as flavonoids and polyphenols, found in herbs like green tea and rosemary, help protect the skin from oxidative stress caused by free radicals. Free radicals are unstable molecules that can damage skin cells, leading to premature aging, inflammation, and various skin disorders. By neutralizing these harmful molecules, antioxidants help maintain a youthful appearance and promote overall skin health.

Anti-Inflammatory Properties

Many herbs have potent anti-inflammatory properties, which are beneficial for soothing irritated or inflamed skin. Compounds such as azulene in chamomile and curcumin in turmeric have been shown to reduce inflammation by inhibiting the production of inflammatory cytokines. This makes them particularly effective in treating conditions like acne, eczema, and rosacea. The anti-inflammatory effects of these herbs can help calm the skin, reduce redness, and promote healing.

Hydration and Moisture Retention

Herbs also contribute to skin hydration and moisture retention. Aloe vera, for instance, contains mucopolysaccharides that help bind moisture to the skin, making it an excellent natural moisturizer. Additionally, the fatty acids found in herbs like calendula and lavender help strengthen the skin's lipid barrier, preventing moisture loss and keeping the skin hydrated and supple.

Stimulation of Collagen Production

Certain herbs are known to stimulate collagen production, which is vital for maintaining skin elasticity and firmness. Gotu kola, for example, contains triterpenoids that promote collagen synthesis. Increased collagen production helps reduce the appearance of fine lines and wrinkles, resulting in smoother, more youthful-looking skin.

Antimicrobial and Antibacterial Properties

Herbs like tea tree, thyme, and neem possess strong antimicrobial and antibacterial properties, which can help prevent and treat skin infections. These properties make them effective in managing acne by reducing the bacteria that cause breakouts. Furthermore, their ability to cleanse the skin without stripping it of its natural oils makes them ideal for maintaining a healthy skin microbiome.

Detoxification

Herbs such as dandelion and burdock root have detoxifying properties that can help purify the skin. These herbs aid in the elimination of toxins and promote lymphatic drainage, which can enhance the skin's clarity and brightness. Detoxification through herbal treatments supports the body's natural ability to cleanse itself, leading to clearer and more vibrant skin.

By leveraging the natural power of these bioactive compounds, herbal beauty treatments offer a scientifically backed, effective approach to skincare and haircare. The integration of these herbs into daily routines not only provides immediate aesthetic benefits but also supports long-term health and vitality of the skin and hair.

3.1.2 Comparison with Conventional Beauty Products

When comparing herbal beauty treatments to conventional beauty products, several key differences emerge. These differences highlight the unique advantages of using herbs for skincare and haircare, including natural ingredients, fewer side effects, and environmental sustainability.

Natural Ingredients

Herbal beauty treatments primarily utilize natural ingredients derived from plants. These ingredients are often minimally processed, retaining their natural bioactive compounds, which provide various therapeutic benefits. For example, chamomile is known for its soothing and anti-inflammatory properties, while aloe vera is celebrated for its hydrating and healing effects. In contrast, conventional beauty products frequently contain synthetic chemicals, preservatives, and artificial fragrances. These additives can sometimes cause irritation, allergic reactions, or long-term health concerns. The use of natural ingredients in herbal treatments ensures that the skin and hair are nourished with wholesome, beneficial substances without the risk of harmful side effects.

Fewer Side Effects

One of the significant advantages of herbal beauty treatments is the reduced likelihood of adverse side effects. Herbs have been used for centuries, with a wealth of historical data supporting their safety and efficacy. For instance, lavender oil is widely used for its calming and antiseptic properties, with minimal risk of irritation. Conventional beauty products, however, may contain harsh chemicals such as parabens, sulfates, and phthalates, which have been linked to various health issues, including endocrine disruption and skin sensitivities. By choosing herbal beauty treatments, individuals can avoid exposure to these potentially harmful substances, leading to gentler and safer skincare and haircare routines.

Environmental Sustainability

Herbal beauty treatments also offer significant environmental benefits compared to their conventional counterparts. The production of herbal products often involves sustainable farming practices, organic cultivation, and minimal processing, reducing the environmental footprint. For example, herbs like calendula and rosemary can be grown organically without the need for harmful pesticides or synthetic fertilizers. On the other hand, the production of conventional beauty products often relies on petrochemical-derived ingredients, extensive use of plastics, and energy-intensive manufacturing processes. These practices contribute to environmental pollution and depletion of natural resources. Additionally, many conventional beauty products are tested on animals, raising ethical concerns. Herbal beauty treatments, especially those certified as organic or cruelty-free, support a more sustainable and ethical approach to beauty care.

Effectiveness and Long-Term Benefits

While conventional beauty products may offer quick fixes or immediate results, herbal treatments provide long-term benefits by addressing the root causes of skin and hair issues. For instance, instead of using a silicone-based serum to mask hair damage, a herbal hair oil infused with rosemary and nettle can nourish and strengthen the hair from within, promoting healthier growth over time. Similarly, herbal face masks with ingredients like turmeric and honey can provide anti-inflammatory and antioxidant benefits, improving skin health naturally and sustainably.

Cost and Accessibility

Herbal beauty treatments can also be more cost-effective and accessible. Many herbs used in beauty care, such as mint, lavender, and aloe vera, can be easily grown at home or purchased at local markets. This accessibility allows individuals to create their own beauty treatments without relying on expensive, store-bought products. Conventional beauty products, especially high-end brands, can be costly and may not be readily available to everyone. By utilizing herbs, individuals can achieve effective beauty care solutions that are both affordable and sustainable.

In summary, herbal beauty treatments offer numerous advantages over conventional beauty products. They provide natural, gentle, and effective care for the skin and hair, with fewer side effects and a more sustainable environmental impact. By choosing herbal treatments, individuals can embrace a holistic approach to beauty that benefits both their well-being and the planet.

3.1.3 Long-Term Benefits of Herbal Beauty Routines

Consistent use of herbal beauty treatments can offer significant long-term benefits for skin and hair health. These benefits go beyond the immediate improvements and provide lasting enhancements through natural and gentle care. Here are some key long-term advantages of incorporating herbs into your beauty routine:

Enhanced Hydration

Herbal beauty treatments often include ingredients known for their hydrating properties. For example, aloe vera is renowned for its ability to deeply moisturize the skin without leaving a greasy residue. Regular use of aloe vera can help maintain the skin's moisture balance, leading to a more hydrated and plump appearance over time. Similarly, herbs like rose and chamomile can be infused into toners and facial mists to provide continuous hydration throughout the day. Over the long term, consistent use of these herbal hydrators can improve the skin's ability to retain moisture, reducing the likelihood of dryness and flakiness.

Reduced Inflammation

Many herbs possess anti-inflammatory properties that can help soothe irritated skin and reduce redness. Calendula, for instance, is known for its calming effects on the skin and is often used to treat conditions like eczema and dermatitis. Turmeric, another powerful anti-inflammatory herb, can help diminish acne and other inflammatory skin issues. By regularly incorporating these herbs into your skincare routine, you can achieve a more even and calm complexion. Over time, this can result in fewer flare-ups and a reduction in chronic skin conditions, leading to healthier, more resilient skin.

Improved Skin Texture and Tone

Herbs such as green tea and witch hazel are rich in antioxidants that protect the skin from environmental stressors and promote cell regeneration. Consistent use of products containing these herbs can help improve skin texture and tone. Green tea, for example, can help minimize the appearance of pores and reduce the occurrence of acne, while witch hazel can tighten the skin and improve its elasticity. Over time, the regular application of these antioxidant-rich herbs can lead to smoother, more youthful-looking skin.

Strengthened Hair Health

Herbal treatments can also provide long-term benefits for hair health. Rosemary, for instance, is known to stimulate hair growth and improve circulation to the scalp. Nettle is another herb that strengthens hair shafts and reduces hair fall. Consistent use of herbal hair oils and rinses can lead to thicker, healthier hair with increased shine and reduced breakage. Over time, incorporating these herbs into your hair care routine can result in stronger, more resilient hair that is less prone to damage.

Natural Glow and Radiance

Herbal beauty routines can enhance your skin's natural glow and radiance. Herbs like rosehip and hibiscus are packed with vitamins and antioxidants that nourish the skin from within. Rosehip oil, for example, is rich in vitamin C and essential fatty acids, which help brighten the skin and improve its overall appearance. Hibiscus, often referred to as the "botox plant," helps increase skin elasticity and provides a natural lift. Regular use of these herbs can lead to a naturally radiant complexion that glows with health.

Long-Term Sustainability

Another benefit of herbal beauty routines is their long-term sustainability. Herbal products are generally more environmentally friendly compared to conventional beauty products, as they often involve sustainable farming practices and minimal processing. By choosing herbs over synthetic ingredients, you are supporting eco-friendly practices that benefit both your health and the planet.

Holistic Wellness

The holistic nature of herbal beauty routines contributes to overall well-being. Many herbs used in beauty treatments have aromatherapeutic benefits that can improve mood and reduce stress. Lavender, for example, is known for its calming scent, which can help alleviate anxiety and promote relaxation. By incorporating these herbs into your daily routine, you not only enhance your physical appearance but also support your mental and emotional health.

The consistent use of herbal beauty treatments offers a multitude of long-term benefits. From enhanced hydration and reduced inflammation to improved skin texture and hair health, herbs provide a natural and effective way to achieve and maintain beauty. By embracing herbal beauty routines, you can enjoy a holistic approach to self-care that promotes lasting health and well-being.

3.2 Herbs for Skin Care

Hydration is key to maintaining healthy, glowing skin. Various herbs are renowned for their ability to enhance skin moisture, offering natural and effective solutions for dry and dehydrated skin. These herbs work by binding moisture into the skin and providing soothing and nourishing effects. Below are some of the most effective hydrating herbs and how they can be used for optimal skin moisture.

3.2.1 Hydrating Herbs for Skin Moisture

Aloe Vera

Aloe vera is a powerhouse herb for skin hydration, revered for its ability to soothe, moisturize, and heal the skin. This succulent plant contains a gel-like substance in its leaves that is rich in vitamins, minerals, amino acids, and antioxidants. Here's a deeper look into the benefits of aloe vera and how to use it for optimal skin hydration:

Hydrating Properties: Aloe vera gel is composed of 99% water, making it an excellent natural moisturizer. The gel contains mucopolysaccharides, which are long chains of sugar molecules that help retain moisture in the skin. This hydrating effect helps to keep the skin plump and supple.

Soothing and Healing: Aloe vera is known for its anti-inflammatory and cooling properties, which make it ideal for soothing irritated or sunburned skin. It also promotes wound healing and can help reduce redness and inflammation, providing relief for various skin conditions such as eczema and psoriasis.

Nutrient-Rich: Aloe vera is packed with essential nutrients that benefit the skin, including vitamins A, C, E, and B12, as well as minerals like magnesium and zinc. These nutrients help nourish the skin and support its natural healing processes.

Usage Tips:

• 	*Direct Application*: For immediate hydration, cut a leaf from the aloe vera plant, scoop out the gel, and apply it directly to your skin. This pure form of aloe vera provides the maximum benefits without any added chemicals.

• 	*Aloe Vera Gel Products:* Look for products that contain a high percentage of aloe vera gel. These can be used as daily moisturizers to keep your skin hydrated throughout the day.

- **DIY Aloe Vera Mask**: Mix aloe vera gel with honey and a few drops of essential oil (like lavender or tea tree) to create a hydrating and soothing face mask. Apply the mixture to your face, leave it on for 15-20 minutes, then rinse off with lukewarm water.

- **After-Sun Care:** Use aloe vera gel as an after-sun treatment to cool and soothe sunburned skin. Its anti-inflammatory properties help reduce redness and promote healing.

Incorporating aloe vera into your skincare routine can significantly improve your skin's hydration and overall health, making it an essential herb for those seeking natural and effective skin care solutions.

Calendula

Calendula, also known as pot marigold, is a vibrant, golden-yellow flower renowned for its soothing and healing properties. This herb has been used for centuries in skincare for its ability to hydrate, heal, and protect the skin. Here's an in-depth look at the benefits of calendula and how to utilize it for optimal skin moisture:

Hydrating Properties: Calendula is rich in flavonoids, saponins, and polysaccharides, which contribute to its moisturizing effects. These compounds help retain moisture in the skin, making it an excellent choice for dry and dehydrated skin.

Soothing and Anti-Inflammatory: Calendula is highly valued for its anti-inflammatory properties. It can help calm irritated skin, reduce redness, and soothe conditions like eczema, dermatitis, and psoriasis. Its soothing nature makes it ideal for sensitive skin types.

Healing and Regenerative: Calendula promotes wound healing and skin regeneration. It stimulates collagen production, which is essential for maintaining skin elasticity and firmness. This makes it useful for healing minor cuts, burns, and abrasions, as well as for reducing the appearance of scars.

Antioxidant-Rich: The antioxidants in calendula protect the skin from free radical damage, which can lead to premature aging. By neutralizing these harmful molecules, calendula helps maintain youthful, healthy skin.

Usage Tips:

- **Calendula-Infused Oil:** Create your own calendula oil by infusing dried calendula petals in a carrier oil, such as olive or almond oil. This can be applied directly to the skin as a moisturizer or used in DIY skincare recipes.

- **Calendula Cream:** Use calendula cream to treat dry, irritated, or inflamed skin. These creams are often available in natural health stores and can be applied as needed to affected areas.

- **_DIY Calendula Balm_**: Make a soothing balm by mixing calendula-infused oil with beeswax. This balm can be used to treat dry patches, minor cuts, and burns. Melt the beeswax, mix with the calendula oil, and pour into small containers to cool and solidify.

- **_Calendula Facial Mist_**: Prepare a refreshing facial mist by steeping calendula petals in hot water, then straining and cooling the liquid. Pour it into a spray bottle and use it throughout the day to hydrate and soothe your skin.

Incorporating calendula into your skincare routine can provide substantial benefits, particularly for those with dry, sensitive, or irritated skin. Its natural hydrating, soothing, and healing properties make it an invaluable herb for maintaining healthy, moisturized skin.

Cucumber

Cucumber is a well-known and widely used natural remedy for hydrating and soothing the skin. With its high water content and beneficial nutrients, cucumber is a versatile ingredient in skincare routines aimed at enhancing skin moisture and overall health. Here's a detailed look at the benefits of cucumber for skin hydration and how to incorporate it into your beauty regimen:

Hydrating Properties: Cucumbers are composed of about 96% water, making them an excellent natural hydrator. When applied to the skin, cucumber helps to replenish moisture levels, providing immediate and lasting hydration.

Cooling and Soothing: Cucumber has a naturally cooling effect on the skin, which can help reduce puffiness, inflammation, and irritation. This makes it especially beneficial for soothing sunburned skin or calming sensitive skin.

Rich in Nutrients: Cucumber is packed with vitamins and minerals such as vitamin C, vitamin K, and potassium. These nutrients contribute to maintaining healthy skin by promoting collagen production, reducing dark circles, and improving skin elasticity.

Antioxidant Benefits: The antioxidants in cucumber, including beta-carotene and flavonoids, help protect the skin from environmental stressors and free radical damage. This can prevent premature aging and keep the skin looking youthful and vibrant.

Usage Tips:

- **_Cucumber Slices:_** The simplest way to use cucumber is by applying fresh slices directly to the skin. Place cucumber slices over your eyes to reduce puffiness and dark circles, or apply them to other areas of the face for a refreshing and hydrating treatment.

- **Cucumber Juice:** Extract the juice from a fresh cucumber using a blender or juicer. Apply the juice to your skin with a cotton pad or add it to your favorite toner or facial mist for an extra boost of hydration.

- **Cucumber Face Mask**: Blend cucumber with other hydrating ingredients like yogurt or honey to create a nourishing face mask. Apply the mask to your face and leave it on for 15-20 minutes before rinsing off with cool water.

- **Cucumber Gel:** Make a soothing gel by blending cucumber with aloe vera gel. This combination enhances the hydrating and cooling effects, making it perfect for treating sunburns or irritated skin. Store the gel in the refrigerator for an added cooling sensation when applied.

- **DIY Cucumber Toner:** Create a refreshing toner by mixing cucumber juice with rose water. This toner can be used after cleansing to hydrate and balance the skin, preparing it for moisturizer.

Incorporating cucumber into your skincare routine can provide immediate and long-term benefits for hydration and skin health. Its natural cooling, soothing, and hydrating properties make cucumber an essential ingredient for achieving and maintaining well-moisturized, healthy skin.

3.2.2 Anti-Aging Herbs for Skin Vitality

Rosehip

Rosehip, derived from the seeds of the wild rose bush, is renowned for its potent anti-aging properties. Packed with essential fatty acids, vitamins, and antioxidants, rosehip offers numerous benefits for maintaining youthful, vibrant skin. Here's a comprehensive look at how rosehip can enhance skin vitality and reduce the signs of aging:

Anti-Aging Properties: Rosehip oil is rich in vitamins A and C, which are crucial for maintaining skin health. Vitamin A (retinol) helps to improve skin texture, reduce the appearance of wrinkles, and promote cell regeneration. Vitamin C is essential for collagen production, which keeps the skin firm and elastic.

Hydration and Moisture: The essential fatty acids in rosehip oil, including omega-3 and omega-6, help to lock in moisture and keep the skin hydrated. These fatty acids also strengthen the skin barrier, preventing moisture loss and maintaining skin suppleness.

Antioxidant Protection: Rosehip is a powerhouse of antioxidants, such as lycopene and beta-carotene, which protect the skin from free radical damage. This helps to prevent premature aging caused by environmental stressors like pollution and UV rays.

Brightening and Even Skin Tone: The high concentration of vitamin C in rosehip oil aids in brightening the skin and reducing hyperpigmentation. Regular use can help to fade dark spots, even out skin tone, and give the skin a radiant glow.

Healing and Regeneration: Rosehip oil is known for its healing properties. It can help to reduce the appearance of scars, stretch marks, and fine lines. The oil promotes skin regeneration, making it effective for repairing damaged skin and enhancing overall skin health.

Usage Tips:

• ***Rosehip Oil:*** Apply a few drops of pure rosehip oil to your face and neck after cleansing and toning. Gently massage the oil into your skin using upward, circular motions. Use it as part of your nightly skincare routine to reap its anti-aging benefits.

• ***DIY Rosehip Serum:*** Create a nourishing serum by combining rosehip oil with other beneficial oils like jojoba oil or argan oil. Add a few drops of essential oils such as frankincense or lavender for added skin benefits. Apply the serum before your moisturizer to lock in hydration and promote youthful skin.

• ***Rosehip Face Mask:*** Make a rejuvenating face mask by mixing rosehip oil with natural ingredients like honey, yogurt, or oatmeal. Apply the mask to your face and leave it on for 15-20 minutes before rinsing off with lukewarm water. This mask will help to hydrate, brighten, and revitalize your skin.

• ***Rosehip and Aloe Vera Gel:*** Blend rosehip oil with aloe vera gel to create a soothing and hydrating gel. This combination is perfect for calming irritated skin and providing intense moisture. Apply the gel to your face and let it absorb fully before applying your regular moisturizer.

• ***Rosehip Eye Cream:*** Create a gentle eye cream by mixing rosehip oil with a carrier oil like sweet almond oil and adding a few drops of vitamin E oil. Apply this mixture around the delicate eye area to reduce the appearance of fine lines and dark circles.

Incorporating rosehip into your skincare routine can provide powerful anti-aging benefits, helping to reduce wrinkles, improve skin texture, and promote a youthful, radiant complexion. Its natural properties make it an invaluable ingredient for maintaining skin vitality and health.

Green Tea

Green tea is celebrated not only as a soothing beverage but also for its remarkable benefits in skincare, particularly for its anti-aging properties. Rich in antioxidants and nutrients, green tea can help protect and rejuvenate the skin, making it an essential herb for maintaining youthful vitality.

Anti-Aging Properties: Green tea is packed with catechins, a type of antioxidant that helps fight free radicals, which are responsible for aging the skin. One of the most potent catechins in green tea is epigallocatechin gallate (EGCG), known for its anti-aging and anti-inflammatory effects. EGCG helps to protect the skin from UV damage, reduce the formation of wrinkles, and improve skin elasticity.

Reduction of Fine Lines and Wrinkles: The antioxidants in green tea help to neutralize free radicals, preventing them from breaking down collagen and elastin in the skin. This preservation of collagen and elastin helps to maintain the skin's firmness and elasticity, reducing the appearance of fine lines and wrinkles.

Anti-Inflammatory Benefits: Green tea has strong anti-inflammatory properties that help to calm irritated skin and reduce redness. This makes it particularly beneficial for those with sensitive or acne-prone skin, as it can help to soothe and heal the skin.

Detoxification and Skin Brightening: Green tea helps to detoxify the skin by eliminating toxins and impurities, resulting in a clearer complexion. Its astringent properties help to shrink pores and reduce excess oil, giving the skin a smooth and even appearance. Regular use of green tea in skincare can also help to brighten the skin, giving it a natural, healthy glow.

Protection Against UV Damage: The polyphenols in green tea offer protection against UV-induced skin damage. Applying green tea topically can help to reduce the harmful effects of UV rays, such as sunburn and long-term photoaging. This makes green tea an excellent ingredient for sunscreen formulations and after-sun care products.

Usage Tips:

• **Green Tea Toner:** Brew a strong cup of green tea and let it cool. Use it as a toner by applying it to your face with a cotton pad after cleansing. This toner will help to tighten pores, reduce redness, and refresh the skin.

• **Green Tea Face Mask:** Create a rejuvenating face mask by mixing green tea powder (matcha) with yogurt and honey. Apply the mask to your face and leave it on for 15-20 minutes before rinsing off with lukewarm water. This mask will help to hydrate, brighten, and soothe the skin.

• **Green Tea Serum:** Infuse green tea in a carrier oil such as jojoba or sweet almond oil. After straining the tea leaves, use the oil as a serum to apply to your face before moisturizing. This will provide your skin with potent antioxidants and anti-aging benefits.

• **Green Tea Eye Compress:** Soak cotton pads in cooled green tea and place them over your eyes for 10-15 minutes. This compress will help to reduce puffiness, dark circles, and soothe tired eyes.

• **Green Tea Steam Facial:** Add a few green tea bags to a bowl of hot water and steam your face for 5-10 minutes. The steam will open up your pores, allowing the antioxidants to penetrate deeply and detoxify your skin.

Incorporating green tea into your skincare routine can significantly enhance your skin's health and appearance. Its potent antioxidants and anti-inflammatory properties make it a powerful ally in the fight against aging, helping to maintain a youthful, radiant complexion.

Ginseng

Ginseng is renowned for its rejuvenating properties and is a staple in traditional medicine, especially in East Asian cultures. Its benefits extend to skincare, where it is prized for its anti-aging properties and ability to enhance skin vitality.

Anti-Aging Properties: Ginseng is rich in phytonutrients, which help to stimulate and activate the skin's metabolism and blood flow to regenerate and tone. These compounds help to reduce the appearance of fine lines and wrinkles by boosting collagen production and promoting skin elasticity.

Skin Firming and Tightening: Ginseng contains natural ingredients that can help to firm and tighten the skin, making it appear more youthful. Its ability to enhance collagen synthesis supports the skin's structure, leading to a smoother and more toned appearance.

Brightening and Even Skin Tone: Ginseng helps to brighten the skin and improve its overall tone. It works by inhibiting melanin production, which helps to reduce hyperpigmentation and dark spots. Regular use of ginseng can result in a more even and radiant complexion.

Anti-Inflammatory and Calming Effects: The anti-inflammatory properties of ginseng make it ideal for calming irritated or sensitive skin. It helps to reduce redness and puffiness, making it a beneficial ingredient for those with sensitive or acne-prone skin.

Protection Against Environmental Stressors: Ginseng is packed with antioxidants that protect the skin from environmental stressors such as pollution and UV radiation. These antioxidants help to neutralize free radicals, preventing them from causing damage that leads to premature aging.

Usage Tips:

•   *Ginseng Face Serum:* Create a rejuvenating face serum by infusing ginseng root in a carrier oil like jojoba or argan oil. Apply a few drops to your face and gently massage it into your skin. This will help to firm and brighten your complexion.

•   *Ginseng Face Mask:* Mix ginseng powder with honey and yogurt to create a nourishing face mask. Apply the mask to your face and leave it on for 15-20 minutes before rinsing off with warm water. This mask will hydrate, brighten, and revitalize your skin.

- **_Ginseng Toner:_** Brew a cup of ginseng tea and let it cool. Use it as a toner by applying it to your face with a cotton pad after cleansing. This toner will help to tighten pores, reduce inflammation, and refresh your skin.

- **_Ginseng Eye Cream:_** Combine ginseng extract with aloe vera gel and a few drops of vitamin E oil to create an eye cream. Apply it around your eyes before bed to reduce puffiness and dark circles.

- **_Ginseng Steam Facial:_** Add a few slices of fresh ginseng root to a bowl of hot water and steam your face for 5-10 minutes. The steam will open up your pores, allowing the ginseng to penetrate deeply and detoxify your skin.

Incorporating ginseng into your skincare routine can provide a multitude of benefits, from firming and tightening the skin to brightening and evening out the complexion. Its powerful antioxidants and anti-inflammatory properties make it a versatile and valuable ingredient for maintaining youthful, healthy skin.

3.2.3 Herbs for Treating Skin Conditions

Chamomile

Chamomile is a well-known herb celebrated for its soothing and anti-inflammatory properties. It has been used for centuries to treat a variety of skin conditions, making it a valuable addition to any skincare regimen.

Anti-Inflammatory Properties: Chamomile contains several active compounds, including bisabolol and chamazulene, which have potent anti-inflammatory effects. These compounds help to reduce redness, swelling, and irritation, making chamomile an excellent treatment for inflammatory skin conditions such as eczema and dermatitis.

Soothing and Calming: The soothing nature of chamomile makes it ideal for sensitive skin and for calming irritated areas. It can provide immediate relief to inflamed skin, helping to soothe conditions like rosacea and sunburn.

Antioxidant Benefits: Chamomile is rich in antioxidants, which help to protect the skin from damage caused by free radicals. These antioxidants can prevent premature aging and promote healthy, glowing skin.

Antibacterial and Antifungal: Chamomile possesses antibacterial and antifungal properties, making it effective in treating acne and other bacterial skin infections. It helps to cleanse the skin, reduce bacteria, and prevent breakouts.

Promotes Healing: Chamomile accelerates the healing process of minor wounds and scars. Its anti-inflammatory and soothing properties help to repair and regenerate damaged skin tissues, reducing the appearance of scars and promoting smooth, healthy skin.

Usage Tips:

• ***Chamomile Infused Oil:*** Create a soothing chamomile-infused oil by steeping dried chamomile flowers in a carrier oil like olive or jojoba oil for a few weeks. Apply the oil to irritated or inflamed skin to calm and heal.

• ***Chamomile Face Mask:*** Mix chamomile tea with honey and oatmeal to create a gentle face mask. Apply it to your face, leave it on for 15-20 minutes, then rinse off with lukewarm water. This mask will soothe and hydrate your skin.

• ***Chamomile Toner:*** Brew a strong cup of chamomile tea and let it cool. Use it as a toner by applying it to your face with a cotton pad after cleansing. This toner will reduce redness and calm your skin.

• ***Chamomile Compress:*** Soak a cloth in chamomile tea and apply it to affected areas for 10-15 minutes. This compress can relieve the symptoms of eczema, dermatitis, and other inflammatory skin conditions.

• ***Chamomile Bath:*** Add a few chamomile tea bags or dried chamomile flowers to your bathwater for a calming and skin-soothing soak. This is particularly beneficial for treating widespread skin conditions like eczema.

Incorporating chamomile into your skincare routine can help manage and treat various skin conditions. Its anti-inflammatory, soothing, and antibacterial properties make it a versatile herb for maintaining healthy, calm, and clear skin.

Witch Hazel

Witch hazel is a powerful herb known for its astringent and anti-inflammatory properties, making it a popular choice for treating a variety of skin conditions. Derived from the bark and leaves of the witch hazel shrub (Hamamelis virginiana), it has been used for centuries in skincare remedies.

Astringent Properties: Witch hazel is a natural astringent, which means it can tighten and tone the skin. This helps to reduce the appearance of pores, control excess oil production, and give the skin a smoother, more refined texture. It's particularly beneficial for oily and acne-prone skin.

Anti-Inflammatory Effects: The tannins and flavonoids in witch hazel have strong anti-inflammatory properties. This makes it effective in reducing redness, swelling, and irritation associated with conditions such as acne, eczema, and psoriasis. It can calm inflamed skin and provide relief from itching and discomfort.

Antimicrobial Benefits: Witch hazel has natural antimicrobial properties, which help to cleanse the skin and prevent bacterial infections. It can be used to treat minor cuts, scrapes, and insect bites, reducing the risk of infection and promoting healing.

Soothing Irritated Skin: Witch hazel is excellent for soothing and calming irritated skin. It can be used to relieve sunburn, razor burn, and other forms of skin irritation. Its cooling effect provides immediate comfort and helps to restore the skin's natural balance.

Antioxidant Protection: Rich in antioxidants, witch hazel helps to protect the skin from environmental stressors and free radical damage. This can prevent premature aging and maintain the skin's youthful appearance.

Usage Tips:

•   ***Witch Hazel Toner:*** Use witch hazel as a toner by applying it to your face with a cotton pad after cleansing. This will tighten pores, control oil, and reduce inflammation.

•   ***Acne Treatment:*** Apply witch hazel directly to acne-prone areas with a cotton ball. Its astringent and antimicrobial properties will help to clear up blemishes and prevent new breakouts.

•   ***Soothing Compress:*** Soak a clean cloth in witch hazel and apply it to sunburned or irritated skin for 10-15 minutes. This will reduce redness and soothe discomfort.

•   ***Razor Burn Relief:*** Apply witch hazel to areas affected by razor burn. It will calm the skin and reduce redness and irritation.

•   ***Healing Solution:*** Mix witch hazel with aloe vera gel and apply it to minor cuts and insect bites. This combination will cleanse the area, prevent infection, and promote healing.

Incorporating witch hazel into your skincare routine can provide numerous benefits, particularly for those with oily, acne-prone, or irritated skin. Its astringent, anti-inflammatory, and antimicrobial properties make it a versatile and effective herb for maintaining clear, healthy skin.

Neem

Neem, also known as Azadirachta indica, is a versatile herb renowned for its potent medicinal properties. Originating from the Indian subcontinent, neem has been used for thousands of years in traditional Ayurvedic medicine. It's particularly effective in treating various skin conditions due to its anti-inflammatory, antimicrobial, and healing properties.

Anti-Inflammatory Properties: Neem is rich in compounds like nimbidin and nimbin, which have strong anti-inflammatory effects. These properties make neem effective in reducing redness, swelling, and irritation caused by conditions such as eczema, psoriasis, and dermatitis. Regular use can help calm inflamed skin and provide relief from discomfort.

Antimicrobial and Antifungal Benefits: Neem's powerful antimicrobial properties make it highly effective against bacteria, viruses, and fungi. This is especially beneficial for treating acne, as neem can help eliminate the bacteria that cause breakouts. Its antifungal properties also make it useful for treating fungal infections like ringworm and athlete's foot.

Healing and Regenerative Effects: Neem is rich in antioxidants and essential fatty acids, which promote skin healing and regeneration. It helps to repair damaged skin, reduce scarring, and improve overall skin health. Neem oil can be used to treat minor cuts, wounds, and abrasions, accelerating the healing process.

Detoxifying and Purifying: Neem has detoxifying properties that help purify the skin by removing toxins and impurities. This can lead to a clearer complexion and improved skin tone. Neem's ability to regulate oil production makes it particularly beneficial for oily and acne-prone skin types.

Anti-Aging Benefits: Neem is packed with antioxidants, which protect the skin from free radical damage and environmental stressors. This helps prevent premature aging, reduces the appearance of fine lines and wrinkles, and maintains youthful, healthy skin.

Usage Tips:

•   ***Neem Oil:*** Apply neem oil directly to the skin to treat acne, eczema, and psoriasis. It's also effective for healing minor cuts and wounds. Dilute neem oil with a carrier oil like coconut or jojoba oil to reduce its potency if you have sensitive skin.

•   ***Neem Face Mask:*** Mix neem powder with water or yogurt to create a paste. Apply this mask to the face and leave it on for 10-15 minutes before rinsing off. This will help detoxify the skin, reduce acne, and improve overall complexion.

•   ***Neem Cleanser:*** Use neem-infused cleansers or soaps to cleanse the skin daily. This will help control oil production, prevent breakouts, and keep the skin clear and healthy.

•   ***Neem Bath:*** Add neem leaves or neem powder to your bathwater to soothe and treat skin conditions over the entire body. This is particularly beneficial for eczema and other widespread skin irritations.

•   ***Neem Spot Treatment:*** Apply a small amount of neem oil or neem paste directly to acne spots or other areas of concern. Leave it on overnight to reduce inflammation and speed up healing.

Incorporating neem into your skincare routine can provide numerous benefits, particularly for those with acne-prone, inflamed, or irritated skin. Its anti-inflammatory, antimicrobial, and healing properties make it a powerful and versatile herb for maintaining healthy, clear skin.

3.3 Herbs for Hair Care

Herbs have been utilized for centuries to maintain and enhance hair health, offering natural solutions to common hair problems. These botanical wonders are packed with essential nutrients, vitamins, and minerals that promote hair growth, strengthen strands, and improve overall scalp health. Incorporating herbs into your hair care routine can lead to stronger, shinier, and more resilient hair. In this section, we will explore herbs specifically beneficial for strengthening hair, maintaining scalp health, and enhancing hair shine and texture.

3.3.1 Herbs for Strengthening Hair

Nettle

Nettle, also known as stinging nettle, is a powerful herb packed with a wide range of nutrients that contribute to hair health. Rich in vitamins A, C, and K, as well as essential minerals like iron, magnesium, and calcium, nettle helps to strengthen hair, promote growth, and improve overall scalp health. Nettle's anti-inflammatory properties also make it effective in soothing the scalp and reducing dandruff. Here's an in-depth look at how nettle can benefit your hair:

Nutritional Benefits:

• **Vitamins:** Nettle is rich in vitamins A, C, and K, which are vital for healthy hair growth. Vitamin A helps to produce sebum, an oily substance that moisturizes the scalp. Vitamin C is crucial for collagen production, which strengthens hair strands. Vitamin K supports hair growth and prevents hair loss.

• **Minerals:** The high mineral content, including iron and magnesium, helps to improve blood circulation to the scalp, ensuring that hair follicles receive essential nutrients. Iron is particularly important as it helps to prevent hair loss by supporting red blood cell production.

Usage Tips:

•   ***Nettle Tea:*** Nettle tea can be consumed daily to nourish your hair from the inside out. To make nettle tea, steep 1-2 teaspoons of dried nettle leaves in hot water for about 10-15 minutes. Strain and enjoy. The nutrients in the tea help to strengthen hair and promote healthy growth.

•   ***Nettle Hair Rinse:*** A nettle hair rinse can be used to enhance hair strength and shine. To prepare, boil a handful of fresh nettle leaves in water for about 15 minutes. Let the mixture cool, strain, and use it as a final rinse after shampooing. This rinse can also help to reduce dandruff and soothe an irritated scalp.

•   ***Nettle Oil:*** Nettle oil can be applied directly to the scalp to promote hair growth and strength. To make nettle oil, infuse dried nettle leaves in a carrier oil like olive or coconut oil for several weeks. Massage the infused oil into your scalp and leave it on for at least 30 minutes before washing it out. Regular use can help to prevent hair loss and improve overall hair health.

General Application:

•   ***Nettle Shampoo:*** Look for shampoos and conditioners that contain nettle extract. Using these products regularly can help to strengthen hair and maintain scalp health.

•   ***Nettle Supplements:*** Nettle is also available in supplement form, which can be taken daily to support hair health. Consult with a healthcare provider before starting any new supplement regimen.

Nettle is a versatile herb that can be easily incorporated into your hair care routine. Its high nutrient content makes it an excellent choice for those looking to strengthen their hair, reduce hair loss, and improve scalp health. Whether consumed as a tea, used as a rinse, or applied as an oil, nettle offers a natural and effective way to enhance the vitality of your hair.

Horsetail

Horsetail, a plant with a rich history of use in traditional herbal medicine, is renowned for its ability to strengthen hair and promote healthy growth. This herb is particularly valued for its high silica content, which is essential for hair strength and elasticity. Here's a detailed look at how horsetail can benefit your hair:

Nutritional Benefits:

•   ***Silica:*** Horsetail is one of the richest plant sources of silica, a mineral that strengthens hair and prevents brittleness. Silica helps to maintain hair elasticity, reduces breakage, and enhances shine.

•   ***Antioxidants:*** Horsetail contains antioxidants such as flavonoids and phenolic acids, which protect hair follicles from oxidative stress and damage caused by free radicals.

- **Minerals:** Besides silica, horsetail is also rich in other essential minerals like calcium, potassium, and manganese, which support overall hair health.

Usage Tips:

- **Horsetail Tea:** Drinking horsetail tea regularly can provide your body with the silica and other minerals needed to strengthen hair from within. To prepare horsetail tea, steep 1-2 teaspoons of dried horsetail in hot water for about 10-15 minutes. Strain and enjoy. Consuming this tea can help improve hair texture and reduce hair fall.

- **Horsetail Hair Rinse**: A horsetail hair rinse can be used to strengthen hair and add shine. Boil a handful of fresh or dried horsetail in water for about 15 minutes. Let the mixture cool, strain, and use it as a final rinse after shampooing. This rinse can also help to reduce dandruff and soothe an irritated scalp.

- **Horsetail Extract:** Horsetail extract, available in liquid or capsule form, can be added to your hair care routine. Mix a few drops of liquid horsetail extract into your shampoo or conditioner, or take it as a supplement to support hair health from the inside out.

General Application:

- **Horsetail-Infused Oil:** Infuse horsetail in a carrier oil like jojoba or coconut oil to create a nourishing scalp treatment. Apply the infused oil to your scalp, massage it in, and leave it on for at least 30 minutes before washing it out. Regular use can help to strengthen hair and promote growth.

- **Horsetail Hair Masks:** Incorporate horsetail into homemade hair masks. Mix powdered horsetail with ingredients like yogurt, honey, or avocado to create a strengthening hair mask. Apply the mask to your hair, leave it on for 20-30 minutes, and then rinse thoroughly.

- **Horsetail Supplements:** Horsetail is available in supplement form, which can be taken daily to support hair health. Always consult with a healthcare provider before starting any new supplement regimen.

Horsetail is a powerful ally in the quest for strong, healthy hair. Its high silica content makes it particularly effective in preventing hair breakage, enhancing shine, and improving overall hair strength. Whether consumed as a tea, used as a rinse, or applied as an oil, horsetail offers a natural and effective way to boost hair health and vitality.

Fenugreek

Fenugreek, a popular herb in traditional medicine, is celebrated for its numerous health benefits, particularly for strengthening hair. Rich in proteins, vitamins, and phytonutrients, fenugreek helps nourish hair follicles, promote hair growth, and improve overall hair health. Here's an in-depth look at the benefits of fenugreek for hair:

Nutritional Benefits:

• ***Proteins and Amino Acids***: Fenugreek seeds are packed with proteins and amino acids, which are essential for strengthening the hair shaft and promoting healthy hair growth. These nutrients help repair damaged hair and reduce hair breakage.

• ***Iron and Nicotinic Acid:*** Fenugreek is a good source of iron and nicotinic acid (vitamin B3), which improve blood circulation to the scalp, nourish hair follicles, and stimulate hair growth.

• ***Phytoestrogens:*** These plant-based compounds mimic estrogen and can help balance hormones, potentially reducing hair loss related to hormonal imbalances.

• ***Lecithin:*** Fenugreek contains lecithin, a natural emollient that hydrates and strengthens hair, making it more manageable and less prone to damage.

Usage Tips:

• ***Fenugreek Paste***: A fenugreek paste can be used as a hair mask to nourish and strengthen hair. Soak 2-3 tablespoons of fenugreek seeds in water overnight. Grind the soaked seeds into a fine paste the next morning. Apply the paste to your scalp and hair, leave it on for 30-45 minutes, and then rinse thoroughly with water. This treatment helps reduce hair fall and dandruff while promoting hair growth.

• ***Fenugreek Infused Oil:*** Infuse fenugreek seeds in a carrier oil like coconut or olive oil to create a potent hair oil. Heat the oil slightly, add fenugreek seeds, and let it simmer for a few minutes. Allow the oil to cool, strain, and store it in a bottle. Massage the infused oil into your scalp and hair, leave it on for at least an hour (or overnight), and then wash it out. This oil treatment strengthens hair, adds shine, and promotes growth.

• ***Fenugreek Hair Rinse:*** Prepare a fenugreek hair rinse by boiling a handful of fenugreek seeds in water for 10-15 minutes. Let the mixture cool, strain, and use it as a final rinse after shampooing. This rinse helps condition the hair, making it smooth and manageable.

General Application:

• ***Fenugreek Powder:*** Fenugreek powder can be mixed with other hair-friendly ingredients to create nourishing hair masks. Combine fenugreek powder with yogurt, honey, or aloe vera gel to make a strengthening hair mask. Apply the mask to your hair and scalp, leave it on for 20-30 minutes, and then rinse thoroughly.

•   ***Fenugreek Sprouts:*** Consuming fenugreek sprouts can provide internal nourishment that supports hair health. Fenugreek sprouts are rich in nutrients that promote healthy hair growth and improve overall hair vitality. Add them to your salads, smoothies, or meals for a nutritional boost.

•   ***Fenugreek Supplements:*** Fenugreek supplements are available in capsule form and can be taken daily to support hair health. Always consult with a healthcare provider before starting any new supplement regimen.

Fenugreek is a versatile and powerful herb for hair care. Its rich nutritional profile makes it an excellent natural remedy for strengthening hair, promoting growth, and improving scalp health. Whether used as a paste, infused oil, rinse, or supplement, fenugreek offers numerous benefits for achieving strong, healthy, and vibrant hair.

3.3.2 Scalp Health and Detoxifying Herbs

Peppermint

Peppermint is a well-known herb with a multitude of benefits for scalp health and detoxification. Its cooling and soothing properties make it an ideal choice for addressing various scalp issues such as itching, dryness, and dandruff. Here's a detailed exploration of peppermint's benefits and uses for scalp health:

Benefits:

•   ***Cooling and Soothing***: Peppermint contains menthol, which provides a cooling sensation that can soothe irritated and itchy scalps. This makes it particularly effective in relieving discomfort caused by conditions like dandruff and scalp inflammation.

•   ***Antimicrobial Properties:*** The antimicrobial and antifungal properties of peppermint help cleanse the scalp of bacteria, fungi, and other pathogens that can cause scalp infections and dandruff.

•   ***Improves Blood Circulation:*** Peppermint oil can stimulate blood circulation to the scalp, promoting healthy hair growth by ensuring that hair follicles receive the nutrients and oxygen they need.

•   ***Balances Scalp Oils***: Peppermint helps regulate the production of sebum (natural scalp oil), making it beneficial for both dry and oily scalps. It can moisturize a dry scalp while also preventing excess oil buildup.

Usage Tips:

•   ***Peppermint Oil Scalp Massage:*** Dilute a few drops of peppermint essential oil in a carrier oil like coconut or jojoba oil. Massage this mixture into your scalp using gentle circular motions. This can help stimulate blood flow, reduce scalp irritation, and promote hair growth. Leave it on for at least 15-20 minutes before washing it out with shampoo.

• **Peppermint Hair Rinse:** Prepare a peppermint hair rinse by adding a few drops of peppermint essential oil to a bowl of water. After shampooing and conditioning, pour this mixture over your scalp and hair as a final rinse. This rinse will leave your scalp feeling refreshed and invigorated.

• **Peppermint Infused Shampoo:** Add a few drops of peppermint essential oil to your regular shampoo to enhance its cleansing and invigorating properties. This can help keep your scalp clean and healthy while providing a refreshing sensation with each wash.

• **DIY Peppermint Scalp Spray**: Create a peppermint scalp spray by mixing water, a few drops of peppermint essential oil, and a tablespoon of witch hazel in a spray bottle. Shake well and spritz this mixture onto your scalp to refresh and soothe it throughout the day. This is particularly useful during hot weather or after intense physical activities.

General Application:

• **Peppermint Tea Rinse:** Brew a strong peppermint tea by steeping peppermint leaves in boiling water for 10-15 minutes. Allow the tea to cool and use it as a hair rinse after shampooing. This not only helps cleanse the scalp but also adds a pleasant fragrance to your hair.

• **Peppermint Scalp Scrub:** Mix peppermint oil with sugar and a carrier oil to create a scalp scrub. Gently massage this scrub into your scalp to exfoliate and remove dead skin cells, promoting a healthy scalp environment.

• **Peppermint and Aloe Vera Gel:** Combine peppermint oil with aloe vera gel to create a soothing scalp treatment. Apply this mixture to your scalp to calm irritation and provide hydration.

Peppermint is a powerful herb for maintaining a healthy scalp. Its cooling, antimicrobial, and circulation-boosting properties make it a versatile ingredient in various scalp treatments. Regular use of peppermint in your hair care routine can lead to a refreshed, balanced, and healthy scalp environment, ultimately supporting better hair growth and overall scalp health.

Tea Tree

Tea tree oil, derived from the leaves of the Melaleuca alternifolia plant, is renowned for its potent antiseptic and anti-inflammatory properties. It is widely used in hair and scalp care for its ability to treat various scalp conditions and promote a healthy environment for hair growth. Here's an in-depth look at tea tree oil's benefits and uses for scalp health and detoxification:

enefits:

• **_Antimicrobial Properties:_** Tea tree oil is highly effective against bacteria, fungi, and viruses, making it an excellent choice for treating scalp infections, dandruff, and seborrheic dermatitis.

• **_Reduces Inflammation:_** Its anti-inflammatory properties help soothe irritated and inflamed scalps, providing relief from itching and discomfort.

• **_Cleanses and Unclogs Hair Follicles:_** Tea tree oil helps remove excess oil, dirt, and dead skin cells from the scalp, which can clog hair follicles and hinder hair growth.

• **_Balances Scalp Oil Production:_** It regulates the production of sebum, ensuring the scalp is neither too dry nor too oily, which helps maintain a balanced and healthy scalp environment.

Usage Tips:

• **_Tea Tree Oil Scalp Treatment:_** Mix a few drops of tea tree oil with a carrier oil such as coconut or olive oil. Apply this mixture to your scalp and massage gently. Leave it on for 20-30 minutes before washing it out with a mild shampoo. This treatment helps combat dandruff and soothe scalp irritation.

• **_Tea Tree Oil Shampoo:_** Add a few drops of tea tree oil to your regular shampoo to enhance its cleansing properties. Use this shampoo to wash your hair as usual. This can help keep your scalp free from infections and reduce dandruff.

• **_Tea Tree Hair Rinse_**: Prepare a hair rinse by adding a few drops of tea tree oil to a bowl of water. After shampooing, pour this rinse over your scalp and hair. This can help cleanse your scalp and leave it feeling refreshed.

• **_Tea Tree Oil Scalp Spray:_** Create a scalp spray by mixing water, a few drops of tea tree oil, and a tablespoon of witch hazel in a spray bottle. Shake well and spritz this mixture onto your scalp to refresh and soothe it throughout the day.

General Application:

• **_Tea Tree and Aloe Vera Gel:_** Combine tea tree oil with aloe vera gel to create a soothing and hydrating scalp treatment. Apply this mixture to your scalp to calm irritation and provide moisture.

• **_Tea Tree Oil Hair Mask:_** Mix tea tree oil with yogurt or honey to create a nourishing hair mask. Apply this mask to your scalp and hair, leave it on for 20-30 minutes, and then rinse thoroughly. This mask helps cleanse the scalp and promotes healthy hair growth.

• **_Tea Tree and Apple Cider Vinegar Rinse:_** Combine tea tree oil with apple cider vinegar and water to create a detoxifying scalp rinse. Use this rinse after shampooing to help balance the scalp's pH and remove buildup.

General Use:

• **_Tea Tree Oil and Baking Soda Scrub:_** Create a scalp scrub by mixing tea tree oil with baking soda and water. Gently massage this scrub into your scalp to exfoliate and remove dead skin cells, promoting a clean and healthy scalp environment.

• **_Tea Tree Oil Infused Conditioner:_** Add a few drops of tea tree oil to your conditioner for an extra boost of antimicrobial and soothing benefits. Use this conditioner regularly to maintain a healthy scalp.

Tea tree oil is a powerful ally in scalp health and detoxification. Its antimicrobial, anti-inflammatory, and cleansing properties make it a versatile ingredient for treating various scalp conditions and promoting overall scalp health. Regular use of tea tree oil in your hair care routine can lead to a clean, balanced, and healthy scalp, which supports optimal hair growth and reduces common scalp issues.

Sage

Sage, scientifically known as Salvia officinalis, is a versatile herb with a long history of medicinal and culinary uses. In hair and scalp care, sage is celebrated for its detoxifying, antimicrobial, and soothing properties. It is particularly beneficial for maintaining a healthy scalp environment and promoting hair growth. Here's an in-depth look at sage's benefits and uses for scalp health and detoxification:

Benefits:

• **_Antimicrobial Properties:_** Sage has natural antimicrobial properties that help combat bacteria and fungi on the scalp, reducing the risk of infections and dandruff.

• **_Anti-Inflammatory Effects:_** It helps soothe scalp inflammation and irritation, providing relief from itching and discomfort associated with various scalp conditions.

• **_Detoxifying Action:_** Sage aids in detoxifying the scalp by removing excess oils, dirt, and product buildup, which can clog hair follicles and impede hair growth.

• **_Stimulates Hair Growth:_** The stimulating properties of sage improve blood circulation to the scalp, encouraging hair follicles to produce stronger and healthier hair.

• **_Balances Oil Production:_** Sage helps regulate sebum production, ensuring the scalp remains balanced and not overly greasy or dry.

Usage Tips:

• **_Sage Infused Rinse:_** Prepare a sage rinse by steeping fresh or dried sage leaves in hot water for 15-20 minutes. Once cooled, strain the liquid and use it as a final rinse after shampooing. This rinse helps cleanse the scalp, reduce dandruff, and leave the hair with a healthy shine.

- ***Sage and Apple Cider Vinegar Scalp Toner***: Mix sage tea with apple cider vinegar in equal parts. Apply this toner to your scalp using a cotton ball or spray bottle. This combination helps balance the scalp's pH, reduce dandruff, and detoxify the scalp.

- ***Sage Oil Massage:*** Dilute a few drops of sage essential oil in a carrier oil, such as jojoba or olive oil. Massage this mixture into your scalp and leave it on for at least 30 minutes before washing it out. This treatment helps improve blood circulation, stimulate hair growth, and detoxify the scalp.

General Application:

- ***Sage Hair Mask:*** Combine sage leaves with yogurt or honey to create a nourishing hair mask. Apply this mask to your scalp and hair, leave it on for 20-30 minutes, and then rinse thoroughly. This mask helps soothe and detoxify the scalp while providing moisture to the hair.

- ***Sage and Rosemary Scalp Spray:*** Prepare a scalp spray by mixing sage tea with rosemary essential oil and water. Use this spray to refresh and cleanse your scalp between washes, reducing oiliness and promoting a healthy scalp environment.

- ***Sage and Tea Tree Oil Scrub:*** Create an exfoliating scalp scrub by mixing sage leaves, tea tree oil, and sugar. Gently massage this scrub into your scalp to remove dead skin cells and buildup, promoting a clean and healthy scalp.

General Use:

- ***Sage and Mint Scalp Refresh:*** Combine sage leaves with mint leaves and steep them in hot water. Once cooled, use this infusion as a scalp refresh spray to invigorate the scalp and reduce itchiness.

- ***Sage-Infused Shampoo:*** Add sage tea to your regular shampoo to enhance its cleansing properties. Use this shampoo to wash your hair as usual, benefiting from sage's antimicrobial and detoxifying effects.

- ***Sage and Lemon Hair Rinse:*** Prepare a hair rinse by mixing sage tea with lemon juice. After shampooing, pour this rinse over your scalp and hair to cleanse and detoxify. The lemon juice adds an extra boost of clarifying properties, leaving your scalp feeling fresh and clean.

Sage is a powerful herb for maintaining scalp health and detoxification. Its antimicrobial, anti-inflammatory, and detoxifying properties make it an excellent choice for treating various scalp issues and promoting a healthy environment for hair growth. Incorporating sage into your hair care routine can lead to a balanced, clean, and healthy scalp, supporting strong and vibrant hair.

3.3.3 Herbs for Enhancing Hair Shine and Texture

Hibiscus

Hibiscus, known for its vibrant flowers, is more than just a beautiful plant; it is a powerful herb for hair care. Scientifically known as Hibiscus rosa-sinensis, this herb is renowned for its ability to enhance hair shine, improve texture, and promote overall hair health. Here's an in-depth look at the benefits and uses of hibiscus for hair care:

Benefits:

• *Enhances Hair Shine:* Hibiscus flowers are rich in vitamins and antioxidants that help to restore the natural luster of hair, making it appear shiny and vibrant.

• *Improves Hair Texture:* The mucilage content in hibiscus acts as a natural conditioner, smoothing the hair cuticle and improving hair texture.

• *Strengthens Hair:* Hibiscus is packed with amino acids that nourish hair roots, strengthen hair strands, and reduce breakage.

• *Promotes Hair Growth:* The nourishing properties of hibiscus stimulate blood circulation to the scalp, encouraging the growth of healthy, strong hair.

• *Reduces Dandruff and Itchiness:* Its antimicrobial properties help to combat dandruff and soothe an itchy scalp, promoting a healthier scalp environment.

Usage Tips:

• *Hibiscus Hair Rinse:* Prepare a hair rinse by steeping hibiscus petals in hot water for 15-20 minutes. Allow the mixture to cool, then strain and use it as a final rinse after shampooing. This rinse will add shine and softness to your hair.

• *Hibiscus Hair Mask:* Make a hair mask by grinding fresh hibiscus petals into a paste and mixing it with yogurt or coconut milk. Apply the mask to your hair and scalp, leave it on for 30-45 minutes, and then rinse thoroughly. This mask helps to deeply condition and nourish your hair.

• *Hibiscus Oil:* Infuse hibiscus petals in a carrier oil such as coconut or olive oil. Massage the infused oil into your scalp and hair, leave it on for at least 30 minutes (or overnight for better results), and then wash it out. This oil treatment enhances shine, improves texture, and strengthens hair.

General Application:

• *Hibiscus and Aloe Vera Gel:* Combine hibiscus powder with aloe vera gel to create a soothing and hydrating hair treatment. Apply this mixture to your hair and scalp, leave it on for 20-30 minutes, and then rinse thoroughly. This treatment helps to smooth the hair cuticle and add shine.

- *Hibiscus and Henna Pack:* Mix hibiscus powder with henna powder and water to create a conditioning hair pack. Apply the pack to your hair, leave it on for 1-2 hours, and then rinse thoroughly. This pack not only conditions the hair but also enhances its natural color and shine.

- *Hibiscus Tea Hair Spray:* Prepare a strong hibiscus tea and pour it into a spray bottle. Use this spray on damp hair as a leave-in conditioner to add shine and improve hair texture throughout the day.

General Use:

- *Hibiscus and Honey Hair Mask:* Mix hibiscus powder with honey to create a moisturizing hair mask. Apply the mask to your hair and scalp, leave it on for 20-30 minutes, and then rinse thoroughly. This mask helps to hydrate and soften hair, leaving it shiny and smooth.

- *Hibiscus and Coconut Oil Treatment:* Combine hibiscus powder with coconut oil to create a nourishing hair treatment. Apply the mixture to your hair and scalp, leave it on for 30-45 minutes, and then rinse thoroughly. This treatment helps to condition and add shine to the hair.

- *Hibiscus and Rice Water Rinse*: Prepare a hair rinse by mixing hibiscus tea with rice water. Use this rinse after shampooing to enhance shine and improve hair texture. The combination of hibiscus and rice water provides a powerful boost of nutrients for your hair.

Hibiscus is a versatile herb that offers numerous benefits for hair care. Its ability to enhance shine, improve texture, and promote overall hair health makes it an excellent addition to any hair care routine. By incorporating hibiscus into your hair care regimen, you can achieve lustrous, healthy, and beautiful hair.

Rosemary

Rosemary, scientifically known as Rosmarinus officinalis, is a fragrant herb commonly used in culinary dishes, but it also offers significant benefits for hair care. Known for its invigorating properties, rosemary is a powerful herb that enhances hair shine, improves texture, and promotes overall hair health. Here's an in-depth look at the benefits and uses of rosemary for hair care:

Benefits:

- *Enhances Hair Shine:* Rosemary stimulates blood circulation in the scalp, which helps to rejuvenate hair follicles and add a natural shine to the hair.

- *Improves Hair Texture:* The herb contains ursolic acid, which strengthens hair strands, making them smoother and more manageable.

- *Promotes Hair Growth:* Rosemary has been shown to encourage hair growth by stimulating blood flow to the scalp, which helps in delivering essential nutrients to hair follicles.

- **Reduces Dandruff and Scalp Irritation:** Its anti-inflammatory and antimicrobial properties help to combat dandruff and soothe an itchy scalp, creating a healthier environment for hair growth.

- **Prevents Premature Graying:** Regular use of rosemary can help in preventing premature graying of hair due to its antioxidant properties.

Usage Tips:

- **Rosemary Hair Rinse:** Prepare a hair rinse by steeping fresh or dried rosemary leaves in hot water for 15-20 minutes. Allow the mixture to cool, then strain and use it as a final rinse after shampooing. This rinse will add shine and vitality to your hair.

- **Rosemary Oil:** Infuse rosemary leaves in a carrier oil such as olive or coconut oil. Massage the infused oil into your scalp and hair, leave it on for at least 30 minutes (or overnight for better results), and then wash it out. This oil treatment enhances shine, improves texture, and strengthens hair.

- **Rosemary Hair Mask:** Create a hair mask by mixing rosemary powder with yogurt or honey. Apply the mask to your hair and scalp, leave it on for 30-45 minutes, and then rinse thoroughly. This mask helps to condition and nourish your hair, making it shinier and healthier.

General Application:

- **Rosemary and Aloe Vera Gel:** Combine rosemary essential oil with aloe vera gel to create a soothing and hydrating hair treatment. Apply this mixture to your hair and scalp, leave it on for 20-30 minutes, and then rinse thoroughly. This treatment helps to smooth the hair cuticle and add shine.

- **Rosemary and Henna Pack:** Mix rosemary powder with henna powder and water to create a conditioning hair pack. Apply the pack to your hair, leave it on for 1-2 hours, and then rinse thoroughly. This pack not only conditions the hair but also enhances its natural color and shine.

- **Rosemary Tea Hair Spray:** Prepare a strong rosemary tea and pour it into a spray bottle. Use this spray on damp hair as a leave-in conditioner to add shine and improve hair texture throughout the day.

General Use:

- **Rosemary and Honey Hair Mask**: Mix rosemary essential oil with honey to create a moisturizing hair mask. Apply the mask to your hair and scalp, leave it on for 20-30 minutes, and then rinse thoroughly. This mask helps to hydrate and soften hair, leaving it shiny and smooth.

- **Rosemary and Coconut Oil Treatment:** Combine rosemary essential oil with coconut oil to create a nourishing hair treatment. Apply the mixture to your hair and scalp, leave it on for 30-45 minutes, and then rinse thoroughly. This treatment helps to condition and add shine to the hair.

- ***Rosemary and Rice Water Rinse:*** Prepare a hair rinse by mixing rosemary tea with rice water. Use this rinse after shampooing to enhance shine and improve hair texture. The combination of rosemary and rice water provides a powerful boost of nutrients for your hair.

Rosemary is a versatile herb that offers numerous benefits for hair care. Its ability to enhance shine, improve texture, and promote overall hair health makes it an excellent addition to any hair care routine. By incorporating rosemary into your hair care regimen, you can achieve lustrous, healthy, and beautiful hair.

Lavender

Lavender, scientifically known as Lavandula angustifolia, is a well-known herb famed for its calming fragrance and therapeutic properties. When it comes to hair care, lavender offers a range of benefits that enhance hair shine, improve texture, and promote overall scalp health. Here's an in-depth look at the benefits and uses of lavender for hair care:

Benefits:

- ***Enhances Hair Shine:*** Lavender oil helps to smooth the hair cuticle, adding a natural shine and making the hair look healthier and more vibrant.

- ***Improves Hair Texture:*** Its moisturizing properties help to soften the hair, improving its texture and making it more manageable.

- ***Promotes Hair Growth:*** Lavender oil has been shown to promote hair growth by increasing blood circulation to the scalp, which helps deliver nutrients to the hair follicles.

- ***Reduces Dandruff and Itchy Scalp:*** Its antimicrobial and anti-inflammatory properties help to reduce dandruff and soothe an itchy scalp, promoting a healthier scalp environment.

- ***Calms and Relaxes:*** The calming scent of lavender can help reduce stress and anxiety, which are often linked to hair loss and poor hair health.

Usage Tips:

- ***Lavender Hair Rinse:*** Prepare a hair rinse by steeping fresh or dried lavender flowers in hot water for 15-20 minutes. Allow the mixture to cool, then strain and use it as a final rinse after shampooing. This rinse will add shine and fragrance to your hair.

- ***Lavender Oil Massage:*** Mix a few drops of lavender essential oil with a carrier oil such as jojoba or coconut oil. Massage the mixture into your scalp and hair, leave it on for at least 30 minutes (or overnight for better results), and then wash it out. This oil treatment enhances shine, improves texture, and promotes relaxation.

• **_Lavender Infused Conditioner:_** Add a few drops of lavender essential oil to your regular conditioner to boost its moisturizing and soothing properties. Use this enhanced conditioner as usual to leave your hair soft, shiny, and fragrant.

General Application:

• **_Lavender and Aloe Vera Gel_**: Combine lavender essential oil with aloe vera gel to create a soothing and hydrating hair treatment. Apply this mixture to your hair and scalp, leave it on for 20-30 minutes, and then rinse thoroughly. This treatment helps to smooth the hair cuticle and add shine.

• **_Lavender and Honey Hair Mask:_** Mix lavender essential oil with honey to create a moisturizing hair mask. Apply the mask to your hair and scalp, leave it on for 20-30 minutes, and then rinse thoroughly. This mask helps to hydrate and soften hair, leaving it shiny and smooth.

• **_Lavender Hair Mist:_** Prepare a lavender hair mist by mixing lavender essential oil with distilled water in a spray bottle. Use this mist on damp or dry hair to add shine, fragrance, and improve hair texture throughout the day.

General Use:

• **_Lavender and Coconut Oil Treatment:_** Combine lavender essential oil with coconut oil to create a nourishing hair treatment. Apply the mixture to your hair and scalp, leave it on for 30-45 minutes, and then rinse thoroughly. This treatment helps to condition and add shine to the hair.

• **_Lavender and Rice Water Rinse:_** Prepare a hair rinse by mixing lavender tea with rice water. Use this rinse after shampooing to enhance shine and improve hair texture. The combination of lavender and rice water provides a powerful boost of nutrients for your hair.

• **_Lavender and Yogurt Hair Mask:_** Mix lavender essential oil with yogurt to create a conditioning hair mask. Apply the mask to your hair and scalp, leave it on for 20-30 minutes, and then rinse thoroughly. This mask helps to nourish and hydrate your hair, leaving it shiny and healthy.

Lavender is a versatile herb that offers numerous benefits for hair care. Its ability to enhance shine, improve texture, and promote overall scalp health makes it an excellent addition to any hair care routine. By incorporating lavender into your hair care regimen, you can achieve lustrous, healthy, and beautiful hair.

Chapter 4: Step-by-Step Guides for Creating Herbal Beauty Treatments

4.1 Making Herbal Infusions for Beauty Products

Herbal infusions are a cornerstone of natural beauty routines, harnessing the therapeutic properties of herbs to create potent, effective beauty treatments. By soaking herbs in a carrier liquid, you can extract their beneficial compounds and use them to enhance your skincare and haircare products. This process allows you to customize your beauty regimen with natural ingredients tailored to your specific needs. In this section, we'll explore the fundamentals of making herbal infusions, from the basics of the process to specific methods for creating oil-based and water-based infusions.

4.1.1 Basics of Herbal Infusion Making

Herbal infusions are a simple yet powerful way to incorporate the benefits of herbs into your beauty routine. Here's a step-by-step guide to get you started:

Choosing the Right Herbs

The first step in making an effective herbal infusion is selecting the appropriate herbs. Different herbs offer various benefits, so it's important to choose based on your specific needs:

• **Chamomile:** Known for its soothing and anti-inflammatory properties, chamomile is excellent for calming irritated skin and reducing redness.

• **Rosemary:** This herb is great for stimulating hair growth and improving scalp health due to its circulation-boosting properties.

• **Lavender:** With its calming scent and antibacterial properties, lavender is ideal for treating acne-prone skin and promoting relaxation.

• **Calendula:** Famous for its healing and moisturizing benefits, calendula is perfect for dry or damaged skin.

- **Peppermint**: This herb is known for its cooling and refreshing properties, making it ideal for oily or acne-prone skin.

Preparation

Proper preparation is crucial for maximizing the benefits of your herbal infusion:

1. **Use Dried Herbs**: Dried herbs are preferred because they have a more concentrated amount of active compounds and are less likely to introduce moisture that could cause mold growth.

2. **Crush or Chop the Herbs**: Breaking down the herbs increases their surface area, allowing for better extraction of their beneficial compounds. You can use a mortar and pestle or simply chop them finely with a knife.

Infusing the Herbs

The process of infusing herbs involves soaking them in a carrier liquid to extract their beneficial properties:

1. **Place Herbs in a Jar:** Put the prepared herbs in a clean, dry glass jar. The amount of herbs you use can vary, but a good rule of thumb is to fill the jar about halfway with herbs.

2. **Add the Carrier Liquid:** Cover the herbs completely with your chosen carrier liquid. This can be oil (like jojoba, olive, or coconut) for oil-based infusions, or water (preferably distilled or purified) for water-based infusions. Ensure that all the herbs are submerged to prevent mold growth.

3. **Seal the Jar Tightly:** Use a lid to seal the jar tightly, ensuring no air can get in.

Steeping

The steeping process allows the herbs to infuse their beneficial compounds into the carrier liquid:

1. **Steep Time:** Allow the herbs to steep in the liquid for a period ranging from a few hours to several weeks. The duration depends on the type of herbs and the desired strength of the infusion. For a quicker infusion, you can gently heat the mixture using a double boiler method for a few hours.

2. **Storage Conditions: Keep** the jar in a cool, dark place during the steeping period. This helps to preserve the potency of the herbs and prevents the breakdown of beneficial compounds due to light exposure.

3. **Occasional Shaking:** Shake the jar gently every few days to help mix the contents and promote even extraction.

Straining and Storage

Once your infusion has reached the desired strength, it's time to strain and store it:

1.   ***Strain the Herbs:*** Use a fine mesh strainer or cheesecloth to strain out the herbs from the liquid. Make sure to press or squeeze the herbs to extract as much liquid as possible.

2.   ***Storage:*** Pour the strained infusion into a clean, airtight container. Dark glass bottles are ideal for storage as they protect the infusion from light, which can degrade its quality.

3.   ***Label and Date:*** Always label your infusions with the date they were made and the type of herbs used. This helps you keep track of their shelf life and potency. Generally, oil-based infusions can last up to a year, while water-based infusions should be used within a week and stored in the refrigerator.

By following these steps, you can create effective and personalized herbal infusions that enhance your beauty routine naturally and effectively.

4.1.2 Infusing Herbs into Oils

Herb-infused oils are a versatile base for many beauty products, providing nourishing and healing properties for skin and hair. The process of making these oils is straightforward and can be easily done at home. Here's a detailed guide to help you create your own herb-infused oils:

Selecting the Oil

Choosing the right carrier oil is crucial for the effectiveness of your infusion. Here are some popular options:

•   ***Jojoba Oil:*** Known for its similarity to the natural oils of the skin, jojoba oil is excellent for all skin types, particularly oily and acne-prone skin. It absorbs quickly and doesn't clog pores.

•   ***Coconut Oil:*** Rich in fatty acids, coconut oil is highly moisturizing and antibacterial, making it ideal for dry skin and hair. It solidifies at cooler temperatures, which can affect the infusion process.

•   ***Olive Oil:*** This oil is deeply nourishing and has anti-inflammatory properties. It's suitable for most skin types but is especially beneficial for dry and mature skin.

Preparing the Herbs

Using dried herbs is essential to prevent mold and bacteria growth in your infused oil. Here's how to prepare them:

1.   ***Dry the Herbs:*** Ensure your herbs are completely dried before using them. Fresh herbs contain water, which can lead to spoilage.

2.   ***Crush or Chop the Herbs***: Breaking down the herbs increases their surface area, helping to release their beneficial oils and compounds more effectively. Use a mortar and pestle or simply chop them finely.

Infusion Process

The infusion process involves soaking the prepared herbs in the chosen oil to extract their beneficial properties:

1.   ***Place the Herbs in a Jar:*** Fill a clean, dry glass jar about halfway with the crushed or chopped herbs.

2.   ***Cover with Carrier Oil:*** Pour the carrier oil over the herbs, making sure they are fully submerged. This helps to prevent any mold from forming.

3.   ***Seal the Jar:*** Close the jar tightly with a lid to prevent any air from entering, which could lead to oxidation and spoilage of the oil.

4.   ***Choose Your Infusion Method:***

- Sunlight Method: Place the sealed jar in a sunny spot for 2-6 weeks. The warmth from the sun helps to infuse the herbs into the oil gradually. Shake the jar every few days to mix the contents.
- Gentle Heat Method: If you prefer a quicker method, use a double boiler to gently heat the jar of oil and herbs. Simmer on low heat for a few hours, ensuring the oil doesn't get too hot, as excessive heat can destroy the beneficial properties of the herbs.

Straining and Storing

Once your infusion has reached the desired strength, it's time to strain and store it:

1.   ***Strain the Herbs:*** Using a fine mesh strainer or cheesecloth, strain the herbs out of the oil. Make sure to press or squeeze the herbs to extract as much oil as possible.

2.   ***Store the Infused Oil:*** Pour the strained oil into a clean, dark glass bottle. Dark glass helps to protect the oil from light, which can degrade its quality. Seal the bottle tightly.

3.   ***Label and Date:*** Always label your infused oil with the date and the type of herbs used. This helps you keep track of its freshness. Store the bottle in a cool, dry place. Herb-infused oils generally have a shelf life of about six months to a year, depending on the type of oil used.

Uses for Herb-Infused Oils

Herb-infused oils can be used in a variety of beauty products:

- **_Moisturizers:_** Use the infused oil directly on your skin or mix it with other ingredients to create a personalized moisturizer.

- **_Hair Treatments:_** Apply the oil to your scalp and hair for a nourishing treatment that can help with dryness and promote healthy growth.

- **_Massage Oils:_** The infused oils can be used for soothing and therapeutic massages, enhancing relaxation and skin health.

By following these steps, you can create custom herb-infused oils tailored to your beauty needs, harnessing the natural power of herbs to enhance your skin and hair health.

4.2 Creating Custom Herbal Blends for Skincare

Creating custom herbal blends for skincare allows you to tailor your beauty routine to your skin's unique needs. By combining various herbs known for their specific properties, you can address a range of skin concerns and enhance your skin's health and appearance. Whether you are dealing with dryness, irritation, or the effects of aging, there's an herbal blend that can help. This section will guide you through the process of creating blends for different skin types, anti-inflammatory blends for irritated skin, and antioxidant-rich blends for anti-aging.

4.2.1 Tailoring Blends for Different Skin Types

Understanding your skin type is crucial when creating custom herbal blends. Each skin type has unique needs that can be addressed with specific herbs. Here are some recommended blends for oily, dry, combination, and sensitive skin:

Oily Skin

Oily skin can benefit from herbs that balance oil production and have astringent properties to tighten pores and reduce shine.

- Witch Hazel: Known for its astringent properties, witch hazel helps to control oil and reduce pore size.

- Lemon Balm: This herb has antibacterial properties and can help regulate sebum production.

- Rosemary: It's excellent for stimulating circulation and balancing oil production.

Suggested Blend: Combine equal parts of dried witch hazel, lemon balm, and rosemary. Infuse the blend in distilled water to create a toner, or infuse it in a light carrier oil like grapeseed oil for a facial serum.

Dry Skin

Dry skin needs herbs that provide hydration and nourishment, helping to lock in moisture and soothe flaky patches.

- Calendula: With its moisturizing and healing properties, calendula is perfect for dry skin.

- Aloe Vera: Known for its hydrating properties, aloe vera helps to soothe and moisturize dry skin.

- Chamomile: This soothing herb helps to calm and hydrate dry, irritated skin.

Suggested Blend: Mix equal parts of dried calendula, aloe vera, and chamomile. Infuse in a gentle carrier oil like almond oil for a hydrating facial oil, or use as a base for a moisturizing cream.

Combination Skin

Combination skin benefits from herbs that balance oil production in the T-zone while providing hydration to dry areas.

- Lavender: Balances oil production and soothes dry areas.

- Green Tea: Rich in antioxidants, green tea helps to reduce oiliness and prevent breakouts.

- Rose: Hydrates and soothes dry patches while balancing the skin.

Suggested Blend: Combine equal parts of dried lavender, green tea, and rose petals. Infuse in witch hazel to create a balancing toner, or infuse in jojoba oil for a lightweight facial oil.

Sensitive Skin

Sensitive skin requires gentle, soothing herbs that calm irritation and reduce redness without causing further sensitivity.

- Chamomile: Extremely gentle and soothing, chamomile is perfect for sensitive skin.

- Calendula: Known for its healing and anti-inflammatory properties, calendula helps to calm sensitive skin.

- Oat Straw: This herb is excellent for soothing and reducing irritation.

Suggested Blend: Mix equal parts of dried chamomile, calendula, and oat straw. Infuse in distilled water to create a soothing toner, or infuse in a gentle carrier oil like apricot kernel oil for a calming facial oil.

Tips for Creating and Using Custom Blends

• Patch Test: Always perform a patch test when trying a new herbal blend to ensure you do not have any adverse reactions.

• Consistency: Use your herbal blends consistently to see the best results. Incorporate them into your daily skincare routine.

• Storage: Store your herbal blends in dark, airtight containers to preserve their potency and extend their shelf life.

Creating custom herbal blends tailored to your skin type can transform your skincare routine, providing targeted solutions to meet your specific needs.

4.2.2 Anti-Inflammatory Blends for Irritated Skin

Creating anti-inflammatory blends for irritated skin involves selecting herbs known for their soothing and calming properties. These herbs can help reduce redness, swelling, and discomfort associated with inflammation. Here are detailed descriptions and usage tips for chamomile, calendula, and green tea:

Chamomile

Chamomile is renowned for its anti-inflammatory and soothing properties, making it an excellent choice for irritated skin. Its natural compounds, such as chamazulene and bisabolol, help to calm redness and reduce swelling.

Uses:

• Chamomile Infusion: Prepare a strong chamomile infusion by steeping dried chamomile flowers in boiling water for 15-20 minutes. Once cooled, use the infusion as a facial toner to soothe irritated skin.

• Chamomile Compress: Soak a clean cloth in chamomile tea and apply it as a compress to inflamed areas to reduce redness and swelling.

• Chamomile Face Mask: Mix chamomile powder with honey and apply it to the face as a calming mask. Leave on for 15 minutes before rinsing off with warm water.

Benefits:

• Reduces redness and irritation.

• Soothes inflamed skin.

• Provides gentle hydration.

Calendula

Calendula, also known as marigold, is highly effective in treating various skin conditions due to its anti-inflammatory and healing properties. It is rich in flavonoids and saponins, which help to reduce inflammation and promote skin repair.

Uses:

• Calendula Oil: Infuse dried calendula flowers in a carrier oil such as olive or almond oil. Apply the oil directly to irritated skin to help reduce inflammation and speed up healing.

• Calendula Cream: Add calendula-infused oil to a homemade cream base for a soothing and hydrating skin treatment.

• Calendula Bath Soak: Add dried calendula petals to a warm bath to soothe and calm irritated skin over the entire body.

Benefits:

• Promotes skin healing.

• Reduces redness and irritation.

• Moisturizes and soothes dry, inflamed skin.

Green Tea

Green tea is rich in antioxidants and polyphenols, particularly epigallocatechin gallate (EGCG), which has strong anti-inflammatory and skin-soothing properties. It helps to calm irritated skin and protect it from environmental damage.

Uses:

• Green Tea Toner: Brew a strong green tea and let it cool. Use it as a facial toner to calm irritated skin and reduce redness.

• Green Tea Face Mist: Pour cooled green tea into a spray bottle and mist it onto the face throughout the day for a refreshing and soothing effect.

• Green Tea Face Mask: Mix green tea powder with yogurt and honey to create a calming face mask. Apply to the skin and leave on for 15-20 minutes before rinsing off.

Benefits:

• Reduces inflammation and redness.

• Provides antioxidant protection.

- Calms and soothes irritated skin.

Tips for Creating Anti-Inflammatory Blends

1.   Combine Herbs: For enhanced benefits, consider combining chamomile, calendula, and green tea in your blends. For example, you can create a soothing facial toner by mixing equal parts of chamomile and green tea infusions.

2.   Use Gentle Carriers: When making oil infusions or creams, choose gentle carrier oils like jojoba or almond oil that are less likely to irritate sensitive skin.

3.   Storage: Store your anti-inflammatory blends in dark, airtight containers to preserve their potency and prevent degradation.

By incorporating these herbs into your skincare routine, you can effectively manage inflammation and soothe irritated skin, leading to a healthier, more balanced complexion.

4.2.3 Antioxidant-Rich Blends for Anti-Aging

Antioxidant-rich herbs are powerful allies in the fight against aging, as they help to combat free radicals and promote skin regeneration. Incorporating these herbs into your skincare routine can lead to a more youthful, radiant complexion. Here are detailed descriptions and usage tips for rosehip, pomegranate, and ginkgo biloba:

Rosehip

Rosehip is packed with vitamins A and C, essential fatty acids, and antioxidants, making it an excellent choice for anti-aging skincare. It helps to boost collagen production, reduce fine lines, and improve skin elasticity.

Uses:

- Rosehip Oil: Use cold-pressed rosehip oil as a nightly serum to nourish and regenerate the skin. Apply a few drops to your face and neck before bed.

- Rosehip Face Mask: Mix rosehip powder with aloe vera gel and apply it to the face. Leave on for 15-20 minutes before rinsing off with warm water.

- Rosehip Infusion: Prepare a rosehip infusion and use it as a toner to hydrate and refresh the skin. Steep dried rosehips in boiling water for 15 minutes, then cool and apply.

Benefits:

- Boosts collagen production.

- Reduces the appearance of fine lines and wrinkles.

- Improves skin tone and texture.

Pomegranate

Pomegranate is rich in antioxidants, particularly ellagic acid, which helps to protect the skin from free radical damage and promotes cell regeneration. It is also known for its anti-inflammatory properties.

Uses:

- Pomegranate Seed Oil: Apply pomegranate seed oil directly to the skin as a potent anti-aging treatment. It can be used alone or mixed with other carrier oils.

- Pomegranate Face Scrub: Combine pomegranate seeds with sugar and honey to create a gentle exfoliating scrub. Use it to remove dead skin cells and reveal smoother skin.

- Pomegranate Toner: Make a pomegranate toner by blending pomegranate juice with a few drops of witch hazel. Apply with a cotton pad after cleansing.

Benefits:

- Protects against free radical damage.

- Promotes skin cell regeneration.

- Reduces inflammation and enhances skin radiance.

Ginkgo Biloba

Ginkgo biloba is renowned for its antioxidant properties and ability to improve blood circulation. It helps to protect the skin from oxidative stress and supports a healthy, youthful appearance.

Uses:

- Ginkgo Biloba Extract: Add a few drops of ginkgo biloba extract to your moisturizer or serum to boost its anti-aging benefits.

- Ginkgo Biloba Face Mist: Create a face mist by infusing ginkgo biloba leaves in boiling water, then cooling and transferring to a spray bottle. Mist your face throughout the day to refresh and protect your skin.

- Ginkgo Biloba Mask: Blend ginkgo biloba powder with yogurt and apply as a face mask. Leave on for 15-20 minutes before rinsing off.

Benefits:

- Protects against oxidative stress.

- Improves blood circulation and skin vitality.

- Enhances overall skin health and appearance.

Tips for Creating Antioxidant-Rich Blends

1.   Combine Herbs: Enhance the anti-aging effects by combining rosehip, pomegranate, and ginkgo biloba in your skincare formulations. For example, create a powerful anti-aging serum by blending rosehip oil with pomegranate seed oil and a few drops of ginkgo biloba extract.

2.   Gentle Carriers: When making oil infusions or serums, choose carrier oils that complement the herbs' properties, such as argan oil or jojoba oil, which are also known for their skin-nourishing benefits.

3.   Storage: Store your antioxidant-rich blends in dark glass bottles to protect them from light and preserve their potency. Keep them in a cool, dry place to extend their shelf life.

By incorporating these antioxidant-rich herbs into your skincare routine, you can effectively combat the signs of aging and promote a youthful, glowing complexion.

4.3 Crafting Herbal Hair Treatments

Crafting your own herbal hair treatments allows you to harness the natural benefits of herbs to improve the health and appearance of your hair. By creating customized hair masks, rinses, shampoos, and conditioners, you can address specific hair concerns and enjoy a more natural, holistic hair care routine. This section will guide you through the process of making nourishing hair masks, revitalizing hair rinses, and effective herbal shampoos and conditioners. Let's explore how these treatments can transform your hair care regimen.

4.3.1 Nourishing Hair Masks

Nourishing hair masks are a fantastic way to deliver intense hydration and essential nutrients to your hair. By using ingredients like avocado, rosemary, and honey, you can create treatments that strengthen and hydrate your hair, leaving it soft, shiny, and manageable.

Avocado

Avocado is a superfood for your hair. Rich in vitamins A, D, and E, as well as fatty acids, it provides deep moisture and strengthens the hair shaft.

Uses:

•   Hydrating Mask: Mash a ripe avocado and mix it with a tablespoon of olive oil. Apply the mixture to your hair, focusing on the ends, and leave it on for 30 minutes before rinsing.

•   Protein Boost: Combine mashed avocado with an egg yolk and a tablespoon of honey. Apply to your hair and let it sit for 20-30 minutes before washing out.

•   Scalp Treatment: Blend avocado with coconut milk and massage into the scalp to soothe dryness and flakiness.

Benefits:

•   Deeply hydrates and nourishes the hair.

•   Strengthens the hair shaft, reducing breakage.

•   Adds shine and softness to the hair.

Rosemary

Rosemary is known for its ability to stimulate hair growth and improve scalp health. It also has antioxidant properties that help to protect hair from damage.

Uses:

•   Hair Growth Stimulator: Create a rosemary infusion by steeping fresh rosemary leaves in boiling water. Use the cooled infusion as a hair rinse or add it to your shampoo.

•   Strengthening Mask: Mix a few drops of rosemary essential oil with coconut oil and massage into your scalp. Leave it on for 20 minutes before rinsing.

•   Scalp Health: Add rosemary essential oil to a carrier oil, like jojoba oil, and massage into the scalp to reduce dandruff and improve circulation.

Benefits:

•   Stimulates hair growth by improving circulation to the scalp.

•   Strengthens hair and prevents thinning.

•   Enhances scalp health and reduces dandruff.

Honey

Honey is a natural humectant, meaning it draws moisture into the hair and retains it. It also has antibacterial properties that help to keep the scalp healthy.

Uses:

•   Moisturizing Mask: Mix two tablespoons of honey with a cup of warm water. Apply the mixture to your hair and scalp, leave it on for 20-30 minutes, and then rinse thoroughly.

•   Shine Enhancer: Combine honey with apple cider vinegar for a natural hair shine treatment. Apply to your hair after shampooing and rinse out after 15 minutes.

•   Deep Conditioning: Mix honey with coconut oil and apply it as a deep conditioner. Leave it on for 30 minutes before washing your hair.

Benefits:

•   Adds moisture and shine to the hair.

•   Strengthens hair follicles and reduces breakage.

•   Keeps the scalp healthy with its antibacterial properties.

By incorporating these ingredients into your hair masks, you can enjoy stronger, healthier, and more hydrated hair. The natural properties of avocado, rosemary, and honey make them ideal for crafting effective, nourishing hair treatments

4.3.2 Herbal Hair Rinses

Herbal hair rinses are an excellent way to boost the shine, manageability, and overall health of your hair. By incorporating herbs like chamomile, nettle, and apple cider vinegar, you can create natural treatments that enhance your hair's appearance and texture. Let's explore the benefits and uses of these ingredients.

Chamomile

Chamomile is renowned for its soothing and brightening properties, making it an ideal choice for a hair rinse that adds shine and lightens hair naturally.

Uses:

•   Brightening Rinse: Steep a handful of dried chamomile flowers in boiling water for 30 minutes. Strain the infusion and let it cool. After shampooing, pour the chamomile rinse over your hair, leave it on for a few minutes, and then rinse with cool water.

- Soothing Scalp: Combine chamomile tea with a few drops of lavender essential oil for a calming scalp treatment. Apply after shampooing and rinse out after 5-10 minutes.

- Conditioning Treatment: Mix chamomile infusion with aloe vera gel and use it as a leave-in conditioner to soothe and hydrate the scalp.

Benefits:

- Naturally lightens hair and enhances blonde highlights.

- Adds shine and softness to the hair.

- Soothes and calms an irritated scalp.

Nettle

Nettle is a powerhouse herb for hair health, known for its ability to strengthen hair and improve scalp conditions. It is rich in vitamins and minerals that promote healthy hair growth.

Uses:

- Strengthening Rinse: Steep dried nettle leaves in boiling water for 20 minutes. Strain and cool the infusion. Use it as a final rinse after shampooing to strengthen hair and stimulate growth.

- Anti-Dandruff Treatment: Combine nettle infusion with apple cider vinegar and use it as a scalp rinse to reduce dandruff and improve scalp health.

- Nourishing Rinse: Mix nettle infusion with a few drops of rosemary essential oil to create a nourishing rinse that promotes hair growth and reduces hair loss.

Benefits:

- Strengthens hair follicles and prevents hair loss.

- Reduces dandruff and soothes the scalp.

- Promotes shiny, healthy hair.

Apple Cider Vinegar

Apple cider vinegar (ACV) is a popular natural hair care ingredient known for balancing the scalp's pH, removing buildup, and enhancing hair shine.

Uses:

- Shine-Boosting Rinse: Mix one part ACV with two parts water. After shampooing, pour the mixture over your hair, massage it into the scalp, and rinse thoroughly with cool water.

• Clarifying Rinse: Combine ACV with a herbal infusion (like chamomile or nettle) to create a clarifying rinse that removes product buildup and leaves hair clean and shiny.

• pH Balancing Rinse: Use diluted ACV (1 part ACV to 3 parts water) as a final rinse to restore the natural pH balance of your scalp and hair.

Benefits:

• Balances the scalp's pH and reduces itchiness.

• Removes buildup from hair products, leaving hair clean and shiny.

• Enhances hair manageability and smoothness.

By incorporating chamomile, nettle, and apple cider vinegar into your hair rinses, you can enjoy the natural benefits these ingredients offer, resulting in healthier, shinier, and more manageable hair.

4.3.3 DIY Herbal Shampoos and Conditioners

Creating your own herbal shampoos and conditioners allows you to customize your hair care routine with natural ingredients that cater specifically to your hair's needs. Using herbs like peppermint, lavender, and aloe vera, you can craft products that cleanse, condition, and rejuvenate your hair. Here's a closer look at these ingredients and their benefits:

Peppermint

Peppermint is a refreshing herb known for its stimulating properties, making it an excellent addition to shampoos and conditioners.

Uses:

• Peppermint Shampoo: Add a few drops of peppermint essential oil to your shampoo base to invigorate the scalp and promote hair growth. The menthol in peppermint provides a cooling sensation that can help soothe an itchy scalp.

• Scalp Treatment: Combine peppermint oil with a carrier oil (like jojoba or coconut oil) and massage it into the scalp before washing your hair. This can help to increase blood circulation and stimulate hair follicles.

• Conditioning Rinse: Create a peppermint-infused water by steeping fresh peppermint leaves in boiling water, letting it cool, and using it as a final rinse after conditioning.

Benefits:

- Stimulates the scalp and promotes hair growth.
- Provides a cooling, refreshing sensation.
- Helps to soothe and reduce scalp irritation.

122. Peppermint Stimulating Shampoo

Ingredients:

- 1/2 cup liquid castile soap
- 1/4 cup distilled water
- 1 tsp jojoba oil
- 10 drops peppermint essential oil
- 1 tsp vegetable glycerin

Steps:

1 Mix liquid castile soap and distilled water in a bottle.

2 Add jojoba oil, peppermint essential oil, and vegetable glycerin.

3 Shake well to combine.

4 Use a small amount to lather into wet hair and rinse thoroughly.

Usage Tips: This shampoo invigorates the scalp and promotes hair growth.

123. Peppermint Scalp-Soothing Conditioner

Ingredients:

- 1/2 cup coconut oil
- 1/4 cup shea butter
- 10 drops peppermint essential oil
- 5 drops rosemary essential oil

Lavender

Steps:

1 Melt coconut oil and shea butter in a double boiler.

2 Remove from heat and stir in peppermint and rosemary essential oils.

3 Let it cool until it solidifies.

4 Apply to the hair after shampooing, focusing on the scalp, and leave it on for 5 minutes before rinsing.

Usage Tips: This conditioner soothes and cools the scalp while nourishing the hair.

124. Peppermint & Aloe Vera Hair Rinse

Ingredients:

- 1 cup distilled water
- 1/4 cup aloe vera gel
- 10 drops peppermint essential oil

Steps:

1 Mix distilled water and aloe vera gel in a bottle.

2 Add peppermint essential oil and shake well.

3 Apply to hair after shampooing and conditioning, then rinse thoroughly.

Usage Tips: Use as a final rinse to leave hair feeling refreshed and tingly clean.

Lavender is renowned for its calming and healing properties. It is beneficial for both the scalp and hair, making it a versatile ingredient in hair care products.

Uses:

• Lavender Shampoo: Add lavender essential oil to your shampoo base to help calm the scalp and reduce dandruff. Lavender's antimicrobial properties can help to keep the scalp healthy.

• Soothing Conditioner: Mix lavender oil with a conditioner base or carrier oil to create a soothing conditioner that can help to nourish and repair hair.

• Hair Rinse: Steep dried lavender flowers in boiling water to create a lavender-infused rinse. Use it after shampooing to add a light fragrance and soothing properties to your hair care routine.

Benefits:

• Calms and soothes the scalp.
• Reduces dandruff and scalp irritation.
• Promotes healthy hair growth and adds a pleasant fragrance.

125. Lavender Calming Shampoo

Ingredients:

• 1/2 cup liquid castile soap
• 1/4 cup distilled water
• 1 tsp lavender essential oil
• 1 tsp olive oil

Steps:

1 Combine liquid castile soap and distilled water in a bottle.
2 Add lavender essential oil and olive oil.
3 Shake well to mix.
4 Apply to wet hair, lather, and rinse thoroughly.

Usage Tips: Ideal for calming the scalp and reducing dandruff.

126. Lavender & Chamomile Hair Rinse

Ingredients:

• 1 cup chamomile tea (brewed and cooled)
• 1 tsp lavender essential oil

Steps:

1 Brew chamomile tea and let it cool.
2 Add lavender essential oil and stir.
3 Use as a final rinse after shampooing and conditioning.

Usage Tips: Enhances shine and promotes relaxation.

127. Lavender Moisturizing Conditioner

Ingredients:

• 1/2 cup coconut milk
• 1/4 cup aloe vera gel
• 10 drops lavender essential oil

Steps:

1 Mix coconut milk and aloe vera gel in a bowl.
2 Add lavender essential oil and stir well.

3   Apply to hair after shampooing, leave on for 5-10 minutes, and rinse thoroughly.

Usage Tips: This conditioner hydrates and soothes the hair, leaving it soft and manageable.

Aloe Vera

Aloe vera is a powerhouse ingredient for hair care due to its moisturizing and healing properties. It's especially beneficial in conditioners and hair treatments.

Uses:

•   Aloe Vera Shampoo: Incorporate aloe vera gel into your shampoo base to add moisture and improve the overall health of your hair. Aloe vera helps to cleanse the scalp gently while retaining moisture.

•   Moisturizing Conditioner: Mix aloe vera gel with a conditioner base to create a deeply moisturizing conditioner. Aloe vera helps to detangle hair and reduce frizz.

•   Leave-In Treatment: Use pure aloe vera gel as a leave-in treatment to soothe the scalp, reduce dandruff, and provide a light, non-greasy moisture boost to your hair.

Benefits:

•   Provides deep hydration and moisture to the hair and scalp.

•   Helps to soothe and heal scalp conditions.

•   Promotes smooth, shiny, and frizz-free hair.

128.   Aloe Vera Hydrating Shampoo

Ingredients:

- 1/2 cup aloe vera gel
- 1/2 cup liquid castile soap
- 1 tsp jojoba oil
- 10 drops lavender essential oil

Steps:

1   Combine aloe vera gel and liquid castile soap in a bottle.

2   Add jojoba oil and lavender essential oil.

3   Shake well to blend.

4   Apply to wet hair, lather, and rinse thoroughly.

Usage Tips: Perfect for moisturizing dry and damaged hair.

129.   Aloe Vera & Honey Conditioner

Ingredients:

- 1/2 cup aloe vera gel
- 2 tbsp honey
- 10 drops rosemary essential oil

Steps:

1 Mix aloe vera gel and honey in a bowl.

2 Add rosemary essential oil and stir well.

3 Apply to hair after shampooing, leave on for 5 minutes, and rinse thoroughly.

Usage Tips: This conditioner hydrates and adds shine to hair.

130. Aloe Vera & Mint Hair Rinse

Ingredients:

- 1 cup distilled water
- 1/4 cup aloe vera juice
- 5 drops peppermint essential oil

Steps:

1 Combine distilled water and aloe vera juice in a bottle.

2 Add peppermint essential oil and shake well.

3 Use as a final rinse after shampooing and conditioning.

Usage Tips: Provides a cooling and refreshing finish to your hair care routine.

BOOK 5: Innovations and Sustainability in Herbalism

Chapter 1: Sustainability in Herbal Use

Water-Saving Herbal Garden Techniques

Exploring methods to conserve water in herbal gardening plays a key role in ensuring sustainability and efficient resource use. Implementing strategies like mulching, planting in groups, and using drip irrigation systems can significantly reduce water consumption. Mulching, which involves covering the soil with organic materials such as straw, leaves, or wood chips, helps retain moisture in the soil, thus reducing the frequency of watering. This practice also suppresses weed growth and enriches the soil as the mulch decomposes.

Planting herbs in groups can lessen evaporation and create a microclimate that conserves water. Grouping plants with similar water needs together ensures that each plant receives the right amount of moisture without overwatering. Additionally, using drip irrigation systems targets the root zone directly, avoiding water wastage by delivering water exactly where it is needed, drop by drop. This method is highly efficient compared to traditional overhead watering, which often leads to significant water loss through evaporation and runoff.

Selecting native or drought-tolerant herbs also contributes to water conservation. These plants are naturally adapted to local climate conditions and typically require less water to thrive. Herbs like rosemary, thyme, and sage are excellent choices for water-wise gardening. By adopting these water-saving techniques, gardeners could build a sustainable herbal garden that conserves water and also supports the environment by reducing the demand on local water resources.

Compost Tea for Fertilizing Plants Naturally

Compost tea, a natural fertilizer, can be made by fermenting compost in water for around two to three weeks. This nutrient-rich solution provides essential minerals and beneficial microorganisms to plants, promoting healthier growth. To make compost tea, start by adding a shovel of compost to a 5-gallon bucket of water. Stir this mixture daily to ensure it gets plenty of exposure to air, which aids the fermentation process.

After two to three weeks, strain the mixture to remove solid particles, leaving a nutrient-dense liquid. This compost tea can then be applied directly onto the plants or the soil every two weeks. When applied to the soil, it enriches the root zone, enhancing soil structure and fertility. When sprayed onto plants, it can help boost their resistance to diseases and pests. Using compost tea as a natural fertilizer is a sustainable way to nourish your herbal garden, promoting robust plant health and reducing the need for chemical fertilizers.

Seed Saving Methods for Heirloom Herbs

Saving seeds from heirloom herbs is a simple yet effective technique to preserve plant diversity and sustainability. Heirloom herbs are varieties that have been passed down through generations, valued for their unique characteristics and resilience. To save seeds from these plants, start by choosing a healthy herb plant that is nearing maturation. Allow the plant to flower and set seeds naturally. Once the seeds are mature and dry, usually indicated by a change in color and a hard texture, carefully collect them.

Clean the seeds by removing any chaff or plant debris. This can be done by hand or using a fine mesh sieve. Once cleaned, ensure the seeds are completely dry before storage to prevent mold or rot. Store the dried seeds in labeled envelopes or small jars, keeping them in a cool, dry, and dark place to maintain their viability. Properly stored seeds can last for several years, allowing you to grow your favorite heirloom herbs year after year. By saving seeds, gardeners can contribute to the conservation of biodiversity and ensure the sustainability of their herbal gardens for future generations.

Plant-Based Natural Pest Control Solutions

The use of plant-based solutions for pest control offers a natural and eco-friendly alternative to harmful chemical pesticides. Companion planting is a notable strategy, where specific plants are grown together to naturally deter pests. For example, planting marigolds alongside tomatoes can help repel nematodes, while basil can deter flies and mosquitoes. Additionally, creating organic sprays from plants such as neem, garlic, or eucalyptus can effectively repel pests. Neem oil, in particular, contains azadirachtin, a compound that disrupts the life cycle of insects, reducing their ability to feed and reproduce. These plant-based strategies not only maintain the health of your garden but also protect the environment by avoiding the use of toxic chemicals. Moreover, they contribute to biodiversity, enhancing the resilience and sustainability of your garden ecosystem.

Zero-Waste Herbal Packaging Ideas

Packaging herbs in a zero-waste manner can significantly reduce environmental impact and promote sustainability. Utilizing biodegradable and compostable materials such as hemp, bamboo, or cornstarch-based alternatives can make herbal packaging eco-friendly. For instance, edible wrappers can be used in culinary applications, or fully dissolving bags can leave no trace after use. An innovative idea is seed-infused packaging, which can be planted after use to sprout herbs as it decomposes. These creative solutions not only minimize waste but also engage consumers in sustainable practices. By adopting such packaging methods, we can reduce the environmental footprint of herb packaging while providing practical and beneficial options for consumers.

Herbal Water Filtration System

Creating a natural water filtration system using herbs can provide a simple and effective way to purify water. Begin by selecting water-purifying herbs such as horsetail, peppermint, or fennel seeds. Make an herb pouch using cheesecloth or any natural fabric, filling it with the chosen herbs and securing the ends tightly. Place the herb pouch in a water container, allowing it to steep like tea. The natural properties of these herbs help filter and purify the water, making it safer to drink. Horsetail, for example, contains silica which can bind to impurities, while peppermint has antimicrobial properties. However, it's important to note that this method may not remove all waterborne contaminants or bacteria. Therefore, it is recommended to use this herbal filtration technique in conjunction with other filtration methods for enhanced safety and effectiveness.

Sustainable Wildcrafting Practices

Wildcrafting herbs calls for responsible, ethical, and sustainable practices to minimize the negative impact on natural environments. Gather only what is needed without depleting the plant population, ideally taking no more than 10% of a stand of herbs. Avoid harvesting rare or endangered plants. Always seek permission from landowners or comply with regulations in public lands. Additionally, practices such as removing invasive species, spreading seeds, and caring for habitats contribute to preserving and restoring natural environments. These steps ensure that wildcrafting supports ecosystem health and sustainability.

Community Herb Garden Planning

Creating community herb gardens fosters local sustainability and provides a collective resource for fresh herbs. Begin with thorough planning, including site selection, designing the garden layout, choosing appropriate herbs, and considering budget needs. Establishing the garden involves planting, nurturing, and maintaining it for long-term sustainability. Community herb gardens fulfill household needs, promote environmental stewardship, and become symbols of self-sufficiency. By engaging community members in the cultivation process, these gardens can enhance local food security and strengthen community bonds.

Recycling Herb Residue for Mulch

Recycling herb residue into mulch enriches soil and reduces waste. Collect dried or fresh herb residue and grind it into small pieces. Spread these pieces over your garden, where they will decompose and add nutrients to the soil, improving its fertility and boosting water retention in sandy soils. This method not only utilizes herb leftovers effectively but also supports an eco-friendly approach to waste management. Using recycled herb residue as mulch promotes healthier plants and a more sustainable gardening practice by returning valuable nutrients to the soil.

Biodynamic Herbal Growing Principles

The biodynamic approach to cultivating herbs emphasizes balance and sustainability within nature's rhythms. Grow plants in alignment with lunar cycles, seasonal shifts, and environmental elements such as sunlight and soil quality. Incorporate organic matter into the soil to foster a healthy ecosystem for herbs to flourish optimally. This method enhances the potency and flavors of herbs and contributes to the overall health of the ecosystem. By embracing biodynamic principles, herbal growers can create a harmonious and sustainable environment that supports the vitality of both the plants and the surrounding ecosystem.

Eco-Friendly Herbal Extraction Methods

Eco-friendly extraction of herbal compounds largely focuses on using methods that minimize waste and energy consumption while maximizing yield. Traditional methods like steam distillation and solvent extraction are being replaced by greener alternatives such as supercritical fluid extraction and cold press extraction. Supercritical fluid extraction uses substances like carbon dioxide under extreme pressure and temperature to extract active ingredients without the need for hazardous solvents. This method ensures high purity and preserves the integrity of the compounds, resulting in superior quality extracts.

On the other hand, the cold press method mechanically presses and grinds the plant material, ensuring no heat is used that could degrade the extract. This technique maintains the natural essence and potency of the herbs, providing a pure and unaltered product. Both methods result in less waste and lower energy use, thus significantly reducing environmental impact. By adopting these eco-friendly extraction techniques, we can enjoy the benefits of herbal compounds while promoting sustainability and environmental responsibility.

Chapter 2: Innovations in Herbal Preparation

Solar-Powered Herbal Dehydrator

A solar-powered dehydrator is an innovative method for drying herbs sustainably and efficiently. The design incorporates a solar panel that captures and converts sunlight into heat, which is then directed into a dehydrating chamber to accelerate the evaporation of moisture from the herbs. Additionally, the dehydrator includes vents to allow for airflow, ensuring uniform drying. This method is eco-friendly, reducing dependence on fossil fuels, and cost-effective, as it relies entirely on sunlight. An added benefit of solar dehydrating is its gentleness on herbs, preserving their aroma and medicinal properties better than other drying methods.

Ultrasonic Herb Extraction Technique

Ultrasonic technology has revolutionized the extraction of herbal compounds, enhancing efficiency and effectiveness. It utilizes periodic sound pressure waves that create high-speed, low-pressure microbubbles, which disrupt plant cell walls, making the active compounds more accessible. This technique improves both the quality and quantity of the extracted compounds while saving time and reducing solvent use, making it an environmentally friendly method. Ultrasonic technology provides an innovative, sustainable, and superior alternative for herbal compound extraction compared to traditional methods.

DIY Herbal Encapsulation Machine

Building a homemade machine to encapsulate herbal powders requires basic mechanical skills. Start by obtaining an encapsulation machine kit from a DIY store. The kit typically includes a base, a stand, a powder spreader, and hundreds of different-sized capsules. Set up the base and place the capsules in their designated slots. Fill the capsules with your herbal powder using the provided spatula and powder spreader. Once filled, attach the stand to secure the capsules and gently press to seal. Always ensure cleanliness to maintain the purity of your herbal products. This DIY approach allows for precise control over the encapsulation process, ensuring that your herbal supplements are made to your exact specifications.

Home-Based Herbal Distillation Setup

Setting up a home distillation system for extracting essential oils from herbs involves several crucial steps and careful planning. First, acquire a distillation kit that typically includes a boiler, condenser, and separator. It's essential to ensure that the equipment is of high quality to produce the purest essential oils. Begin by filling the boiler with water and adding the herb of choice into the still. Heat the water to generate steam, which will pass through the herb material. This steam carries the essential oils and travels through the condensation coil, cooling and converting back into a liquid form. The resulting mixture of water and essential oil reaches the separator, where the oil floats on top due to its lower density. Carefully decant the essential oil into a dark glass container to preserve its potency. Safety is paramount during the distillation process; always monitor the heat source and handle hot equipment with care. Additionally, ensure your workspace is well-ventilated to avoid inhaling concentrated vapors. With these steps and precautions, you can efficiently set up a home distillation system to produce your own essential oils.

Portable Herb Grinder and Blender

Portable grinders and blenders are indispensable tools for herb enthusiasts and culinary experts alike, offering numerous benefits and versatile uses. These devices provide a consistent and fine grind, which is crucial for maintaining the full flavor and therapeutic properties of herbs. The portability aspect allows for easy transportation, making them ideal for use at home, in professional kitchens, or even on the go. Many models come with adjustable settings, providing flexibility to achieve various textures and consistencies suitable for different culinary applications. For instance, making a fresh pesto, grinding herbs into fine powders for teas, or creating spice blends for cooking can be done efficiently with a portable grinder or blender. The quick processing time and ease of use significantly expedite preparation, allowing for more creative and spontaneous culinary endeavors. Moreover, these tools help in preserving the aromatic and medicinal qualities of herbs, ensuring that every dish benefits from their full potential. Investing in a high-quality portable grinder or blender enhances your kitchen arsenal, making herb processing a seamless and enjoyable task.

Non-Toxic Herbal Preservation Methods

Preserving herbs effectively is crucial for maintaining their potency, flavor, and therapeutic properties over time. Non-toxic methods are preferred to ensure that the herbs remain safe for consumption and use. One of the simplest and most traditional methods is air-drying. Let the herbs air dry, bunch them into small bundles, tie them with string, and hang them upside down in a room that is warm, dry, and well-ventilated, but not directly exposed to sunlight. This process allows the water to evaporate naturally, preserving the essential oils and flavors. Another excellent method is freezing. After washing and thoroughly drying the herbs, spread them out in a single layer on a baking sheet and freeze them. Once frozen, transfer the herbs to airtight containers or freezer bags to maintain their freshness. Additionally, herbs can be preserved in vinegar or olive oil, both of which are non-toxic and help maintain the herbs' flavor and potency. Infusing herbs in these liquids not only extends their shelf life but also creates flavorful additions for culinary uses. These non-toxic preservation methods ensure that your herbs remain potent and fresh, ready to enhance your dishes and remedies whenever needed.

Automated Herbal Plant Watering System

Creating an automated system for watering herb plants can significantly streamline your gardening routine and ensure consistent care for your plants. Start by selecting an appropriate automatic watering system, such as a drip irrigation system, self-watering pots, or a smart garden system. Drip irrigation systems are particularly efficient, as they deliver water to the plant roots, diminishing evaporation and water trash. Self-watering pots are convenient for individual plants, while smart garden systems offer advanced features like moisture sensors and programmable timers. Once you have chosen your system, install it according to the manufacturer's instructions, ensuring that it covers all your herb plants adequately. Adapt the frequency and amount of water to suit the unique needs of each herb variety, as different herbs have varying water requirements. Incorporating a moisture sensor can further optimize the system by providing real-time feedback on soil moisture levels, preventing both under-watering and over-watering. With a well-designed automated watering system, you can ensure your herbs receive consistent care, promoting healthy growth with minimal daily intervention.

Precision Dosing for Herbal Remedies

Achieving precise dosing of herbal remedies is essential for their optimal effectiveness and safety. Several methods can ensure accuracy in dosing, starting with measuring by weight using a digital scale for dry herbs. This approach guarantees consistency and accuracy, particularly for remedies requiring precise amounts. For tinctures, drops can be calculated using a dropper, with attention to the recommended dosage per drop specified on the tincture bottle. Encapsulated herbs offer another method, where counting capsules ensures the exact dosage. It is crucial to know the right dosage instructions given on the packaging or prescribed by a healthcare professional, considering factors such as the individual's age, health condition, and overall tolerance. Consistency in administering the dosage at regular intervals without skipping doses is vital for maintaining the remedy's effectiveness. Additionally, understanding how different factors like diet, lifestyle, and other medications might interact with the herbal remedies can further optimize their efficacy. By adhering to these methods, you can ensure the safe and effective use of herbal remedies, maximizing their therapeutic benefits.

Cold Brew Herbal Infusion Device

The Cold Brew Herbal Infusion Device is an innovative tool designed to preserve the delicate compounds in herbs by steeping them in cold water over several hours. This method, known for preventing the breakdown of sensitive compounds that can occur with hot water extraction, maintains the herbs' full therapeutic potential. The device features a durable container that holds the herbs and water, a fine filter to separate the herbs after infusion, and a secure lid to maintain freshness throughout the process. Its user-friendly design ensures convenience, making it easy to prepare cold brew herbal infusions without hassle. By steeping herbs in cold water, this device allows for the extraction of a broad spectrum of beneficial compounds, providing a rich, flavorful, and potent infusion. For herbal enthusiasts, the Cold Brew Herbal Infusion Device is indispensable, offering a simple yet effective way to enjoy the full benefits and natural flavors of their favorite herbs.

High-Efficiency Herbal Oil Press

The high-efficiency herbal oil press is a cutting-edge tool revolutionizing the extraction of oils from herbs. This advanced machinery utilizes superior technology and engineering to efficiently press oils from herbs such as lavender, rosemary, and peppermint. The process ensures maximum extraction, yielding high-quality, pure oils free from harmful chemicals and preservatives. The oil press operates with remarkable efficiency, saving energy and reducing waste, making it an environmentally friendly option. By optimizing the extraction process, this device delivers potent, pure herbal oils that retain their natural therapeutic properties. The high-efficiency oil press not only benefits commercial producers by increasing productivity and reducing costs but also appeals to home users seeking to create their own essential oils with ease. This innovation represents a significant advancement in the herbal oil industry, enhancing both the quality and accessibility of herbal oils for various applications, from aromatherapy to natural skincare.

Smart Herb Drying Racks with Humidity Control

Smart drying racks with humidity control provide an advanced solution for drying herbs, ensuring optimal preservation of their medicinal properties and flavors. These high-tech racks allow for precise regulation of humidity levels, ensuring that herbs dry evenly and thoroughly while maintaining their natural color and aroma. Automated temperature controls prevent overheating, which can cause the loss of essential oils and diminish the herbs' therapeutic effectiveness. By eliminating the need for constant manual monitoring and adjustments, these smart drying racks streamline the drying process, making it more efficient and less labor-intensive. The ability to set and maintain ideal drying conditions means that herbs retain their maximum potency and have a longer shelf life. This technology enhances the quality and consistency of dried herbs, making them more effective for both culinary and medicinal uses. Smart drying racks with humidity control are a valuable investment for anyone serious about herb preservation, from small-scale home gardeners to large commercial operations.

Chapter 3: Herbs for a Sustainable Future

Drought-Resistant Herbal Varieties for Arid Climates

Arid climates are ideal for certain herbs that thrive under dry conditions and require minimal water. Among these, oregano, thyme, sage, and rosemary are particularly well-suited, thanks to their adaptation to dry heat and poor soil quality. Lavender, known for its strong and pleasant aroma, is another excellent drought-resistant herb that flourishes in full sun. Additionally, herbs like sorrel and yarrow survive with very little moisture, making them perfect for desert or drought-prone home gardens. These herbs not only tolerate arid conditions but also provide valuable flavors and medicinal properties to households. They can be cultivated in garden beds or containers, offering versatile options for enhancing the sustainability of home gardens in arid regions.

Fast-Growing Herbs for Rapid Harvest Cycles

Sustainable gardening benefits significantly from herbs that grow quickly and can be harvested frequently. Herbs such as mint, basil, parsley, chives, and dill are prime examples of fast-growing plants that provide abundant harvests. Their rapid growth rate ensures a consistent supply, reducing the need for store-bought alternatives and promoting self-sufficiency. These herbs are often perennials, meaning they return each year, contributing to a sustainable cycle of growth and harvest. Their ability to thrive in containers allows for indoor and outdoor cultivation, making them accessible for urban gardeners and those with limited space. By integrating these fast-growing herbs into your garden, you can enjoy fresh, homegrown produce throughout the growing season, enhancing the sustainability and productivity of your gardening efforts.

Carbon-Capturing Plant Species

Certain plant species are very important in mitigating climate change by capturing carbon dioxide (CO_2) from the atmosphere. During photosynthesis, plants absorb CO_2 and store it in their biomass, effectively offsetting greenhouse gas emissions. Fast-growing trees like poplars and willows are particularly effective at capturing carbon due to their rapid growth and substantial biomass. Grasses such as Miscanthus and bamboo also excel in sequestering carbon, thanks to their extensive root systems and fast growth rates. Additionally, marine plants like seaweed and phytoplankton are potent CO_2 absorbers, contributing significantly to carbon sequestration in aquatic environments. Promoting the growth of these carbon-capturing species can become instrumental in our fight against climate change. By incorporating them into landscapes and agricultural practices, we can enhance their role in reducing atmospheric CO_2 levels and supporting a healthier planet.

Herbs that Improve Soil Fertility

Certain herbs are highly beneficial for enhancing soil fertility and overall health, supporting sustainable agricultural practices. Comfrey, with its deep root system, draws up nutrients from the subsoil and enriches the topsoil with essential elements like potassium, phosphorus, and trace minerals. Dandelion, similarly, improves soil health by releasing nutrients that are otherwise locked up in the soil and promoting microbial activity. Nettle is another nutrient-rich herb, containing high amounts of nitrogen, iron, and other beneficial minerals, which help boost soil health and fertility. Using these herbs in gardening and farming practices offers a sustainable approach to improving soil quality. They reduce the dependence on synthetic fertilizers, encourage beneficial insects, and add organic matter to the soil. This natural method of enhancing soil fertility supports the principles of sustainable agriculture and contributes to a healthier, more resilient ecosystem.

Urban Adapted Herbal Species for Roof Gardens

Urban gardening presents a unique opportunity to cultivate green spaces in cities, transforming rooftops into thriving herb gardens. Herbs are particularly suited for roof gardens due to their resilience and low maintenance requirements. Ideal choices for these urban green spaces include basil, mint, rosemary, and thyme, all of which thrive in well-drained containers and can tolerate full sun exposure. These herbs not only add a decorative touch to urban environments but also provide fresh, aromatic ingredients for culinary use. Basil, with its vibrant green leaves, is perfect for adding a splash of color and flavor to dishes. Mint, known for its refreshing scent, can be used in beverages and desserts. Rosemary and thyme are excellent for seasoning a variety of meals, from roasted vegetables to grilled meats. By carefully selecting and caring for these herbs, urban gardeners can create a sustainable and productive green space on their rooftops, enhancing both the aesthetics and the functionality of their living environments.

Herbs that Require Minimal Fertilizer

Certain herbs are naturally adapted to thrive with minimal or no fertilizer, making them an environmentally friendly choice for gardeners. Oregano, rosemary, thyme, and sage are prime examples of herbs that originated from the Mediterranean region, where they grew in non-fertile, dry soils. These resilient herbs require very little intervention, making them ideal for sustainable gardening practices. Similarly, parsley and coriander can flourish without the need for chemical fertilizers, especially when grown in compost-rich soil. By opting for these low-maintenance herbs, gardeners can enjoy a bountiful harvest while minimizing their environmental impact. These herbs not only reduce the need for synthetic fertilizers but also support a healthier garden ecosystem. Their robust nature ensures that they can thrive even in less-than-ideal soil conditions, making them a practical choice for both novice and experienced gardeners aiming to cultivate a sustainable and eco-friendly garden.

Native Plant Promotion for Biodiversity

Promoting the use of native plants is crucial for supporting local biodiversity. Native plants have evolved in harmony with the local ecosystem, forming essential symbiotic relationships with the surrounding wildlife. They provide vital resources such as shelter and food for a wide range of species, including insects, birds, and mammals. A landscape rich in native plants fosters a diverse and balanced ecosystem, enhancing the resilience of local fauna. Additionally, native plants are well adapted to the local soil and climate conditions, requiring less water and maintenance. This makes them a sustainable choice for gardening, as they can thrive without extensive human intervention. By preserving and encouraging the growth of native flora, gardeners can play a significant role in maintaining and enhancing local biodiversity. This practice supports wildlife and aids the overall health and sustainability of the environment.

High-Yield Herbs for Small Spaces

For those with limited gardening space, high-yield herbs such as basil, parsley, mint, chives, and cilantro are excellent choices. These herbs can be grown in small pots, making them perfect for windowsills, balconies, or compact garden spaces. Basil is a particularly abundant herb, known for its ease of care and prolific growth. Parsley is versatile and thrives in various lighting conditions, whether in full sunlight or partial shade. Mint is an incredibly robust herb that can spread rapidly, making it ideal for container gardening to control its growth. Chives and cilantro also offer high yields with minimal space and maintenance requirements. These herbs not only provide a steady supply of fresh ingredients but also add greenery and fragrance to small living spaces. By choosing high-yield herbs, urban gardeners can maximize their harvest even in confined areas, ensuring a constant supply of fresh, home-grown flavors for their culinary needs.

Perennial Herbs for Long-Term Cultivation

Growing perennial herbs offers numerous benefits for sustainability, making them a valuable addition to any garden. Perennial herbs, such as rosemary, thyme, and mint, have lifespans extending beyond two years, which significantly reduces the need for regular replanting. This longevity conserves resources, facilitating a better sustainable gardening practice. These herbs also require less water and fertilizer compared to annual plants, promoting efficient resource use. Their deep root systems aid augment soil health by diminishing erosion and enhancing nutrient content, fostering a more stable and fertile garden environment. Furthermore, perennial herbs act as natural pest deterrents, which minimizes the need for harmful chemical pesticides, supporting a healthier ecosystem. By incorporating perennial herbs into your garden, you can create a more sustainable, eco-friendly space that benefits both the environment and biodiversity.

Pollution-Absorbing Plants for City Environments

In urban areas, certain herbs and plants have been identified for their remarkable ability to absorb pollutants, thereby improving air quality. Spider Plants are particularly effective at removing formaldehyde and xylene from the atmosphere, making them ideal for indoor and outdoor urban settings. English Ivy and Peace Lily excel at reducing levels of benzene and trichloroethylene, which are common pollutants in city environments. Additionally, the Snake Plant, also known as Mother-In-Law's Tongue, is renowned for its capacity to filter out formaldehyde, a common indoor air pollutant. These plants not only enhance the aesthetic appeal of urban spaces but also serve a critical function in purifying the air we breathe. By integrating pollution-absorbing plants into urban landscaping and indoor environments, cities can take a significant step toward reducing air pollution and promoting a healthier living atmosphere for their inhabitants.

Herbal Contributions to Wildlife Habitats

Herbs play a crucial role in creating and maintaining habitats for wildlife, thereby supporting biodiversity. Flowering herbs, for instance, attract pollinators such as bees, butterflies, and birds, which are essential for the reproduction of many plants. Herbs like lavender and fennel provide nectar and pollen that these pollinators need to thrive. Additionally, the seeds and leaves of various herbs serve as food sources for numerous animals, including insects and small mammals. Some herbs, such as dill and parsley, offer cover or nesting sites for insects like ladybugs and caterpillars, which are beneficial for pest control. By fostering a diverse range of herbs in our gardens and landscapes, we can create a rich and supportive environment for local wildlife.

Chapter 4: Education and Modern Herbalism

Virtual Reality Herbal Garden Tours

Virtual Reality (VR) technology has revolutionized the way we explore and learn about herbal gardens. Through the immersive experience provided by VR, users can navigate digital renditions of herbal gardens, interact with various plants, and gain a deep understanding of their characteristics and uses. With VR goggles, learners can virtually touch, harvest, and study different herbs, receiving detailed information on their biological features, medicinal properties, and growth patterns. This innovative approach makes learning about herbs not only accessible and convenient but also engaging and enjoyable, significantly enhancing knowledge retention. VR herbal garden tours are particularly beneficial for those who cannot physically visit such gardens, offering a unique and comprehensive educational experience from the comfort of their homes.

Online Herbalist Certification Courses

Aspiring herbalists now have access to a wide range of online certification courses designed to enhance their knowledge and skills in herbal medicine. These courses cover essential areas such as herbal medicine preparation, anatomy, physiology, and clinical herbalism, aiming to develop professionals capable of supporting wellness through natural remedies. Reputable institutions like the Herbal Academy and the School of Natural Healing offer courses ranging from foundational to advanced levels, including specialized programs in clinical herbalism. Upon completion, participants receive certifications that are highly regarded in the wellness industry. These courses are structured with flexible, self-paced modules, allowing learners to progress at their own convenience while gaining a comprehensive and in-depth education in herbalism.

Augmented Reality App for Plant Identification

Augmented reality (AR) apps are transforming the way we identify and learn about various herbs and plants. By simply pointing a phone camera at a plant, users can instantly identify it and access detailed information about its uses, medicinal benefits, and potential risks. These apps provide an interactive and educational experience, encouraging users to explore and engage with the natural world around them. The integration of AR technology bridges the gap between digital information and real-world exploration, fostering a new level of environmental awareness and appreciation. These apps are invaluable tools for both novice and experienced herbalists, botanists, and nature enthusiasts, enhancing their ability to recognize and understand the plants they encounter.

E-Learning Modules on Herbal Medicine Making

E-learning modules focused on herbal medicine making provide a comprehensive education for individuals interested in natural medicine production. These interactive courses cover a wide range of topics, including the identification of medicinal plants, proper harvesting techniques, and various methods for creating herbal remedies such as tinctures, salves, and teas. Participants learn the fundamental principles of herbalism through multimedia content that combines theoretical knowledge with practical instructions. These modules are designed to be engaging and informative, offering step-by-step guidance on making effective herbal medicines. By completing these e-learning courses, individuals can develop the skills needed to create their own natural treatments, promoting holistic health and wellness in their communities.

Interactive Herbal Workshops Online

Interactive online workshops offer participants the unique opportunity to learn about various herbs and their beneficial uses from the comfort of their own homes. These sessions are conducted live, enabling individuals to engage directly with hosts and experts in real-time discussions. Topics covered in these workshops range widely, including the health benefits of different herbs, their culinary applications, and methods for incorporating them into daily life. Participants also receive practical guidance on growing and harvesting herbs at home, which enhances their understanding of sustainable gardening practices. Supported by expert instructors, these workshops not only provide valuable knowledge but also empower participants to apply their newfound skills, transforming their lifestyles into more sustainable and wellness-focused routines. The interactive nature of these workshops ensures a dynamic learning experience, fostering a community of herb enthusiasts who can share insights and support each other's herbal journeys.

Digital Herbal Recipe Booklets

Digital herbal recipe booklets offer a wealth of information on preparing a wide variety of herbal concoctions, from everyday remedies and tinctures to more complex medicinal preparations. These comprehensively designed guides provide clear, step-by-step instructions, making it easy for anyone to follow and create their own herbal products. The digital format allows for easy access and reference, ensuring that users can quickly find and utilize the recipes they need. These booklets cover not only the recipes themselves but also include detailed information on the benefits of each herb, proper dosages, and tips for safe usage. For those looking to incorporate more natural, herbal elements into their daily lives for both culinary and health purposes, digital herbal recipe booklets are an invaluable resource. They offer a convenient way to explore the world of herbalism, empowering individuals to take control of their health and well-being using natural remedies.

AI-Based Herbal Remedy Customization Tool

AI-based tools are revolutionizing the way we customize herbal remedies to meet individual healthcare needs. By leveraging advanced algorithms, these tools analyze a range of factors including a person's current health status, genetic background, lifestyle habits, and specific health complaints. With this comprehensive data, the AI tool can suggest personalized herbal remedies tailored to the individual's unique needs. These technologies often include AI chatbots that interact with users to gather detailed health information or AI healthcare platforms that integrate with wearable devices to monitor real-time health data. This personalized approach ensures that the herbal remedies recommended are not only effective but also safe and suited to the user's specific conditions. The integration of AI in herbal medicine represents a significant step towards personalized healthcare solutions, making it easier for individuals to receive targeted and efficient treatments that align with their personal health goals.

Webinars on Sustainable Herbal Practices

Webinars that focus on teaching sustainable practices in herbalism are invaluable for traditional healers, professional herbalists, and horticulture enthusiasts alike. These interactive online seminars cover a wide array of topics, including responsible wildcrafting, ethical harvesting, cultivating beneficial plants, and making herbal preparations. Participants gain essential skills such as proper identification of medicinal plants, understanding their uses, and learning effective preservation methods. These webinars often feature experienced herbalists who share their wisdom and practical knowledge, providing both newcomers and seasoned practitioners with valuable insights. By attending these webinars, participants can enhance their understanding of sustainable herbal practices, ensuring that their use of herbs supports environmental health and promotes biodiversity. The knowledge gained from these sessions empowers individuals to practice herbalism in a way that is both ecologically responsible and highly effective.

Online Forum for Herbalists Worldwide

Online forums serve as invaluable platforms for herbalists from around the world to exchange knowledge, experiences, and insights. Renowned forums such as The Grow Network, The Herb Society, and Herb Mentor are vibrant with discussions on a wide array of topics, from plant identification to the therapeutic uses of various herbs. These forums cater to both seasoned professionals and newcomers, providing a space where questions can be asked, personal success stories can be shared, and advice on tackling challenges can be sought. The sense of community and camaraderie fostered in these online spaces is immense, creating a global network of herbalists united by their passion for plant-based healing. Such platforms not only facilitate ongoing learning and professional growth but also help in building relationships and partnerships across geographical boundaries, enriching the collective knowledge and practices in the field of herbalism.

Distance Learning Programs in Ethnobotany

Distance learning programs focused on ethnobotany offer a flexible and comprehensive approach to studying the intricate relationships between people and plants across different cultures. These programs are designed to accommodate students' unique learning paces, providing a versatile educational experience. They cover a broad spectrum of ethnobotanical subjects, including plant identification, the medicinal uses of various plants, and the cultural significance of specific flora. Students have access to a wealth of materials from field experts, engage in interactive discussions, and participate in practical assessments. This robust curriculum ensures a deep understanding of how different societies utilize plants for medicinal, nutritional, and ceremonial purposes. By offering detailed insights into the cultural importance of plants, these programs equip learners with the knowledge to apply ethnobotanical principles in diverse professional contexts, fostering a greater appreciation for the interconnectedness of human and plant life.

Smart Phone Apps for Herbal Remedies Tracking

Smartphone apps designed to track and manage the use of herbal remedies are at the forefront of the integration of technology and natural health care. These apps are incredibly beneficial for individuals who incorporate herbal remedies into their wellness routines. Many of these apps provide access to extensive databases containing detailed information on herbs, including their uses, potential side effects, and interactions with other herbs or medications. Additionally, they offer features like reminders for taking herbs at scheduled times and tools for monitoring progress over time. These functionalities make it easier for users to adhere to their herbal treatment plans and to make informed decisions about their health. By streamlining the process of managing herbal remedies, these apps enhance accessibility to herbal medicine, ensuring that users can harness the full benefits of natural treatments in a convenient and efficient manner.

Chapter 5: The Importance of Roots in Natural Healing

Turmeric Root Anti-Inflammatory Paste

Making and using turmeric root paste for its anti-inflammatory properties is simple and effective. Start by peeling and grating a medium-sized piece of fresh turmeric root. Mix it with equal parts of water and gently heat it in a pan until it forms a thick paste. Allow this mixture to cool. Once cooled, apply it directly to the inflamed areas, leaving it on for about 20-30 minutes before washing it off. The anti-inflammatory compounds in turmeric, particularly curcumin, work wonders in reducing inflammation and soothing the skin.

Turmeric root paste can also be added to foods for its health benefits. Incorporate it into soups, stews, or smoothies to take advantage of its anti-inflammatory properties when consumed orally. Regular consumption of turmeric can help manage chronic inflammation and provide relief from conditions like arthritis. As a precaution, always perform a patch test on your skin before applying the paste to ensure there are no allergic reactions.

Ginger Root Digestive Aid Syrup

To prepare ginger root syrup, begin by peeling and finely slicing about 5 tbsp of fresh ginger root. Combine the sliced ginger with one cup of water and one cup of honey in a saucepan. Heat the mixture until it boils, then diminish the heat and let it simmer for 38-40 min. After simmering, strain the mixture and preserve the syrup in a jar. This syrup can be consumed directly or mixed with warm water or tea.

Ginger is well-known for its digestive benefits, including reducing nausea, easing indigestion, and promoting healthy bowel movements. This natural remedy is quick to prepare, taking less than an hour, and can be stored in the refrigerator for up to a month. Regular use of ginger syrup can help maintain a healthy digestive system and alleviate common digestive issues.

Licorice Root Soothing Tea

Licorice root tea has been a staple in natural remedies for centuries, cherished for its soothing properties for the throat and digestive system. To prepare this tea, steep dried licorice root in boiling water for about 12-14 min. Strain the liquid and enjoy the warm, sweet tea. Licorice root contains glycyrrhizin, a compound that has anti-inflammatory and soothing effects.

For throat health, licorice root tea can help reduce inflammation and pain caused by coughs and sore throats. It acts as a demulcent, coating the throat and providing relief from irritation. For the digestive system, licorice root tea functions as a mild laxative, promoting intestinal health and aiding digestion. It can also soothe conditions like heartburn or gastrointestinal discomfort, making it an effective natural aid for overall digestive wellness.

Dandelion Root Liver Detox Tonic

Preparing a liver detox tonic using dandelion root is straightforward and beneficial for liver health. Start by collecting fresh dandelion roots or purchasing dried ones from health stores. Thoroughly clean the fresh roots and grind them into a powdered form if desired. Boil one quart of water and add two tablespoons of the dandelion root powder to the boiling water. Let the mixture simmer for 15 minutes before straining it into a glass.

For added flavor and detox benefits, consider adding a touch of fresh lemon juice or raw honey. Drink this tonic every morning before breakfast to support liver detoxification. Dandelion root is rich in antioxidants and has diuretic properties, helping to flush out toxins and promote healthy liver function. Regular consumption of this tonic can enhance liver health and improve overall well-being.

Burdock Root Skin Clearing Decoction

Clear skin is a benefit of taking burdock root decoction due to its anti-inflammatory and antibacterial properties. To prepare this decoction, begin by simmering one part burdock root in four parts water for approximately 30 minutes. This simmering process extracts the beneficial compounds from the root. After the decoction has steeped, strain out the roots to obtain a clear liquid. This decoction can be consumed internally to help cleanse the blood and support overall skin health. Additionally, it can be used externally as a skin toner. Allow the decoction to cool, then apply it to the skin with a clean cloth or cotton pad. Regular use of burdock root decoction, both internally and externally, can help reduce pimples, soothe eczema, and improve overall skin clarity. For maximum benefit, it is recommended to intake or apply this decoction consistently for several weeks.

Valerian Root Sleep Tincture

Valerian root tincture is a natural remedy known for its ability to promote restful sleep. To make the tincture, start by finely chopping 3grams tbsp of fresh or dried valerian root. Place the chopped root in a glass jar and cover it with 1 cup of high-proof vodka or rum. Seal the jar tightly and stir well to ensure the root is fully immersed in the alcohol. Allow the mixture to steep for about 12-14 days, shaking it daily to enhance the extraction process. After two weeks, strain the liquid using a cheesecloth, squeezing out as much liquid as possible from the valerian root. The resulting tincture can be stored in a dark glass bottle.

To use, begin with small gramsdoses, such as a few drops under the tongue before bedtime, and gradually increase the dosage as needed. Valerian root tincture can help improve sleep quality by reducing anxiety and promoting relaxation. Always consult a health professional before starting any new remedy to assure it is secure and suitable for your needs.

Maca Root Energy Booster

Maca root, a traditional Peruvian plant, is renowned for its energy-boosting properties. Rich in essential nutrients, including protein, fiber, vitamins, and minerals like Vitamin C, copper, and iron, maca root provides a natural and sustained energy increase. Unlike the quick jolt from caffeine, maca root offers a steady boost in energy and stamina. Maca root typically comes in powder form, making it easy to incorporate into your diet. You can add 1-3 teaspoons of maca root powder to smoothies, oatmeal, or snack bars for a nutritional boost. It is also available in capsules or liquid form, offering a convenient way to consume this powerful adaptogen. Regular intake of maca root can help improve endurance, enhance mental clarity, and support overall vitality. As with any supplement, it's best to start with a lower dose and gradually increase it, paying attention to how your body responds.

Astragalus Root Immune Enhancer

Astragalus root, an ancient Chinese herb, is highly regarded for its immune-boosting properties. The active components of astragalus root, such as polysaccharides, flavonoids, and saponins, help promote white blood cells' production, crucial for defending the body against harmful bacteria and viruses. Additionally, astragalus root may increase the activity of natural killer cells, enhancing the body's ability to combat illness. This herb also has adaptogenic properties, helping the body manage physical and mental stress, which indirectly supports immune health. Astragalus root can be consumed in various forms, including supplements, tea, or powdered form. To prepare your tea, steep some slices of dried astragalus root in hot water for 18-20 min. Regular consumption of astragalus root can strengthen the immune system, reduce the risk of infections, and improve overall health. As with any herbal remedy, it is advisable to consult with a healthcare professional to determine the appropriate dosage and ensure its suitability for your individual health needs.

Beetroot Cardio Health Juice

This recipe for beetroot juice delivers a potent mix of nutrients that promote cardiovascular health. Begin by sourcing two medium-sized beets, one apple, half a lemon, and a small piece of ginger. Thoroughly wash these ingredients, peel the beets, and core the apple. Cut all the produce into manageable portions. Using a juicer, extract the juice and combine it until the mixture is uniform. Consume this juice regularly to reap its benefits. Beets are rich in nitrates, which help lower blood pressure and improve blood flow. Apples add antioxidants and fiber, lemon provides a vitamin C boost, and ginger brings anti-inflammatory benefits. This vibrant, health-infused beetroot juice supports heart health, aids in digestion, and boosts overall vitality.

Rhodiola Rosea Stress Relief Extract

Rhodiola Rosea extract is a powerful adaptogen known for its ability to help the body cope with stress and anxiety. Research shows that Rhodiola Rosea balances hormones and neurotransmitters like cortisol and adrenaline, enhancing the body's stress response system. Regular consumption can improve mental performance under stress and reduce fatigue. Rhodiola Rosea's antioxidant properties also protect cells from oxidative stress. To use Rhodiola Rosea extract, know the dosage instructions on the container or refer to a healthcare provider for personalized advice. This herbal supplement supports mental functioning, maintains energy levels, and promotes a sense of overall well-being, so it's a good natural remedy for stress relief.

Horseradish Respiratory Remedy

Preparing a horseradish remedy for respiratory health is simple and effective. Start by grinding one fresh horseradish root. Mix the ground root with an equal amount of honey. Honey not only sweetens the remedy but also acts as an expectorant to help clear mucus. Let the mixture infuse for about a day. Consume one tablespoon twice daily or as needed. Horseradish contains sulfur compounds that act as natural antibiotics, fighting respiratory infections and reducing congestion. This pungent root can cause heartburn or digestive issues in large amounts, so start with small doses and monitor your body's reaction. This remedy can provide relief from colds, sinusitis, and other respiratory ailments.

Marshmallow Root Digestive Soothe

Marshmallow root has been used for centuries to soothe the digestive system due to its potent anti-inflammatory properties. The mucilage content in the root forms a protective layer inside the gut lining when consumed, easing discomfort from conditions like stomach ulcers and acid reflux. Additionally, it aids in restoring the intestinal wall by promoting cell growth and reducing the inflammatory response. The high fiber content in marshmallow root also helps boost digestion and alleviate constipation. To incorporate marshmallow root into your diet, you can prepare your tea by steeping dried marshmallow root in hot water for 13-15 min. Drinking this tea regularly can significantly improve digestive health and comfort, providing a natural remedy for various digestive issues.

Chapter 6: Practical Applications and Recipes for Herbal Innovations

6.1 Sustainability in Herbal Use

1. WATER-SVING HERBAL GARDEN TECHNIQUES

Ingredients:

- Drip irrigation system
- Mulch
- Native herbs

Steps:

1. Install a drip irrigation system to minimize water waste.
2. Apply a layer of mulch around herbs to retain soil moisture.
3. Choose native herbs that are adapted to local climate conditions and require less water.

Usage Tips: Implement these techniques to conserve water in your herbal garden. Drip irrigation and mulch help retain moisture, while native herbs are naturally drought-resistant.

2. COMPOST TEA FOR FERTILIZING PLANTS NATURALLY

Ingredients:

- Compost
- Water
- Bucket
- Aeration device

Steps:

1. Fill a bucket with water and add compost.
2. Use an aeration device to oxygenate the mixture.
3. Let the mixture steep for 2 days.

4. Strain the liquid and use it to water your plants.

Usage Tips: Use compost tea to provide a natural boost of nutrients to your plants. Regular application can improve soil health and plant growth, making your garden more sustainable.

3. SEED SAVING METHODS FOR HEIRLOOM HERBS

Ingredients:

- Heirloom herb plants
- Paper bags
- Glass jars

Steps:

1. Allow herb plants to flower and set seed.
2. Collect seeds in paper bags once they are mature.
3. Dry seeds thoroughly before storing them in glass jars.

Usage Tips: Save seeds from heirloom herbs to preserve genetic diversity and ensure a sustainable supply of plants for future planting seasons.

4. SUSTAINABLE WILDCRAFTING PRACTICES

Ingredients:

- Foraging guide
- Sustainable harvesting tools

Steps:

1 Learn about local plants and their sustainable harvesting methods.
2 Use appropriate tools to minimize plant damage.
3 Harvest only a small portion of each plant to ensure its continued growth.

Usage Tips: Practice sustainable wildcrafting to gather herbs responsibly. Always respect nature, follow ethical guidelines, and harvest in a way that promotes plant regeneration.

5. ZERO-WASTE HERBAL PACKAGING IDEAS

Ingredients:

- Reusable glass jars
- Cloth bags
- Biodegradable labels

Steps:

1 Store dried herbs in reusable glass jars.
2 Use cloth bags for gifting or selling herbs.
3 Label jars and bags with biodegradable labels.

Usage Tips: Adopt zero-waste packaging practices to reduce your environmental footprint. Reusable and biodegradable materials help minimize waste and promote sustainability.

6. RECYCLING HERB RESIDUE FOR MULCH

Ingredients:

- Herb trimmings
- Compost pile

Steps:

1 Collect herb trimmings and plant residues.
2 Add the trimmings to your compost pile.
3 Allow the material to break down into mulch.

Usage Tips: Recycle herb residues by composting them into nutrient-rich mulch. This practice reduces waste and provides valuable organic matter for your garden.

7. HERBAL WATER FILTRATION SYSTEM

Ingredients:

- Charcoal
- Sand
- Gravel
- Herbs (e.g., mint, basil)
- Container

Steps:

1 Layer charcoal, sand, and gravel in a container.
2 Place herbs on top of the gravel layer.
3 Pour water through the system to filter and infuse it with herbal benefits.

Usage Tips: Create a simple herbal water filtration system to purify and flavor your water naturally. The herbs add a refreshing taste, while the layers help filter out impurities.

8. COMMUNITY HERB GARDEN PLANNING

Ingredients:

- Community members
- Herb seeds and plants
- Garden tools
- Compost

Steps:

1 Organize a group of community members interested in gardening.
2 Select a suitable location for the herb garden.
3 Prepare the soil with compost and plant herb seeds and plants.
4 Assign garden maintenance tasks to community members.

Usage Tips: Develop a community herb garden to promote local food production and community engagement. Sharing the responsibilities and benefits helps build a stronger community.

9. ECO-FRIENDLY HERBAL EXTRACTION METHODS

Ingredients:

- Herbs
- Ethanol
- Vegetable glycerin
- Distilled water

Steps:

1 Select an eco-friendly solvent such as ethanol, vegetable glycerin, or distilled water.
2 Combine herbs with the chosen solvent in a jar.
3 Let the jar sit for a few weeks and shake it occasionally.
4 Strain the liquid and store it in a glass bottle.

Usage Tips: Use eco-friendly extraction methods to create herbal tinctures and extracts. These methods minimize environmental impact while preserving the beneficial properties of the herbs.

10. BIODYNAMIC HERBAL GROWING PRINCIPLES

Ingredients:

- Biodynamic planting calendar
- Herb seeds and plants
- Compost

Steps:

1 Consult the biodynamic planting calendar to determine the best times for planting and harvesting herbs.
2 Prepare the soil with biodynamic compost.
3 Plant and care for herbs according to biodynamic principles.

Usage Tips: Incorporate biodynamic principles into your herb gardening to enhance plant health and soil fertility. Following the natural rhythms of the earth can lead to more robust growth.

11. PLANT-BASED NATURAL PEST CONTROL SOLUTIONS

Ingredients:

- Neem oil
- Garlic
- Soap
- Water
- Spray bottle

Steps:

1 Mix neem oil, crushed garlic, a few drops of soap, and water in a spray bottle.
2 Stir to combine.
3 Spray the solution on affected plants to deter pests.

Usage Tips: Use this natural pest control solution to protect your plants without harmful chemicals. Neem oil and garlic are effective against many common garden pest

6.2 Innovations in Heral Preparation

12. SOLAR-POWERED HERBAL DEHYDRATOR

Ingredients:

- Solar dehydrator kit
- Fresh herbs

Steps:

1 Assemble the solar dehydrator according to the kit instructions.
2 Place fresh herbs on the drying racks.
3 Position the dehydrator in a sunny location.
4 Allow herbs to dry completely before storing them in airtight containers.

Usage Tips: Use a solar-powered dehydrator to preserve herbs sustainably. This method uses renewable energy, reducing your carbon footprint and maintaining the herbs' potency.

13. NON-TOXIC HERBAL PRESERVATION METHODS

Ingredients:

- Herbs
- Natural preservatives (e.g., vitamin E oil, rosemary extract)

Steps:

1 Add natural preservatives to herbal preparations to extend their shelf life.
2 Store the preparations in airtight containers to maintain freshness.

Usage Tips: Employ non-toxic preservation methods to ensure the safety and longevity of your herbal products. Natural preservatives like vitamin E oil and rosemary extract are effective and safe.

14. HIGH-EFFICIENCY HERBAL OIL PRESS

Ingredients:

- Herbs
- High-efficiency oil press

Steps:

1 Load herbs into the oil press.
2 Operate the press described in the manufacturer's instructions to extract the oil.
3 Collect the extracted oil and preserve it in a glass bottle.

Usage Tips: Utilize a high-efficiency oil press to extract pure, high-quality herbal oils. This tool maximizes yield and maintains the integrity of the herbs' beneficial compounds.

15. PRECISION DOSING FOR HERBAL REMEDIES

Ingredients:

- Herbal extracts
- Precision dropper or dosing device

Steps:

1 Measure the exact dosage of herbal extract using a precision dropper or dosing device.

2 Administer the measured dose as needed.

Usage Tips: Utilize precision dosing tools to ensure accurate and consistent administration of herbal remedies. This is especially important for potent extracts that require careful measurement.

16. AUTOMATED HERBAL PLANT WATERING SYSTEM

Ingredients:

- Automated watering system
- Water source
- Herbal garden

Steps:

1 Install the automated watering system in your herbal garden.
2 Connect the system to a water source.
3 Set the timer and watering schedule according to your plants' needs.

Usage Tips: Use an automated watering system to ensure consistent hydration for your herbs. This innovation saves time and water while promoting healthy plant growth.

17. PORTABLE HERB GRINDER AND BLENDER

Ingredients:

- Dried herbs
- Portable herb grinder and blender

Steps:

1 Place dried herbs in the grinder and blend until finely ground.
2 Transfer the ground herbs to an airtight container.

Usage Tips: Use a portable herb grinder and blender to prepare herbal powders on the go. This tool is convenient for creating fresh herbal blends anytime, anywhere.

18. DIY HERBAL ENCAPSULATION MACHINE

Ingredients:

- Herbal powder
- Empty gelatin capsules

- Encapsulation machine

Steps:

1 Fill the encapsulation machine with empty gelatin capsules.
2 Add herbal powder to the machine.
3 Operate the machine to fill and seal the capsules.
4 Preserve the capsules in an airtight container.

Usage Tips: Utilize a DIY encapsulation machine to create your own herbal supplements. This allows for precise dosing and ensures the quality of the ingredients used.

19. COLD BREW HERBAL INFUSION DEVICE

Ingredients:

- Herbs
- Cold brew infusion device
- Water

Steps:

1 Place herbs in the infusion chamber of the cold brew device.
2 Fill the device with water.
3 Refrigerate and let steep for 8-12 hours.
4 Serve the cold brew herbal infusion over ice.

Usage Tips: Enjoy refreshing herbal infusions with a cold brew device. This method preserves delicate flavors and nutrients, providing a smooth and flavorful beverage.

20. HOME-BASED HERBAL DISTILLATION SETUP

Ingredients:

- Herbs
- Distillation equipment
- Water

Steps:

1 Set up the distillation equipment described in the manufacturer's instructions.
2 Add herbs and water to the distillation chamber.

3 Heat the mixture to produce steam and collect the distilled herbal essence.
4 Store the distilled essence in a glass bottle.

Usage Tips: Create your own essential oils and hydrosols with a home-based distillation setup. This method allows you to capture the pure essence of herbs for various uses.

21. ULTRASONIC HERB EXTRACTION TECHNIQUE

Ingredients:

- Fresh herbs
- Solvent (e.g., ethanol)
- Ultrasonic extractor

Steps:

1 Place fresh herbs and solvent in the ultrasonic extractor.
2 Set the machine to the appropriate settings.
3 Run the extraction process as per the machine's instructions.
4 Strain the liquid and store it in a glass bottle.

Usage Tips: Employ ultrasonic extraction to efficiently extract herbal compounds. This advanced technique enhances the yield and purity of the extracts while being environmentally friendly.

6.3 Herbs for a Sustainable Future

22. POLLUTION-ABSORBING PLANTS FOR CITY ENVIRONMENTS

Ingredients:

- Seeds or seedlings of pollution-absorbing plants (e.g., spider plant, English ivy, peace lily)

Steps:

1 Plant pollution-absorbing plants in containers or garden beds.
2 Place the plants in areas with high pollution levels.
3 Water and care for the plants regularly.

Usage Tips: Use pollution-absorbing plants to improve air quality in urban environments. These plants help to filter and clean the air, creating a healthier living space.

23. FAST-GROWING HERBS FOR RAPID HARVEST CYCLES

Ingredients:

- Seeds or seedlings of fast-growing herbs (e.g., basil, cilantro, mint)

Steps:

1 Plant fast-growing herbs in nutrient-rich soil.
2 Water regularly and ensure adequate sunlight.
3 Harvest herbs frequently to encourage continuous growth.

Usage Tips: Grow fast-growing herbs for quick harvests and continuous supply. These herbs are ideal for home gardens and can be harvested multiple times in a single season.

24. HERBS THAT IMPROVE SOIL FERTILITY

Ingredients:

- Seeds or seedlings of soil-enhancing herbs (e.g., comfrey, clover, alfalfa)

Steps:

1 Plant soil-enhancing herbs in nutrient-poor areas.
2 Water and care for the herbs as they grow.
3 Use the herbs as green manure by cutting and incorporating them into the soil.

Usage Tips: Grow herbs that improve soil fertility to enhance garden productivity. These herbs add organic matter and nutrients to the soil, promoting healthy plant growth.

25. URBAN ADAPTED HERBAL SPECIES FOR ROOF GARDENS

Ingredients:

- Seeds or seedlings of urban-adapted herbs (e.g., chives, oregano, parsley)

Steps:

1 Prepare the roof garden with suitable soil and containers.
2 Plant urban-adapted herbs in the containers.
3 Water and maintain the herbs regularly.

Usage Tips: Create a roof garden with herbs adapted to urban environments. These herbs are well-suited for container gardening and can thrive in the unique conditions of rooftop gardens.

26. HERBS THAT REQUIRE MINIMAL FERTILIZER

Ingredients:

- Seeds or seedlings of low-fertilizer herbs (e.g., lavender, sage, thyme)

Steps:

1. Plant low-fertilizer herbs in well-draining soil.
2. Water and care for the herbs with minimal fertilizer application.
3. Monitor the plants for healthy growth.

Usage Tips: Grow herbs that require minimal fertilizer to reduce environmental impact. These herbs are naturally resilient and can thrive with little to no additional nutrients.

27. NATIVE PLANT PROMOTION FOR BIODIVERSITY

Ingredients:

- Seeds or seedlings of native herbs (varies by region)

Steps:

1. Research and select native herbs for your region.
2. Plant the herbs in suitable locations.
3. Water and care for the herbs to promote growth.

Usage Tips: Promote biodiversity by growing native herbs in your garden. Native plants support local ecosystems and provide habitat for beneficial wildlife.

28. HIGH-YIELD HERBS FOR SMALL SPACES

Ingredients:

- Seeds or seedlings of high-yield herbs (e.g., basil, parsley, chives)

Steps:

1. Plant high-yield herbs in containers or small garden beds.
2. Water and fertilize regularly to promote growth.
3. Harvest frequently to encourage continuous production.

Usage Tips: Maximize productivity in small spaces by growing high-yield herbs. These herbs provide abundant harvests even in limited areas, making them ideal for urban gardening.

29. PERENNIAL HERBS FOR LONG-TERM CULTIVATION

Ingredients:

- Seeds or seedlings of perennial herbs (e.g., rosemary, mint, thyme)

Steps:

1. Plant perennial herbs in well-prepared garden beds.
2. Water and care for the herbs as they establish.
3. Prune and maintain the plants to encourage healthy growth.

Usage Tips: Cultivate perennial herbs for long-term gardening success. These herbs come back year after year, providing a reliable source of fresh herbs with minimal replanting.

30. ROUGHT-RESISTANT HERBAL VARIETIES FOR ARID CLIMATES

Ingredients:

- Seeds or seedlings of drought-resistant herbs (e.g., rosemary, thyme, sage)

Steps:

1. Select drought-resistant herbs suited for arid climates.
2. Plant the herbs in well-draining soil.
3. Water sparingly and mulch to retain moisture.

Usage Tips: Choose drought-resistant herbs for sustainable gardening in arid regions. These herbs thrive with minimal water, reducing the strain on water resources.

31. CARBON-CAPTURING PLANT SPECIES

Ingredients:

- Seeds or seedlings of carbon-capturing plants (e.g., bamboo, grasses)

Steps:

1. Plant carbon-capturing species in suitable locations.

2 Ensure proper spacing and care to promote healthy growth.

3 Monitor and maintain plants to maximize carbon sequestration.

Usage Tips: Incorporate carbon-capturing plants into your garden to help mitigate climate change. These plants absorb and store carbon dioxide, reducing greenhouse gases in the atmosphere.

32. HERBAL CONTRIBUTIONS TO WILDLIFE HABITATS

Ingredients:

- Seeds or seedlings of wildlife-friendly herbs (e.g., echinacea, milkweed, lavender)

Steps:

1 Plant wildlife-friendly herbs in your garden.

2 Provide water and shelter for local wildlife.

3 Avoid using pesticides and herbicides to create a safe habitat.

Usage Tips: Enhance your garden's contribution to local wildlife by growing herbs that provide food and habitat. These plants support pollinators and other beneficial creatures, promoting biodiversity.

6.4 Education and Modern Herbalism

33. SMART PHONE APPS FOR HERBAL REMEDIES TRACKING

Ingredients:

- Smartphone
- Herbal remedies tracking app

Steps:

1 Download and install the herbal remedies tracking app.

2 Input your herbal remedy usage and track your progress.

3 Use the app to monitor and adjust your herbal regimen.

Usage Tips: Manage and track your herbal remedies with smartphone apps. These tools help you stay organized and ensure consistent use of your herbal treatments.

34. DIGITAL HERBAL RECIPE BOOKLETS

Ingredients:

- Computer
- Access to digital herbal recipe booklets

Steps:

1 Download digital herbal recipe booklets from reputable sources.

2 Read through the recipes and gather the necessary ingredients.

3 Follow the recipes to create herbal remedies and dishes.

Usage Tips: Expand your herbal repertoire with digital recipe booklets. These resources provide a wealth of herbal recipes that you can easily access and use in your daily life.

35. VIRTUAL REALITY HERBAL GARDEN TOURS

Ingredients:

- VR headset
- Access to virtual garden tours

Steps:

1 Set up your VR headset according to the manufacturer's instructions.

2 Select a virtual herbal garden tour from the available options.

3 Explore the virtual garden to learn about different herbs and their uses.

Usage Tips: Experience herbal gardens from around the world with virtual reality tours. This immersive technology allows you to learn about herbs and gardening techniques in a unique and engaging way.

36. ONLINE FORUM FOR HERBALISTS WORLDWIDE

Ingredients:

- Computer or smartphone
- Access to an online herbalist forum

Steps:

1 Join an online forum dedicated to herbalism.
2 Participate in discussions and share your knowledge.
3 Learn from the experiences and expertise of other herbalists around the world.

Usage Tips: Connect with a global community of herbalists through online forums. These platforms offer a space to exchange ideas, seek advice, and expand your herbal knowledge.

37. AI-BASED HERBAL REMEDY CUSTOMIZATION TOOL

Ingredients:

- Computer or smartphone
- Access to an AI-based herbal remedy tool

Steps:

1 Input your specific health needs and preferences into the tool.
2 The AI will generate customized herbal remedy recommendations.
3 Follow the recommendations to create personalized herbal remedies.

Usage Tips: Leverage AI technology to customize herbal remedies for your unique needs. This tool provides personalized recommendations based on your health profile and preferences.

38. E-LEARNING MODULES ON HERBAL MEDICINE MAKING

Ingredients:

- Computer + Internet connection
- Access to e-learning modules

Steps:

1 Find e-learning modules on herbal medicine making from reputable sources.
2 Enroll in the modules and complete the lessons at your own pace.
3 Practice making herbal remedies using the instructions provided.

Usage Tips: Enhance your herbal medicine-making skills with e-learning modules. These online lessons provide detailed instructions and practical tips for creating effective herbal remedies.

39. INTERACTIVE HERBAL WORKSHOPS ONLINE

Ingredients:

- Computer + Internet connection
- Enrollment in an online herbal workshop

Steps:

1 Register for an interactive herbal workshop online.
2 Participate in live sessions and hands-on activities as instructed.
3 Engage with instructors and fellow participants to enhance your learning.

Usage Tips: Join interactive herbal workshops to learn new skills and connect with other herbal enthusiasts. These workshops offer practical, hands-on learning experiences from the comfort of your home.

40. WEBINARS ON SUSTAINABLE HERBAL PRACTICES

Ingredients:

- Computer
- Internet connection
- Enrollment in webinars

Steps:

1 Find webinars on sustainable herbal practices from reputable sources.
2 Register for the webinars and participate in live sessions.
3 Apply the sustainable practices learned in your own herbal garden.

Usage Tips: Stay informed on sustainable herbal practices by attending webinars. These sessions provide valuable insights and tips for growing and using herbs responsibly and sustainably.

41. INTERACTIVE HERBAL WORKSHOPS ONLINE

Ingredients:

- Computer + Internet connection
- Enrollment in an online herbal workshop

Steps:

4 Register for an interactive herbal workshop online.
5 Participate in live sessions and hands-on activities as instructed.
6 Engage with instructors and fellow participants to enhance your learning.

Usage Tips: Join interactive herbal workshops to learn new skills and connect with other herbal enthusiasts. These workshops offer practical, hands-on learning experiences from the comfort of your home.

42. DISTANCE LEARNING PROGRAMS IN ETHNOBOTANY

Ingredients:

- Computer + Internet connection
- Enrollment in a distance learning program

Steps:

1 Research and select a distance learning program in ethnobotany.
2 Enroll in the program and complete the coursework.
3 Apply the knowledge gained to your herbal practices.

Usage Tips: Deepen your understanding of ethnobotany with distance learning programs. These courses provide comprehensive education on the cultural and historical uses of plants

43. ONLINE HERBALIST CERTIFICATION COURSES

Ingredients:

- Computer + Internet connection
- Enrollment in an online herbalist course

Steps:

1 Research and select a reputable online herbalist certification course.
2 Enroll in the course and complete the required modules.
3 Participate in any hands-on or practical assignments as instructed.

Usage Tips: Advance your knowledge and skills in herbalism with online certification courses. These courses offer flexibility and comprehensive education in herbal medicine and practices.

44. AUGMENTED REALITY APP FOR PLANT IDENTIFICATION

Ingredients:

- Smartphone or tablet
- Augmented reality plant identification app

Steps:

1 Download and install the augmented reality plant identification app on your device.
2 Open the app and use the camera to scan plants in your garden.
3 The app will provide information and identification for each plant.

Usage Tips: Use augmented reality apps to identify and learn about plants in real-time. This technology makes it easy to discover new herbs and understand their uses and benefits

6.5 The Importance of Roots in Natural Healing

45. TURMERIC ROOT ANTI-INFLAMMATORY PASTE

Ingredients:

- 1/3 cup fresh turmeric root, grated
- 1/3 cup water
- 1 tbsp coconut oil

Steps:

1. Combine grated turmeric root and water in a small saucepan.
2. Simmer over low heat until a thick paste forms.
3. Stir in coconut oil and mix.
4. Preserve the paste in a glass jar.

Usage Tips: Apply this anti-inflammatory paste to sore muscles and joints. Turmeric's active compound, curcumin, helps reduce inflammation and relieve pain.

46. ASTRAGALUS ROOT IMMUNE ENHANCER

Ingredients:

- 1 tsp dried astragalus root
- 1 cup boiling water

Steps:

1. Combine dried astragalus root and boiling water in your teapot.
2. Let steep for 8-9 min, then strain.
3. Serve warm.

Usage Tips: Drink this tea regularly to support immune health. Astragalus root is important for its immune-boosting properties, helping the body from illness.

47. GINGER ROOT DIGESTIVE AID SYRUP

Ingredients:

- 1/3 cup fresh ginger root, grated
- 1 cup water
- 1/2 cup honey

Steps:

1. Combine grated ginger root and water in a saucepan.
2. Simmer for 20 minutes, then strain.
3. Add honey to the strained liquid and mix well.
4. Store the syrup in a glass bottle.

Usage Tips: Take a spoonful of this syrup after meals to aid digestion. Ginger is known for its digestive benefits, helping to soothe the stomach and reduce bloating.

48. MARSHMALLOW ROOT DIGESTIVE SOOTHE

Ingredients:

- 1 tsp dried marshmallow root
- 1 cup boiling water

Steps:

1. Combine dried marshmallow root and boiling water in your teapot.
2. Let steep for 8-9 min, then strain.
3. Serve warm.

Usage Tips: Drink this tea to soothe digestive discomfort. Marshmallow root has demulcent properties that help coat and protect the digestive tract, providing relief from irritation.

49. LICORICE ROOT SOOTHING TEA

Ingredients:

- 1 tsp dried licorice root
- 1 cup boiling water
- 1 tbsp honey

Steps:

1. Mix dried licorice root and boiling water in your teapot.
2. Let steep for 8-9 min, then strain.
3. Stir in honey and serve.

Usage Tips: Drink this tea to soothe your throat and support respiratory health. Licorice root has natural demulcent properties that aid to relieve irritation and inflammation.

50. DANDELION ROOT LIVER DETOX TONIC

Ingredients:

- 1 tsp dried dandelion root
- 1 cup boiling water
- 1 tbsp lemon juice

Steps:

1 Combine dried dandelion root and boiling water in your teapot.
2 Let steep for 8-9 min, then strain.
3 Stir in lemon juice and serve.

Usage Tips: Use this tonic to support liver detoxification and overall liver health. Dandelion root is known for its detoxifying properties, helping to cleanse and rejuvenate the liver.

51. BURDOCK ROOT SKIN CLEARING DECOCTION

Ingredients:

- 1 tsp dried burdock root
- 2 cups water

Steps:

1 Combine dried burdock root and water in a saucepan.
2 Simmer for 20 minutes, then strain.
3 Allow the decoction to cool before applying to the skin.

Usage Tips: Use this decoction as a natural remedy for skin issues. Burdock root helps to cleanse the skin and can be used as a topical treatment for acne and other conditions.

52. VALERIAN ROOT SLEEP TINCTURE

Ingredients:

- 1/3 cup dried valerian root
- 1 cup vodka or glycerin

Steps:

1 Combine dried valerian root and vodka or glycerin in a glass jar.
2 Seal the jar and let it sit for about 30 days, shaking occasionally.

3 Strain the liquid and store it in a dark glass bottle.

Usage Tips: Take a few drops of this tincture before bedtime to promote relaxation and improve sleep quality. Valerian root is known for its calming and sedative effects.

53. MACA ROOT ENERGY BOOSTER

Ingredients:

- 1 tbsp maca root powder
- 1 cup almond milk
- 1 tsp honey

Steps:

1 Combine maca root powder, almond milk, and honey in a blender.
2 Mix well.
3 Serve immediately.

Usage Tips: Enjoy this energy-boosting drink in the morning or before a workout. Maca root helps increase stamina and endurance, making it an excellent natural supplement.

54. BEETROOT CARDIO HEALTH JUICE

Ingredients:

- 1 medium beetroot, peeled and chopped
- 1 apple, cored and chopped
- 1/2 lemon, juiced
- 1 cup water

Steps:

1 Combine beetroot, apple, lemon juice, and water in a blender.
2 Mix well.
3 Strain the juice and serve.

Usage Tips: Drink this juice to support cardiovascular health. Beetroot is rich in nitrates, which aid diminish blood pressure and augment blood flow.

55. RHODIOLA ROSEA STRESS RELIEF EXTRACT

Ingredients:

- 1/3 cup dried rhodiola rosea root
- 1 cup vodka or glycerin

Steps:

1. Combine dried rhodiola rosea root and vodka or glycerin in a glass jar.
2. Seal the jar and let it sit for about 30 days, mixing every day.
3. Strain the liquid and store it in a dark glass bottle.

Usage Tips: Take a few drops of this extract during stressful times to promote relaxation and mental clarity. Rhodiola rosea is important for its adaptogenic properties, aiding the body manage stress.

56. HORSERADISH RESPIRATORY REMEDY

Ingredients:

- 1/3 cup freshly grated horseradish root
- 1/3 cup apple cider vinegar
- 1 tbsp honey

Steps:

1. Combine grated horseradish root, apple cider vinegar, and honey in a glass jar.
2. Seal the jar and let it sit for 1-2 weeks, shaking occasionally.
3. Strain the liquid and store it in a glass bottle.

Usage Tips: Take a spoonful of this remedy to clear sinuses and support respiratory health. Horseradish has natural decongestant properties, making it effective for relieving sinus congestion.

Chapter 7: Home Remedies and Preparations

7.1 Creating a Tranquil Home Environment with Plants

57. AIR-PURIFYING HOUSEPLANT MIX

Ingredients:

- 1 Spider plant
- 1 Peace lily
- 1 Boston fern

Steps:

1 Select a pot with good drainage.
2 Place a layer of pebbles at the bottom.
3 Add potting soil and plant the houseplants.
4 Water thoroughly and place in a bright, indirect light.

Usage Tips: Use these houseplants to improve indoor air quality and create a calming environment.

58. RELAXING HERBAL TERRARIUM

Ingredients:

- 1 small glass terrarium
- 1 Lavender plant
- 1 Rosemary plant
- Potting soil
- Pebbles

Steps:

1 Place a layer of pebbles at the bottom of the terrarium.
2 Add potting soil on top.
3 Plant the lavender and rosemary.
4 Water lightly and place in a bright, indirect light.

Usage Tips: Keep this terrarium in your living space to promote relaxation and a pleasant aroma.

59. OXYGEN-BOOSTING BEDROOM PLANT SETUP

Ingredients:

- 1 Snake plant
- 1 Aloe vera plant
- 1 Spider plant
- Potting soil
- Pebbles

Steps:

1 Select pots with good drainage.
2 Place a layer of pebbles at the bottom.
3 Add potting soil and plant the snake plant, aloe vera, and spider plant.
4 Water thoroughly and place in your bedroom.

Usage Tips: These plants boost oxygen levels and improve air quality in your bedroom.

60. FENG SHUI PLANT ARRANGEMENT FOR HARMONY

Ingredients:

- 1 Jade plant
- 1 Bamboo plant
- 1 Peace lily
- Potting soil
- Pebbles

Steps:

1 Choose a pot with good drainage.

2 Place a layer of pebbles at the bottom.

3 Add potting soil and plant the jade, bamboo, and peace lily.

4 Water thoroughly and place in a well-lit area.

Usage Tips: Use this arrangement to balance energy in your home and promote harmony.

---

61. CALMING LAVENDER WINDOW BOXES

Ingredients:

- Lavender plants
- Window box
- Potting soil

Steps:

1 Fill the window box with potting soil.

2 Plant the lavender evenly spaced.

3 Water thoroughly and place in a sunny window.

Usage Tips: Place lavender window boxes in your home to promote relaxation and reduce stress.

---

62. AROMATIC HERB WREATHS FOR PEACEFUL LIVING

Ingredients:

- Fresh rosemary sprigs
- Fresh lavender sprigs
- Fresh thyme sprigs
- Wreath frame
- Floral wire

Steps:

1 Arrange the herb sprigs on the wreath frame.

2 Secure them with floral wire.

3 Continue until the wreath is fully covered.

4 Hang in a well-ventilated area.

Usage Tips: Hang this herb wreath in your home for a pleasant aroma and a touch of natural beauty.

---

63. STRESS-REDUCING INDOOR WATER GARDEN

Ingredients:

- Glass bowl
- Water plants (e.g., water lily, water lettuce)
- Pebbles

Steps:

1 Fill the glass bowl with water.

2 Add pebbles to the bottom.

3 Place the water plants in the bowl.

Usage Tips: Keep this indoor water garden in a quiet space to reduce stress and promote tranquility.

---

64. MOOD-LIFTING KITCHEN HERB GARDEN

Ingredients:

- Basil plant
- Mint plant
- Thyme plant
- Potting soil
- Pebbles
- Window box or pots

Steps:

1 Fill the window box or pots with potting soil.

2 Plant the basil, mint, and thyme.

3 Water thoroughly and place in a sunny kitchen window.

Usage Tips: Use fresh herbs from your kitchen garden to enhance meals and boost your mood.

---

65. SERENE LIVING ROOM IVY PLACEMENT

Ingredients:

- English ivy plant
- Hanging basket or pot
- Potting soil

Steps:

1 Fill the hanging basket or pot with potting soil.

2 Plant the English ivy.

3 Water thoroughly and place in a bright, indirect light.

Usage Tips: Place English ivy in your living room to create a serene and elegant atmosphere.

66. HEALING ALOE CORNER FOR SUNBURN RELIEF

Ingredients:

- Aloe vera plant
- Pot
- Potting soil

Steps:

1 Fill the pot with potting soil.
2 Plant the aloe vera.
3 Water thoroughly and place in a sunny spot.

Usage Tips: Use aloe vera gel from the plant to soothe sunburn and minor skin irritations.

67. PEACEFUL BAMBOO ARRANGEMENT IN HOME OFFICE

Ingredients:

- Bamboo stalks
- Vase
- Pebbles
- Water

Steps:

1 Place pebbles in the vase.
2 Add bamboo stalks.
3 Fill with water to cover the roots.

Usage Tips: Keep bamboo in your home office to promote peace and improve focus.

7.2 Eco-Friendly House Cleaning with Natural Products

68. ALL-PURPOSE CITRUS PEEL CLEANER

Ingredients:

- Peels from 2 oranges
- 2 cups white vinegar
- 1 cup water

Steps:

1 Place citrus peels in a jar.
2 Cover with white vinegar and let sit for 2 weeks.
3 Strain the mixture and dilute with water.
4 Pour into a spray bottle.

Usage Tips: Use this cleaner on countertops, floors, and other surfaces for a natural, fresh scent.

69. BAKING SODA AND VINEGAR DRAIN CLEANER

Ingredients:

- 1/2 cup baking soda
- 1/2 cup white vinegar
- Boiling water

Steps:

1 Pour baking soda down the drain.
2 Follow with white vinegar and let sit for 15 minutes.
3 Flush with boiling water.

Usage Tips: Use this method once a month to keep drains clear and free of odors.

70. LEMON AND ROSEMARY DISINFECTANT SPRAY

Ingredients:

- Peels from 1 lemon
- 2 sprigs fresh rosemary
- 2 cups white vinegar
- 1 cup water

Steps:

1 Place lemon peels and rosemary in a jar.

2 Cover with white vinegar and let sit for 2 weeks.

3 Strain the mixture and dilute with water.

4 Pour into a spray bottle.

Usage Tips: Use this disinfectant spray on surfaces to clean and freshen naturally.

71. ECO-FRIENDLY WINDOW CLEANER WITH CORNSTARCH

Ingredients:

- 1/3 cup white vinegar
- 1/3 cup rubbing alcohol
- 1 tbsp cornstarch
- 2 cups water

Steps:

1 Transfer all ingredients in a spray bottle.

2 Stir well to mix.

3 Spray on windows and wipe clean with a microfiber cloth.

Usage Tips: Use this window cleaner for a streak-free shine on glass surfaces.

72. LAVENDER AND TEA TREE MOLD REMOVER

Ingredients:

- 1/2 cup white vinegar
- 1/2 cup water
- 12 drops lavender essential oil
- 12 drops tea tree essential oil

Steps:

1 Transfer all ingredients in a spray bottle.

2 Stir well to mix.

3 Spray on moldy surfaces and let sit for 15 minutes.

4 Scrub and rinse clean.

Usage Tips: Use this mold remover to naturally eliminate mold and mildew from surfaces.

73. NATURAL CARPET FRESHENER WITH BAKING SODA AND ESSENTIAL OILS

Ingredients:

- 1 cup baking soda
- 12 drops essential oil of your choice (e.g., lavender, lemon)

Steps:

1 Transfer baking soda and essential oil in a jar.

2 Stir well to mix.

3 Sprinkle on carpet and let sit for 30 min.

4 Vacuum thoroughly.

Usage Tips: Use this carpet freshener to remove odors and freshen carpets naturally.

74. HERBAL FLOOR WASH WITH MINT AND LEMON

Ingredients:

- 1 gallon hot water
- 1/3 cup white vinegar
- 1/3 cup baking soda
- 12 drops peppermint essential oil
- 12 drops lemon essential oil

Steps:

1 Transfer all ingredients in a bucket.

2 Stir well to mix.

3 Use a mop to clean floors.

Usage Tips: Use this floor wash to clean and deodorize floors naturally.

75. GREASE-CUTTING DISH SOAP WITH LIME AND BASIL

Ingredients:

- 1 cup liquid castile soap
- 1/3 cup white vinegar
- 12 drops lime essential oil
- 12 drops basil essential oil

Steps:

1 Transfer all ingredients in a bottle.

2 Stir well to mix.

3 Use as regular dish soap.

Usage Tips: Use this dish soap to effectively cut grease and leave dishes sparkling clean.

76. CINNAMON AND CLOVE FRIDGE FRESHENER

Ingredients:

- 1 cup baking soda
- 12 drops cinnamon essential oil
- 12 drops clove essential oil

Steps:

1 Transfer baking soda and essential oils in a jar.
2 Stir well to mix.
3 Place an open jar in the fridge to absorb odors.

Usage Tips: Use this freshener to keep your refrigerator smelling fresh and clean.

77. ANTIBACTERIAL THYME AND LEMON COUNTER SPRAY

Ingredients:

- 1/2 cup white vinegar
- 1/2 cup water
- 12 drops thyme essential oil
- 12 drops lemon essential oil

Steps:

1 Transfer all ingredients in a spray bottle.
2 Stir well to mix.
3 Spray on countertops and wipe clean.

Usage Tips: Use this spray to disinfect countertops and other surfaces naturally.

78. SOFT SCRUB CLEANER WITH LAVENDER AND EUCALYPTUS

Ingredients:

- 1/2 cup baking soda
- 1/3 cup liquid castile soap
- 12 drops lavender essential oil
- 12 drops eucalyptus essential oil

Steps:

1 Transfer all ingredients in a bowl.
2 Mix to form a paste.
3 Apply to surfaces and scrub with a sponge.
4 Rinse clean.

Usage Tips: Use this soft scrub cleaner for tough stains and grime in the kitchen and bathroom.

7.3 DIY Personal Care Products

79. PROTECTIVE SHEA BUTTER SUNSCREEN

Ingredients:

- 1/3 cup shea butter
- 1/3 cup coconut oil
- 2 tbsp zinc oxide
- 12 drops carrot seed essential oil

Steps:

1 Melt shea butter and coconut oil together in a double boiler.
2 Remove from heat and stir in zinc oxide and carrot seed essential oil.
3 Pour the mixture into a jar and let it cool.

Usage Tips: Apply this sunscreen to protect your skin from harmful UV rays.

80. THYME AND WITCH HAZEL AFTERSHAVE

Ingredients:

- 1/2 cup witch hazel
- 1/3 cup dried thyme
- 12 drops tea tree essential oil

Steps:

1 Place dried thyme in a jar.
2 Cover with witch hazel and let sit for 2 weeks.
3 Strain the mixture and add tea tree essential oil.

4 Pour into a bottle.

Usage Tips: Use this aftershave to soothe and disinfect your skin after shaving.

81. HERBAL DEODORANT WITH SAGE AND ROSEMARY

Ingredients:

- 1/3 cup coconut oil
- 1/3 cup baking soda
- 1/3 cup arrowroot powder
- 12 drops sage essential oil
- 12 drops rosemary essential oil

Steps:

1 Transfer all ingredients in a bowl.
2 Stir to form a paste.
3 Transfer to a jar and apply a small amount to underarms.

Usage Tips: Use this deodorant daily for natural odor protection.

82. SOOTHING CALENDULA LIP BALM

Ingredients:

- 1/3 cup coconut oil
- 1/3 cup beeswax pellets
- 1 tbsp calendula oil

Steps:

1 Melt coconut oil and beeswax pellets together in a double boiler.
2 Remove from heat and stir in calendula oil.
3 Pour the mixture into lip balm tubes and let it cool.

Usage Tips: Apply this lip balm to soothe and protect your lips.

83. NATURAL PEPPERMINT TOOTHPASTE

Ingredients:

- 1/3 cup coconut oil
- 1/3 cup baking soda
- 12 drops peppermint essential oil

Steps:

1 Combine all ingredients in a jar.
2 Mix well to form a paste.
3 Utilize a small amount on your toothbrush.

Usage Tips: Use this toothpaste to naturally clean and freshen your teeth.

84. HOMEMADE LAVENDER AND HONEY FACE WASH

Ingredients:

- 1/3 cup liquid castile soap
- 1/3 cup honey
- 12 drops lavender essential oil

Steps:

1 Transfer all ingredients in a bottle.
2 Stir well to mix.
3 Use a small amount to wash your face, then rinse.

Usage Tips: Use this gentle face wash daily to cleanse and soothe your skin.

85. CHAMOMILE AND CUCUMBER EYE CREAM

Ingredients:

- 1/3 cup coconut oil
- 1/3 cup shea butter
- 1 tbsp cucumber juice
- 1 tbsp chamomile tea

Steps:

1 Melt coconut oil and shea butter together in a double boiler.
2 Remove from heat and stir in cucumber juice and chamomile tea.
3 Pour the mixture into a jar and let it cool.

Usage Tips: Apply this eye cream to reduce puffiness and hydrate the delicate skin around your eyes.

86. ROSEWATER AND ALOE VERA FACIAL TONER

Ingredients:

- 1/2 cup rosewater
- 1/3 cup aloe vera gel
- 1/3 cup witch hazel

Steps:

1 Transfer all ingredients in a spray bottle.
2 Stir well to mix.
3 Spray onto your face after cleansing.

Usage Tips: Use this toner to refresh and hydrate your skin.

87. COFFEE AND COCONUT OIL BODY SCRUB

Ingredients:

- 1/2 cup coffee grounds
- 1/3 cup coconut oil
- 1/3 cup brown sugar

Steps:

1 Transfer all ingredients in a bowl.
2 Stir well and transfer to a jar.
3 Apply to damp skin in circular motions, then rinse off.

Usage Tips: Utilize this scrub in the shower to exfoliate and moisturize your skin.

88. ANTIOXIDANT-RICH GREEN TEA MOISTURIZER

Ingredients:

- 1/3 cup green tea
- 1/3 cup shea butter
- 1/3 cup coconut oil

Steps:

1 Melt shea butter and coconut oil together in a double boiler.
2 Remove from heat and stir in green tea.
3 Pour the mixture into a jar and let it cool.

Usage Tips: Use this moisturizer to nourish and protect your skin from environmental damage.

89. HEALING HERBAL HAND CREAM WITH COMFREY AND SHEA

Ingredients:

- 1/3 cup shea butter
- 1/3 cup coconut oil
- 1 tbsp comfrey oil

Steps:

1 Melt shea butter and coconut oil together in a double boiler.
2 Remove from heat and stir in comfrey oil.
3 Pour the mixture into a jar and let it cool.

Usage Tips: Use this hand cream to heal and protect dry, cracked hand.

7.4 Creating a Natural First Aid Kit

90. ANTISEPTIC HERBAL SALVE WITH CALENDULA AND TEA TREE OIL

Ingredients:

- 1/3 cup coconut oil
- 1/3 cup beeswax pellets
- 1 tbsp calendula oil
- 12 drops tea tree essential oil

Steps:

1 Melt coconut oil and beeswax pellets together in a double boiler.
2 Remove from heat and stir in calendula oil and tea tree essential oil.
3 Pour the mixture into a jar and let it cool.

Usage Tips: Apply this salve to cuts and scrapes to prevent infection and promote healing.

91. ERBAL ANTI-ITCH BALM WITH CHICKWEED AND PLANTAIN

Ingredients:

- 1/3 cup coconut oil
- 1/3 cup beeswax pellets
- 1 tbsp chickweed oil
- 1 tbsp plantain oil

Steps:

1. Melt coconut oil and beeswax pellets together in a double boiler.
2. Remove from heat and stir in chickweed oil and plantain oil.
3. Pour the mixture into a jar and let it cool.

Usage Tips: Apply this balm to insect bites, rashes, and other itchy skin conditions for relief.

92. GINGER CAPSULES FOR NAUSEA AND MOTION SICKNESS

Ingredients:

- 1 tbsp dried ginger powder
- Empty gelatin or vegetarian capsules

Steps:

1. Fill the empty capsules with dried ginger powder using a capsule machine or by hand.
2. Store the filled capsules in an airtight container.

Usage Tips: Take one capsule before traveling or at the onset of nausea to ease symptoms.

93. LAVENDER ESSENTIAL OIL FOR STRESS AND SLEEP AID

Ingredients:

- 12 drops lavender essential oil
- 1 tbsp carrier oil (e.g., coconut oil, jojoba oil)

Steps:

1. Transfer lavender essential oil and carrier oil in a small bottle.
2. Stir well to mix.

Usage Tips: Apply a few drops to your wrists or temples to relieve stress and promote sleep.

94. SOOTHING ALOE VERA GEL FOR BURNS AND CUTS

Ingredients:

- 1/3 cup fresh aloe vera gel
- 12 drops lavender essential oil

Steps:

1. Combine aloe vera gel and lavender essential oil in a jar.
2. Mix well and store in the refrigerator.

Usage Tips: Use this gel to soothe burns, cuts, and other skin irritations.

95. NATURAL INSECT REPELLENT WITH CITRONELLA AND EUCALYPTUS

Ingredients:

- 1/3 cup witch hazel
- 1/3 cup water
- 12 drops citronella essential oil
- 12 drops eucalyptus essential oil

Steps:

1. Combine witch hazel, water, citronella essential oil, and eucalyptus essential oil in a spray bottle.
2. Stir well to mix.

Usage Tips: Spray on your skin and clothing to repel insects naturally.

96. ACTIVATED CHARCOAL PASTE FOR POISON ABSORPTION

Ingredients:

- 1 tbsp activated charcoal powder
- 2 tbsp water

Steps:

1. Combine activated charcoal powder and water in a small bowl.
2. Mix well to form a paste.

Usage Tips: Apply it to insect bites, stings, or minor skin irritations to draw out toxins.

---

97. CHAMOMILE EYE COMPRESS FOR RELAXATION

Ingredients:

- 1 tbsp dried chamomile flowers
- 1 cup hot water

Steps:

1 Steep dried chamomile flowers in hot water for 8-9 min.
2 Strain and soak a clean cloth in the chamomile tea.
3 Wring out excess liquid and place the cloth over your eyes.

Usage Tips: Use this compress to relax and soothe tired eyes.

---

98. ARNICA CREAM FOR BRUISES AND SPRAINS

Ingredients:

- 1/3 cup shea butter
- 1/3 cup coconut oil
- 1 tbsp arnica oil

Steps:

1 Melt shea butter and coconut oil together in a double boiler.
2 Remove from heat and stir in arnica oil.
3 Pour the mixture into a jar and let it cool.

Usage Tips: Apply this cream to bruises and sprains to reduce inflammation and pain.

---

99. ECHINACEA TINCTURE FOR IMMUNE SUPPORT

Ingredients:

- 1/3 cup dried echinacea root
- 1 cup vodka or glycerin (for alcohol-free version)

Steps:

1 Place dried echinacea root in a jar.
2 Pour vodka or glycerin over the root, ensuring it is fully submerged.
3 Seal the jar and let it sit for about 30 days, shaking occasionally.
4 Strain the tincture into a dropper bottle.

Usage Tips: Take a few drops of this tincture at the first sign of a cold to boost your immune system.

---

100. PEPPERMINT OIL ROLL-ON FOR HEADACHE RELIEF

Ingredients:

- 12 drops peppermint essential oil
- 1 tbsp carrier oil (e.g., coconut oil, jojoba oil)

Steps:

1 Combine peppermint essential oil and carrier oil in a roll-on bottle.
2 Stir well to mix.

Usage Tips: Apply to your temples and the back of your neck to relieve headaches.

7.5 Therapeutic Gardening: Cultivating Calm

101. HEALING HERB WALKWAY FEATURING LEMON BALM AND ROSEMARY

Ingredients:

- Lemon balm plants
- Rosemary plants
- Pots or garden bed
- Potting soil

Steps:

1 Fill pots or garden bed with potting soil.
2 Plant the lemon balm and rosemary along a garden path.

3 Water thoroughly and mulch to retain moisture.

Usage Tips: Walk along this healing herb path to enjoy the soothing aromas and calming effects.

102. FRAGRANT HERB PILLOWS FOR GARDEN BENCHES

Ingredients:

- Cotton fabric
- Dried lavender
- Dried chamomile
- Needle and thread

Steps:

1 Sew small pillows from the cotton fabric, leaving one side open.
2 Fill with dried lavender and chamomile.
3 Sew the opening closed.

Usage Tips: Place these herb pillows on garden benches for a fragrant and comfortable seating area.

103. STRESS-REDUCING GARDEN LAYOUT PLAN

Ingredients:

- Lavender plants
- Rosemary plants
- Mint plants
- Chamomile plants

Steps:

1 Select a sunny location for your garden.
2 Arrange the plants in a layout that allows for easy access and maintenance.
3 Plant the lavender, rosemary, mint, and chamomile.
4 Water thoroughly and mulch to retain moisture.

Usage Tips: Design your garden to create a peaceful and stress-reducing environment.

104. RELAXATION NOOK WITH CHAMOMILE AND LAVENDER

Ingredients:

- Chamomile plants
- Lavender plants
- Pots or garden bed
- Potting soil

Steps:

1 Fill pots or garden bed with potting soil.
2 Plant the chamomile and lavender.
3 Water thoroughly and place in a sunny, quiet corner.

Usage Tips: Create a cozy nook with these relaxing herbs to unwind and enjoy nature.

105. DIY HERBAL WREATH FOR NATURAL AROMATHERAPY

Ingredients:

- Fresh rosemary sprigs
- Fresh lavender sprigs
- Fresh thyme sprigs
- Wreath frame
- Floral wire

Steps:

1 Arrange the herb sprigs on the wreath frame.
2 Secure them with floral wire.
3 Continue until the wreath is fully covered.
4 Hang in a well-ventilated area.

Usage Tips: Hang this herbal wreath in your home or garden to enjoy natural aromatherapy.

106. SERENITY ROCK GARDEN WITH LOW-MAINTENANCE SUCCULENTS

Ingredients:

- Succulent plants
- Rocks or pebbles
- Sand
- Cactus soil

Steps:

1 Create a design with rocks or pebbles in a shallow tray.
2 Fill with sand and cactus soil.
3 Plant the succulents and arrange rocks or pebbles around them.
4 Water lightly and place in a sunny spot.

Usage Tips: Use this rock garden as a peaceful and low-maintenance addition to your outdoor space.

107. MINDFULNESS HERB SPIRAL WITH VARIED TEXTURES AND SCENTS

Ingredients:

- Thyme plants
- Mint plants
- Basil plants
- Sage plants
- Potting soil
- Pebbles or stones

Steps:

1 Create a spiral design with pebbles or stones.
2 Fill the spiral with potting soil.
3 Plant the thyme, mint, basil, and sage in the spiral.
4 Water thoroughly and place in a sunny location.

Usage Tips: Use this herb spiral to engage your senses and practice mindfulness in the garden.

108. AROMATIC MEDITATION CORNER WITH BASIL AND MINT

Ingredients:

- Basil plant
- Mint plant
- Pots or garden bed
- Potting soil

Steps:

1 Fill pots or garden bed with potting soil.
2 Plant the basil and mint.

3 Water thoroughly and place in a quiet corner of your garden.

Usage Tips: Create a meditation space surrounded by aromatic herbs to enhance your practice.

109. SOOTHING SOUND WIND CHIME WITH BAMBOO AND HERBS

Ingredients:

- Bamboo chime
- Fresh herbs (e.g., rosemary, lavender)
- String

Steps:

1 Tie bundles of fresh herbs to the bamboo chime with string.
2 Hang the chime in a breezy spot in your garden.

Usage Tips: Enjoy the soothing sounds and scents of the wind chime in your garden.

110. HERBAL HANGING BASKETS FOR VISUAL RELAXATION

Ingredients:

- Hanging baskets
- Mint plants
- Thyme plants
- Potting soil

Steps:

1 Fill hanging baskets with potting soil.
2 Plant the mint and thyme in the baskets.
3 Water thoroughly and hang in a sunny location.

Usage Tips: Use these hanging baskets to add greenery and relaxation to your outdoor areas.

111.   CALMING HERBAL TEA GARDEN KIT

Ingredients:

- Mint plant
- Chamomile plant
- Lemon balm plant
- Potting soil
- Pots or garden bed

Steps:

1 Fill pots or garden bed with potting soil.
2 Plant the mint, chamomile, and lemon balm.
3 Water thoroughly and place in a sunny location.

Usage Tips: Use fresh herbs from your garden to make calming herbal teas.

7.6 Plant Care for a Healthy Home

112.   SLOW-RELEASE GARLIC FERTILIZER STAKES

Ingredients:

- Garlic cloves
- Wooden skewers

Steps:

1 Peel and crush garlic cloves.
2 Thread the crushed garlic onto wooden skewers.
3 Insert the skewers into the soil around plants.

Usage Tips: Use these garlic fertilizer stakes to provide slow-release nutrients and repel pests.

113.   ECO-FRIENDLY POTTING MIX WITH COCONUT COIR

Ingredients:

- 1 part coconut coir
- 1 part compost
- 1 part perlite

Steps:

1 Combine coconut coir, compost, and perlite in a large container.
2 Mix well to combine.
3 Use as potting mix for indoor and outdoor plants.

Usage Tips: Use this eco-friendly potting mix to provide excellent drainage and nutrient retention for plants.

114.   NUTRIENT-RICH HERBAL COMPOST FOR INDOOR PLANTS

Ingredients:

- Vegetable scraps
- Coffee grounds
- Eggshells
- Grass clippings
- Leaves
- Water

Steps:

1 Combine all ingredients in a compost bin or pile.
2 Turn the compost regularly to aerate.
3 Add water as needed to keep moist.
4 Once fully decomposed, use the compost to fertilize indoor plants.

Usage Tips: Use this compost to provide indoor plants with essential nutrients for healthy growth.

115.   HOMEMADE INSECTICIDAL SOAP WITH NEEM OIL

Ingredients:

- 1 tsp neem oil
- 1/2 tsp liquid castile soap
- 1 quart water
- Spray bottle

Steps:

1 Combine neem oil, liquid castile soap, and water in a spray bottle.

2 Stir well to mix.

3 Spray on plants to control pests.

Usage Tips: Use this insecticidal soap to naturally control pests on indoor and outdoor plants.

116. ESSENTIAL OIL SPRAY FOR DUST MITES AND ALLERGENS

Ingredients:

- 1 cup water
- 1/3 cup white vinegar
- 12 drops eucalyptus essential oil
- 12 drops lavender essential oil
- Spray bottle

Steps:

1 Combine water, white vinegar, eucalyptus essential oil, and lavender essential oil in a spray bottle.

2 Stir well to mix.

3 Spray on plants and surrounding areas to reduce dust mites and allergens.

Usage Tips: Use this spray to keep your home and plants free from dust mites and allergens.

117. NATURAL ROOTING HORMONE WITH WILLOW WATER

Ingredients:

- 2 cups chopped willow branches
- 1 quart water

Steps:

1 Place chopped willow branches in a jar.

2 Cover with water and let sit for 24-48 hours.

3 Strain the mixture and use as rooting hormone.

Usage Tips: Use willow water to encourage root growth on plant cuttings.

118. DIY HERB-BASED PLANT FOOD

Ingredients:

- 1 cup compost
- 1/3 cup fish emulsion
- 1 tbsp kelp meal
- 1 gallon water

Steps:

1 Combine compost, fish emulsion, and kelp meal in a large container.

2 Add water and stir well to mix.

3 Use as liquid fertilizer for indoor and outdoor plants.

Usage Tips: Use this herb-based plant food to boost plant growth and health naturally.

119. NATURAL LEAF SHINE WITH MILK AND WATER

Ingredients:

- 1/3 cup milk
- 1/3 cup water
- Soft cloth

Steps:

1 Transfer milk and water in a bowl.

2 Dip the cloth in the mixture and wring out excess liquid.

3 Wipe the leaves of indoor plants to clean and shine.

Usage Tips: Use this natural leaf shine to keep your indoor plants looking vibrant and healthy.

120. PLANT-BASED MOLD PREVENTION SPRAY

Ingredients:

- 1 cup water
- 1/3 cup apple cider vinegar
- 12 drops tea tree essential oil
- Spray bottle

Steps:

1 Transfer water, apple cider vinegar, and tea tree essential oil in a spray bottle.

2 Stir well to mix.

3 Spray on plant leaves and soil to prevent mold.

Usage Tips: Use this spray regularly to prevent mold growth on indoor plants and soil.

121. HUMIDITY BOOSTING PEBBLE TRAY FOR HOUSEPLANTS

Ingredients:

- Shallow tray
- Pebbles
- Water

Steps:

1 Fill the shallow tray with pebbles.
2 Add water to cover the pebbles.
3 Place houseplants on top of the pebbles.

Usage Tips: Use this pebble tray to increase humidity around houseplants, especially in dry environments.

122. AIR-PURIFYING INDOOR PLANT MIX

Ingredients:

- Spider plant
- Peace lily
- Boston fern
- Potting soil
- Pots

Steps:

1 Fill pots with potting soil.
2 Plant the spider plant, peace lily, and Boston fern.
3 Water thoroughly and place in bright, indirect light.

Usage Tips: Use this plant mix to purify the air and improve indoor air quality.

7.7 Home Detox with Herbal Remedies

123. HERBAL AIR FRESHENER WITH PURIFYING ESSENTIAL OILS

Ingredients:

- 1 cup distilled water
- 1/3 cup witch hazel
- 12 drops tea tree essential oil
- 12 drops lavender essential oil
- Spray bottle

Steps:

1 Transfer distilled water, witch hazel, tea tree essential oil, and lavender essential oil in a spray bottle.
2 Stir well to mix.
3 Spray around your home as needed.

Usage Tips: Use this air freshener to purify and freshen the air in your home.

124. DETOXIFYING HOUSEPLANT ARRANGEMENT

Ingredients:

- Aloe vera plant
- Spider plant
- Peace lily
- Potting soil
- Pots

Steps:

1 Fill pots with potting soil.
2 Plant the aloe vera, spider plant, and peace lily.
3 Water thoroughly and place in bright, indirect light.

Usage Tips: Use this arrangement to detoxify the air and improve indoor air quality.

125. NATURAL DRAIN CLEANER WITH VINEGAR AND ORANGE PEELS

Ingredients:

- Peels from 2 oranges
- 1/2 cup baking soda
- 1 cup white vinegar

Steps:

1 Place orange peels in a jar.
2 Cover with white vinegar and let sit for 1 week.
3 Pour baking soda down the drain.
4 Follow with the vinegar mixture and let sit for 15 minutes.
5 Flush with boiling water.

Usage Tips: Use this natural drain cleaner to keep drains clear and free of odors.

126. HERBAL LINEN SPRAY FOR FRESHENING FABRICS

Ingredients:

- 1 cup distilled water
- 1/3 cup witch hazel
- 12 drops lavender essential oil
- 12 drops eucalyptus essential oil
- Spray bottle

Steps:

1 Transfer distilled water, witch hazel, lavender essential oil, and eucalyptus essential oil in a spray bottle.
2 Stir well to mix.
3 Spray on linens and fabrics as needed.

Usage Tips: Use this linen spray to freshen and disinfect your bed linens and clothing.

127. DETOXIFYING BENTONITE CLAY AND APPLE CIDER VINEGAR ROOM DEODORIZER

Ingredients:

- 1/3 cup bentonite clay
- 1/3 cup apple cider vinegar
- 12 drops tea tree essential oil

Steps:

1 Transfer bentonite clay, apple cider vinegar, and tea tree essential oil in a bowl.
2 Stir well to form a paste.
3 Place the mixture in a small dish and let it sit in a room.

Usage Tips: Use this room deodorizer to detoxify and freshen the air in your home.

128. GREEN CLEANING SCRUB WITH ROSEMARY AND BAKING SODA

Ingredients:

- 1 cup baking soda
- 1/3 cup liquid castile soap
- 12 drops rosemary essential oil

Steps:

1 Transfer baking soda, liquid castile soap, and rosemary essential oil in a bowl.
2 Stir well to form a paste.
3 Apply to surfaces and scrub with a sponge.
4 Rinse clean.

Usage Tips: Use this green cleaning scrub for tough stains and grime in the kitchen and bathroom.

129. CLEANSING SAGE AND LAVENDER SMUDGE STICKS

Ingredients:

- Fresh sage sprigs
- Fresh lavender sprigs
- Cotton string

Steps:

1 Bundle the sage and lavender sprigs together.
2 Secure the bundle with cotton string.
3 Hang to dry for 1-2 weeks.

Usage Tips: Use these smudge sticks to cleanse and purify the air in your home.

130.   DETOX WATER PITCHER WITH CUCUMBER, MINT, AND LEMON

Ingredients:

- 1 cucumber, sliced
- 1 lemon, sliced
- 1 handful fresh mint leaves
- 1 gallon water

Steps:

1. Combine cucumber, lemon, and mint in a pitcher.
2. Fill with water and let sit for 1 hour.
3. Serve chilled.

Usage Tips: Drink this detox water throughout the day to stay hydrated and flush out toxins.

131.   PURIFYING HIMALAYAN SALT LAMP BOWL

Ingredients:

- Himalayan salt lamp bowl
- Himalayan salt chunks
- Essential oil of your choice (e.g., lavender, eucalyptus)

Steps:

1. Place Himalayan salt chunks in the salt lamp bowl.
2. Add a few drops of essential oil.
3. Turn on the lamp to release the aroma and purify the air.

Usage Tips: Use this salt lamp bowl to improve air quality and add a soothing ambiance to your home.

132.   ANTIMICROBIAL THYME AND LEMON FLOOR CLEANER

Ingredients:

- 1 gallon hot water
- 1/3 cup white vinegar
- 12 drops thyme essential oil
- 12 drops lemon essential oil

Steps:

1. Transfer hot water, white vinegar, thyme essential oil, and lemon essential oil in a bucket.
2. Stir well to mix.
3. Use a mop to clean floors.

Usage Tips: Use this floor cleaner to disinfect and freshen your home naturally.

133.   ECO-FRIENDLY WALL PAINT WITH ESSENTIAL OIL INFUSIONS

Ingredients:

- Eco-friendly paint
- 12 drops essential oil of your choice (e.g., lavender, lemon)

Steps:

1. Stir the essential oil into the paint.
2. Mix well to combine.
3. Use as regular paint to cover walls.

Usage Tips: Use this paint to add a pleasant scent to your home while decorating.

7.8 Herbs to Strengthen Emotional Resilience

134. ADAPTOGENIC HERBAL TEA BLEND WITH ASHWAGANDHA AND HOLY BASIL

Ingredients:

- 1 tsp dried ashwagandha root
- 1 tsp dried holy basil leaves
- 1 tsp dried licorice root
- 1 cup boiling water

Steps:

1. Transfer dried ashwagandha root, holy basil leaves, and licorice root in your teapot.
2. Pour boiling water into the teapot.
3. Let steep for 8-9 min.
4. Strain into a cup and serve.

Usage Tips: Drink this tea daily to support your body's response to stress and enhance emotional resilience.

135. CALMING ESSENTIAL OIL ROLL-ON WITH BERGAMOT AND SANDALWOOD

Ingredients:

- 12 drops bergamot essential oil
- 12 drops sandalwood essential oil
- 1 tbsp carrier oil (e.g., coconut oil, jojoba oil)

Steps:

1. Transfer bergamot essential oil, sandalwood essential oil, and carrier oil in a roll-on bottle.
2. Stir well to mix.

Usage Tips: Apply this roll-on to your wrists or temples to promote calm and emotional balance.

136. EMOTIONAL SUPPORT HERBAL CAPSULES

Ingredients:

- 1 tbsp dried ashwagandha root powder
- 1 tbsp dried holy basil powder
- Empty gelatin or vegetarian capsules

Steps:

1. Combine dried ashwagandha root powder and holy basil powder in a bowl.
2. Fill the empty capsules with the powdered herbs using a capsule machine or by hand.
3. Store the filled capsules in an airtight container.

Usage Tips: Take one capsule daily to support emotional balance and resilience.

137. HERBAL MOOD-BOOSTING SMOOTHIE

Ingredients:

- 1 banana
- 1 cup almond milk
- 1 tbsp raw cacao powder
- 1 tsp maca powder
- 1 tbsp honey

Steps:

1. Transfer all ingredients in a blender.
2. Mix until smooth.
3. Pour into a glass and serve immediately.

Usage Tips: Enjoy this smoothie in the morning to boost your mood and enhance emotional resilience.

138. NOURISHING ST. JOHN'S WORT INFUSED OIL FOR SKIN APPLICATION

Ingredients:

- 1/3 cup dried St. John's Wort flowers
- 1/2 cup olive oil

Steps:

1. Place dried St. John's Wort flowers in a jar.
2. Cover with olive oil and seal the jar.
3. Let sit in a sunny spot for about 30 days, shaking occasionally.

4 Strain the oil into a clean jar.

Usage Tips: Apply this infused oil to your skin to nourish and support emotional well-being.

139. STRESS RELIEF HERBAL INHALER WITH PEPPERMINT AND EUCALYPTUS

Ingredients:

- 12 drops peppermint essential oil
- 12 drops eucalyptus essential oil
- Blank inhaler

Steps:

1 Add peppermint essential oil and eucalyptus essential oil to the blank inhaler.
2 Close the inhaler tightly.

Usage Tips: Inhale deeply from this herbal inhaler to relieve stress and promote emotional balance.

140. DAILY HERBAL TONIC FOR NERVOUS SYSTEM SUPPORT

Ingredients:

- 1 tsp dried lemon balm
- 1 tsp dried chamomile
- 1 tsp dried oatstraw
- 1 cup boiling water

Steps:

1 Combine dried lemon balm, chamomile, and oatstraw in your teapot.
2 Pour boiling water into the teapot.
3 Let steep for 8-9 min.
4 Strain into a cup and serve.

Usage Tips: Drink this tonic daily to support your nervous system and promote emotional resilience.

141. COMFORTING HERBAL PILLOW MIST

Ingredients:

- 1/2 cup distilled water

- 1/3 cup witch hazel
- 12 drops lavender essential oil
- 12 drops chamomile essential oil
- Spray bottle

Steps:

1 Transfer distilled water, witch hazel, lavender essential oil, and chamomile essential oil in a spray bottle.
2 Stir well to mix.

Usage Tips: Spray this mist on your pillow before bed to promote restful sleep and emotional comfort.

142. FLOWER ESSENCE THERAPY FOR EMOTIONAL BALANCING

Ingredients:

- 12 drops Bach Rescue Remedy
- 1 cup water

Steps:

1 Combine Bach Rescue Remedy and water in a bottle.
2 Stir well to mix.

Usage Tips: Take a few drops of this flower essence therapy under your tongue to balance emotions.

143. RESILIENCE-BOOSTING HERBAL BATH SOAK

Ingredients:

- 1 cup Epsom salts
- 1/3 cup dried lavender flowers
- 12 drops lavender essential oil

Steps:

1 Combine Epsom salts, dried lavender flowers, and lavender essential oil in a bowl.
2 Stir well and transfer to a jar.
3 Add 1/2 cup of the mixture to warm bathwater.

Usage Tips: Soak in this bath for 20 minutes to relax and boost emotional resilience.

144. PROTECTIVE AMULET WITH DRIED LAVENDER AND ROSE QUARTZ

Ingredients:

- Small fabric pouch
- 1 tbsp dried lavender flowers
- 1 small rose quartz crystal

Steps:

1. Fill the fabric pouch with dried lavender flowers.
2. Add the rose quartz crystal.
3. Tie or sew the pouch closed.

Usage Tips: Carry this amulet with you for emotional protection and to promote a sense of calm.

7.9 Learning to Make Salves and Balms

145. HEALING CALENDULA SALVE FOR SKIN IRRITATIONS

Ingredients:

- 1/3 cup coconut oil
- 1/3 cup beeswax pellets
- 1 tbsp calendula oil

Steps:

1. Melt coconut oil and beeswax pellets together in a double boiler.
2. Remove from heat and stir in calendula oil.
3. Pour the mixture into a jar and let it cool.

Usage Tips: Apply this salve to cuts, scrapes, and other skin irritations to promote healing.

146. MOISTURIZING BEESWAX LIP BALM WITH PEPPERMINT

Ingredients:

- 1/3 cup coconut oil
- 1/3 cup beeswax pellets
- 12 drops peppermint essential oil

Steps:

1. Melt coconut oil and beeswax pellets together in a double boiler.
2. Remove from heat and stir in peppermint essential oil.
3. Pour it into lip balm tubes and let it cool.

Usage Tips: Use this lip balm to moisturize and protect your lips, especially in dry weather.

147. SOOTHING CHAMOMILE EYE BALM FOR PUFFY EYES

Ingredients:

- 1/3 cup coconut oil
- 1/3 cup shea butter
- 1 tbsp chamomile oil

Steps:

1. Melt coconut oil and shea butter together in a double boiler.
2. Remove from heat and stir in chamomile oil.
3. Pour it into a jar and let it cool.

Usage Tips: Apply this eye balm to reduce puffiness and soothe the delicate skin around your eyes.

148. ANTIFUNGAL TEA TREE AND LAVENDER FOOT BALM

Ingredients:

- 1/3 cup coconut oil
- 1/3 cup shea butter

- 12 drops tea tree essential oil
- 12 drops lavender essential oil

Steps:

1 Melt coconut oil and shea butter together in a double boiler.
2 Remove from heat and stir in tea tree essential oil and lavender essential oil.
3 Pour it into a jar and let it cool.

Usage Tips: Use this foot balm to treat fungal infections and soothe tired feet.

149. ECZEMA RELIEF HERBAL BALM WITH CHICKWEED

Ingredients:

- 1/3 cup coconut oil
- 1/3 cup beeswax pellets
- 1 tbsp chickweed oil

Steps:

1 Melt coconut oil and beeswax pellets together in a double boiler.
2 Remove from heat and stir in chickweed oil.
3 Pour it into a jar and let it cool.

Usage Tips: Apply this balm to eczema-affected areas to reduce itching and inflammation.

150. ARNICA BALM FOR PAIN RELIEF

Ingredients:

- 1/3 cup shea butter
- 1/3 cup coconut oil
- 1 tbsp arnica oil

Steps:

1 Melt shea butter and coconut oil together in a double boiler.
2 Remove from heat and stir in arnica oil.
3 Pour it into a jar and let it cool.

Usage Tips: Apply this balm to bruises, sprains, and sore muscles to relieve pain.

151. DIY HERBAL MUSCLE RUB WITH CAYENNE AND GINGER

Ingredients:

- 1/3 cup coconut oil
- 1/3 cup shea butter
- 1 tbsp cayenne powder
- 1 tbsp ginger powder

Steps:

1 Melt coconut oil and shea butter together in a double boiler.
2 Remove from heat and stir in cayenne powder and ginger powder.
3 Pour it into a jar and let it cool.

Usage Tips: Use this muscle rub to relieve sore muscles and improve circulation.

152. PROTECTIVE HAND SALVE WITH LEMON AND SHEA BUTTER

Ingredients:

- 1/3 cup shea butter
- 1/3 cup coconut oil
- 12 drops lemon essential oil

Steps:

1 Melt shea butter and coconut oil together in a double boiler.
2 Remove from heat and stir in lemon essential oil.
3 Pour it into a jar and let it cool.

Usage Tips: Apply this hand salve to protect and nourish dry, cracked hands.

153. ALL-PURPOSE HERBAL HEALING BALM WITH COMFREY AND PLANTAIN

Ingredients:

- 1/3 cup coconut oil
- 1/3 cup beeswax pellets
- 1 tbsp comfrey oil
- 1 tbsp plantain oil

Steps:

1 Melt coconut oil and beeswax pellets together in a double boiler.
2 Remove from heat and stir in comfrey oil and plantain oil.
3 Pour it into a jar and let it cool.

Usage Tips: Use this healing balm on cuts, scrapes, and other minor skin irritations.

---

154. COOLING ALOE VERA AND MINT AFTER-SUN BALM

Ingredients:

- 1/3 cup coconut oil
- 1/3 cup shea butter
- 1 tbsp aloe vera gel
- 12 drops peppermint essential oil

Steps:

1 Melt coconut oil and shea butter together in a double boiler.
2 Remove from heat and stir in aloe vera gel and peppermint essential oil.
3 Pour it into a jar and let it cool.

Usage Tips: Apply this after-sun balm to soothe and cool sunburned skin.

---

155. NOURISHING ROSEHIP AND VITAMIN E NIGHT BALM

Ingredients:

- 1/3 cup shea butter
- 1/3 cup coconut oil
- 1 tbsp rosehip oil
- 12 drops vitamin E oil

Steps:

1 Melt shea butter and coconut oil together in a double boiler.
2 Remove from heat and stir in rosehip oil and vitamin E oil.
3 Pour it into a jar and let it cool.

Usage Tips: Use this night balm to nourish and rejuvenate your skin while you sleep.

BOOK 6: HERBAL WELLNESS FOR EVERY GENERATION AND FAMILY

Herbal remedies have been a cornerstone of traditional medicine for centuries, offering natural and holistic approaches to health and wellness. In this section, we focus on tailoring these timeless practices to meet the unique needs of children, the elderly, and pregnant women. Each of these groups has distinct physiological requirements and sensitivities, making it essential to approach herbal care with a careful and informed perspective.

Understanding the specific needs of children, the elderly, and pregnant women is crucial for ensuring that herbal remedies are both safe and effective. Children, with their developing bodies, require gentle herbs that promote health without causing adverse effects. The elderly, on the other hand, benefit from herbs that support longevity, enhance cognitive function, and address age-related conditions. Pregnant women need herbs that can safely assist with common pregnancy-related issues like nausea, swelling, and stress, ensuring the well-being of both mother and baby.

This book provides comprehensive guidance on selecting and using herbs to support these special populations. We explore specific herbal remedies tailored to address common health concerns, from soothing colic in infants to alleviating joint pain in seniors and managing morning sickness during pregnancy. Each remedy is crafted with care, ensuring that it meets the unique needs of these groups.

In addition to targeted remedies, this book also offers family-friendly herbal recipes and wellness routines. Holistic health is a family affair, and integrating herbs into daily life can be a delightful and beneficial practice for all ages. From nutritious herbal teas and smoothies to soothing baths and balms, these recipes promote overall wellness and bring families together in their pursuit of health.

By focusing on the specific needs of children, the elderly, and pregnant women, this book empowers readers with the knowledge to use herbs safely and effectively. Through careful selection and preparation, herbs can provide gentle support for various health issues, enhance well-being, and promote a natural, balanced lifestyle for the whole family. Join us as we delve into the art of herbal care tailored to special populations, ensuring that everyone can benefit from the healing power of nature.

Chapter 1: Safe Herbs for Children, Elderly, and Pregnant Women

1.1 Holistic Wellness for Teenagers

1. TEEN STRESS SOOTHE TEA

Ingredients:

- 1 tsp dried chamomile flowers
- 1 tsp dried lemon balm leaves
- 1 cup boiling water
- Honey to taste

Steps:

1 Add chamomile flowers and lemon balm leaves to a teapot.
2 Pour hot water into the teapot.
3 Allow the tea to steep for 8-9 minutes.
4 Strain the infusion into a cup.
5 Sweeten with honey, if desired.

Usage Tips: Drink this tea in the evening to reduce stress and promote relaxation before bedtime.

2. ACNE CLEARING THYME TONIC

Ingredients:

- 1 tbsp dried thyme
- 1 cup boiling water
- 1 tsp apple cider vinegar

Steps:

1 Put dried thyme in a bowl.
2 Pour hot water over the thyme.
3 Steep for 20 minutes, then strain.
4 Mix in apple cider vinegar.

Usage Tips: Apply this tonic to the face with a cotton ball to help clear acne and soothe skin.

3. MIND FOCUS BOOSTER SMOOTHIE

Ingredients:

- 1 banana
- 1 cup almond milk
- 1 tbsp almond butter
- 1 tsp maca powder
- 1/2 cup spinach

Steps:

1 Combine all ingredients in a blender.
2 Blend until smooth.
3 Pour into a glass and serve immediately.

Usage Tips: Drink this smoothie in the morning to enhance focus and mental clarity throughout the day.

4. GENTLE DETOX DANDELION LEMONADE

Ingredients:

- 1 tbsp dried dandelion root
- 1 cup boiling water
- 1 lemon (juice)
- Honey to taste
- Ice

Steps:

1 Put dried dandelion root in a cup.
2 Pour boiling water over the root and steep for 8-9 minutes.
3 Strain the tea into a pitcher and mix in lemon juice and honey.
4 Stir well and serve over ice.

Usage Tips: Drink this lemonade regularly to support gentle detoxification and liver health.

---

5. SLEEP EASY CHAMOMILE LAVENDER SACHETS

Ingredients:

- 1/3 cup dried chamomile flowers
- 1/3 cup dried lavender flowers
- Small fabric sachets

Steps:

1. Combine dried chamomile and lavender flowers in a bowl.
2. Mix well and fill small fabric sachets with the blend.
3. Tie or sew the sachets closed.

Usage Tips: Place these sachets under your pillow to promote restful sleep and relaxation.

---

6. ENERGY BOOSTING BERRY AND SPINACH SHAKE

Ingredients:

- 1/2 cup mixed berries
- 1 banana
- 1 cup spinach
- 1 cup almond milk
- 1 tbsp honey

Steps:

1. Place all ingredients in a blender.
2. Blend until the mixture is smooth.
3. Pour into a glass and serve immediately.

Usage Tips: This shake is perfect for a midday energy boost or a nutritious breakfast.

---

7. EMOTIONAL WELLNESS FLOWER ESSENCE

Ingredients:

- Fresh flower petals (e.g., rose, lavender, chamomile)
- Spring water
- 1/3 cup brandy

Steps:

1. Fill a small bowl with spring water and add fresh flower petals.
2. Place the bowl in direct sunlight for 3-4 hours.
3. Strain the flower water into a dark glass bottle and add brandy.
4. Mix well.

Usage Tips: Take a few drops of this essence under the tongue or in water to support emotional wellness.

---

8. MOOD LIFTING ST. JOHN'S WORT CAPSULES

Ingredients:

- 1/3 cup dried St. John's Wort
- Empty gelatin or vegetarian capsules

Steps:

1. Grind dried St. John's Wort into a fine powder using a coffee grinder.
2. Fill the empty capsules with the powdered herb using a capsule machine or by hand.
3. Store the filled capsules in an airtight container.

Usage Tips: Take one capsule daily to help lift mood and manage symptoms of mild depression.

---

9. HORMONE BALANCING LICORICE ROOT DRINK

Ingredients:

- 1 tsp dried licorice root
- 1 cup boiling water
- Honey to taste

Steps:

1. Place dried licorice root in a cup.
2. Pour hot water over the root.
3. Steep for 12-14 minutes.
4. Strain the tea into a cup.
5. Add honey for sweetness, if desired.

Usage Tips: Drink this tea daily to help balance hormones and reduce symptoms of hormonal imbalance.

10. ANTIOXIDANT RICH ACAI BOWL

Ingredients:

- 1 packet frozen acai puree
- 1 banana
- 1/3 cup almond milk
- 1/2 cup granola
- 1/3 cup fresh berries

Steps:

1 Combine acai puree, banana, and almond milk in a blender.
2 Blend until smooth.
3 Pour into a bowl and garnish with granola and fresh berries.

Usage Tips: Enjoy this acai bowl as a nutritious breakfast or snack packed with antioxidants.

11. SKIN HEALTH HERBAL SALVE

Ingredients:

- 1/3 cup dried calendula flowers
- 1/3 cup dried comfrey leaves
- 1/2 cup olive oil
- 1/3 cup beeswax pellets

Steps:

1 Infuse calendula flowers and comfrey leaves in olive oil by heating on low for 1 hour.
2 Strain the mixture and return to a clean pot.
3 Add beeswax pellets and heat until melted.
4 Transfer the mixture into a jar and let it cool.

Usage Tips: Apply this salve to cuts, scrapes, and dry skin to promote healing and moisturization.

1.2 Safe Herbs for Children

12. MILD IMMUNE SUPPORT ECHINACEA SYRUP

Ingredients:

- 1/3 cup dried echinacea root
- 2 cups water
- 2 cup honey

Steps:

1 Combine echinacea root and water in a pot.
2 Bring to a boil, then reduce heat and let simmer for 20 minutes.
3 Strain the liquid and return it to the pot.
4 Stir in honey until it dissolves.
5 Transfer the syrup to a bottle and store it in the refrigerator.

Usage Tips: Give children 1 tsp daily during cold and flu season to support their immune system.

13. SLEEP INDUCING VALERIAN ROOT DROPS

Ingredients:

- 1/3 cup dried valerian root
- 1 cup vodka or glycerin (for alcohol-free version)

Steps:

1 Place dried valerian root in a jar.
2 Pour vodka or glycerin over the root, ensuring it is fully submerged.
3 Seal the jar and let it sit for about 30 days, shaking occasionally.
4 Strain the tincture into a dropper bottle.

Usage Tips: Give children a few drops of this tincture before bedtime to promote restful sleep.

14. DIGESTIVE AID FENNEL HONEY

Ingredients:

- 1/3 cup fennel seeds
- 1 cup honey

Steps:

1 Crush fennel seeds slightly with a mortar and pestle.
2 Combine fennel seeds and honey in a jar.
3 Seal the jar and let it sit for 2 weeks, shaking occasionally.
4 Strain the honey to remove the seeds.

Usage Tips: Give children 1 tsp of this honey after meals to aid digestion and reduce bloating.

15. SOOTHING CALENDULA SKIN CREAM

Ingredients:

- 1/3 cup dried calendula flowers
- 1/3 cup coconut oil
- 1/3 cup shea butter
- 2 tbsp beeswax pellets

Steps:

1 Infuse calendula flowers in coconut oil by heating on low for 1 hour.
2 Strain the mixture and return to a clean pot.
3 Add shea butter and beeswax pellets and heat until melted.
4 Transfer the mixture into a jar and let it cool.

Usage Tips: Apply this cream to children's skin to soothe and heal minor irritations and dry patches.

16. CALMING LEMON BALM COOKIES

Ingredients:

- 1/2 cup softened butter
- 1/2 cup sugar
- 1 egg
- 1 tbsp dried lemon balm
- 1 1/2 cups flour

Steps:

1 Preheat the oven to 350°F (175°C).

2 Cream butter and sugar together until light and fluffy.
3 Beat in the egg and dried lemon balm.
4 Gradually add flour, mixing until combined.
5 Drop by spoonfuls onto a baking sheet.
6 Bake for 10-12 minutes or until golden brown.

Usage Tips: Serve these cookies as a calming treat to help children relax after a busy day.

17. GENTLE LAVENDER BATH BOMBS

Ingredients:

- 1 cup baking soda
- 1/3 cup citric acid
- 1/3 cup cornstarch
- 1/3 cup Epsom salts
- 2 tbsp dried lavender flowers
- 8 drops lavender essential oil
- Water (as needed)

Steps:

1 In a bowl, combine baking soda, citric acid, cornstarch, and Epsom salts.
2 Add dried lavender flowers and lavender essential oil.
3 Lightly spritz with water and mix until the mixture holds together.
4 Press the mixture into molds and let them dry completely.

Usage Tips: Drop a bath bomb into warm bathwater to create a soothing and relaxing bath for children.

18. COUGH RELIEF MARSHMALLOW ROOT SYRUP

Ingredients:

- 1/3 cup dried marshmallow root
- 2 cups water
- 1 cup honey

Steps:

1 Place marshmallow root and water in a pot.
2 Bring to a boil, then reduce the heat and let it simmer for 20 minutes.

3 Strain the liquid and pour it back into the pot.
4 Stir in honey until it fully dissolves.
5 Transfer the syrup to a bottle and refrigerate.

Usage Tips: Give children 1 tsp of this syrup as needed to relieve cough and soothe the throat.

19. FEVER REDUCING ELDERFLOWER POPSICLES

Ingredients:

- 1/3 cup dried elderflowers
- 2 cups boiling water, 1/3 cup honey
- Juice of 1 lemon
- Popsicle molds

Steps:

1 Put dried elderflowers in a bowl.
2 Pour boiling water over the elderflowers and let steep for 20 minutes.
3 Strain the infusion and mix in honey and lemon juice.
4 Stir well and pour into popsicle molds.
5 Freeze until solid.

Usage Tips: Give children these popsicles to help reduce fever and keep them hydrated during illness.

20. ANTI-ITCH CHICKWEED BALM

Ingredients:

- 1/3 cup dried chickweed, 1/3 cup olive oil
- 1/3 cup beeswax pellets

Steps:

1 Infuse chickweed in olive oil by heating on low for 1 hour.
2 Strain the mixture and return to a clean pot.
3 Add beeswax pellets and heat until melted.

4 Transfer the mixture into a jar and let it cool.

Usage Tips: Apply this balm to itchy skin to soothe and reduce irritation naturally.

21. HAPPY TUMMY GINGER GUMMIES

Ingredients:

- 1/3 cup fresh ginger, grated
- 2 cups water
- 1/3 cup honey
- 2 tbsp gelatin
- Popsicle molds

Steps:

1 Put grated ginger and water in a pot and bring to a boil.
2 Lower the heat and let it simmer for 8-9 minutes, then strain.
3 Stir in honey and gelatin until dissolved.
4 Pour into popsicle molds and let them set in the refrigerator.

Usage Tips: Give children these gummies to soothe upset stomachs and support digestion.

22. ALLERGY EASE NETTLE TEA

Ingredients:

- 1 tsp dried nettle leaves
- 1 cup boiling water
- Honey to taste

Steps:

1 Add dried nettle leaves to a cup.
2 Pour boiling water over the leaves and let them steep for 8-9 minutes.
3 Strain the tea into a cup and sweeten with honey to taste.

Usage Tips: Give children this tea daily during allergy season to ease symptoms naturally.

23. ENERGY ENHANCING SPIRULINA SMOOTHIE

Ingredients:

- 1 banana
- 1 cup almond milk
- 1 tbsp spirulina powder
- 1 tbsp honey

Steps:

1. Transfer all ingredients in a blender.
2. Mix until smooth.
3. Transfer into a glass and serve immediately.

Usage Tips: Drink this smoothie in the morning to enhance energy levels and support overall wellness.

24. IRON-RICH NETTLE INFUSION

Ingredients:

- 1 tbsp dried nettle leaves
- 1 cup boiling water
- Honey to taste

Steps:

1. Add dried nettle leaves to a cup.
2. Pour hot water over the leaves.
3. Let it steep for 12-14 minutes.
4. Strain the tea into a cup and sweeten with honey if you like.

Usage Tips: Drink this infusion daily to boost iron levels and support overall health during pregnancy.

25. PREGNANCY SAFE SKIN ELASTICITY OIL

Ingredients:

- 1/3 cup almond oil
- 1/3 cup coconut oil
- 12 drops lavender essential oil
- 12 drops frankincense essential oil

Steps:

1. Transfer all ingredients in a small bottle.
2. Shake well to blend.

3. Massage the oil onto your belly, thighs, and breasts daily.

Usage Tips: Use this oil to improve skin elasticity and prevent stretch marks during pregnancy.

26. CALMING PREGNANCY BATH SOAK

Ingredients:

- 1 cup Epsom salts
- 1/3 cup baking soda
- 1/3 cup dried lavender flowers
- 12 drops lavender essential oil

Steps:

1. Mix all ingredients in a bowl until well combined.
2. Transfer the mixture to a jar or airtight container.
3. Add 1/2 cup of the mixture to warm bathwater and soak for 20 minutes.

Usage Tips: Use this bath soak to relax and soothe sore muscles during pregnancy.

27. NAUSEA RELIEF GINGER MINT TEA

Ingredients:

- 1-inch piece fresh ginger, sliced
- 1 tbsp fresh mint leaves
- 1 cup boiling water
- Honey to taste

Steps:

1. Combine ginger slices and mint leaves in a cup.
2. Pour hot water into the cup.
3. Steep for 12-14 minutes.
4. Strain into a cup and sweeten with honey if desired.

Usage Tips: Drink this tea as needed to relieve nausea and promote digestive comfort during pregnancy.

28.   PRENATAL RASPBERRY LEAF TONIC

Ingredients:

- 1 tbsp dried raspberry leaves
- 1 cup boiling water
- Honey to taste

Steps:

1. Add dried raspberry leaves to a cup.
2. Pour hot water over the leaves.
3. Allow to steep for 12-14 minutes.
4. Strain into a cup and add honey to taste.

Usage Tips: Drink this tonic daily to strengthen the uterus and support a healthy pregnancy.

---

29.   RELAXING BELLY BALM

Ingredients:

- 1/3 cup shea butter
- 1/3 cup coconut oil
- 12 drops lavender essential oil
- 6 drops chamomile essential oil

Steps:

1. Melt shea butter and coconut oil together using a double boiler.
2. Take off the heat and mix in lavender and chamomile essential oils.
3. Transfer the mixture to a jar and let it cool.

Usage Tips: Massage this balm onto your belly to soothe and moisturize skin during pregnancy.

---

30.   ANTIOXIDANT BOOST DATE AND WALNUT SNACK

Ingredients:

- 1 cup pitted dates
- 1/2 cup walnuts
- 1 tbsp chia seeds
- 1 tbsp cocoa powder

Steps:

1. Mix all ingredients in a food processor.
2. Blend until a sticky dough forms.
3. Roll into small balls and store in the refrigerator.

Usage Tips: Enjoy these snacks for a healthy, antioxidant-rich boost of energy during pregnancy.

---

31. CRAMP SOOTHING MAGNESIUM SPRAY

Ingredients:

- 1/2 cup magnesium chloride flakes
- 1/2 cup distilled water
- 12 drops lavender essential oil

Steps:

1. Dissolve magnesium chloride flakes in distilled water.
2. Mix with lavender essential oil.
3. Pour into a spray bottle.

Usage Tips: Spray this mixture onto sore muscles to relieve cramps and promote relaxation.

---

32.   HYDRATION BOOST CUCUMBER AND ALOE DRINK

Ingredients:

- 1 cucumber, peeled and sliced
- 1/3 cup fresh aloe vera gel
- 2 cups water
- Juice of 1 lemon
- Honey to taste

Steps:

1. Combine cucumber slices, aloe vera gel, water, and lemon juice in a blender.
2. Mix until smooth.
3. Strain the mixture and add honey to taste.
4. Serve over ice.

Usage Tips: Drink this refreshing beverage to stay hydrated and support skin health during pregnancy.

---

33.   STRETCH MARK MINIMIZING LAVENDER CREAM

Ingredients:

- 1/3 cup cocoa butter
- 1/3 cup shea butter

- 1/3 cup coconut oil
- 12 drops lavender essential oil

Steps:

1 Melt cocoa butter, shea butter, and coconut oil together in a double boiler.
2 Remove from heat and mix in lavender essential oil.
3 Pour the mixture into a jar and allow it to cool.

Usage Tips: Apply this cream daily to areas prone to stretch marks to keep skin hydrated and elastic.

Chapter 2: Health and Personal Care

2.1 Herbal Remedies for Seasonal Wellness

34. SEASONAL HEADACHE RELIEF PEPPERMINT AND LAVENDER ROLL-ON

Ingredients:

- 12 drops peppermint essential oil
- 12 drops lavender essential oil
- 1 tbsp carrier oil (such as jojoba or almond oil)
- Roll-on bottle

Steps:

1 Combine peppermint and lavender essential oils with the carrier oil in a roll-on bottle.
2 Stir well to mix.

Usage Tips: Apply this roll-on blend to your temples and neck to relieve headaches. Peppermint provides a cooling sensation that helps to alleviate pain, while lavender calms and relaxes.

35. RAINY SEASON MOOD LIFT ST. JOHN'S WORT TINCTURE

Ingredients:

- 1/2 cup dried St. John's wort
- 1 cup vodka or brandy

Steps:

1 Combine dried St. John's wort and vodka or brandy in a jar.
2 Seal the jar and let sit for about 1 month, shaking daily.
3 Strain the mixture and store the liquid in a glass bottle.

Usage Tips: Take 1 tsp of this tincture daily to improve your mood. St. John's wort is known for its natural antidepressant properties, helping to alleviate symptoms of depression and anxiety.

36. SEASONAL AFFECTIVE DISORDER (SAD) RELIEF

ROSEMARY AND LAVENDER OIL DIFFUSER

Ingredients:

- 12 drops rosemary essential oil
- 12 drops lavender essential oil
- Water
- Diffuser

Steps:

1 Fill your diffuser with water according to the manufacturer's instructions.
2 Add rosemary and lavender essential oils.
3 Turn on the diffuser and enjoy.

Usage Tips: Use this diffuser blend to lift your mood and reduce symptoms of Seasonal Affective Disorder (SAD). Rosemary and lavender both have mood-enhancing and calming properties.

37. AUTUMN IMMUNE BOOST ELDERBERRY SYRUP

Ingredients:

- 1 cup dried elderberries
- 1 tbsp dried echinacea root
- 4 cups water
- 1 cup honey

Steps:

1 Combine dried elderberries, dried echinacea root, and water in a pot.
2 Bring to a boil, then simmer for 45 min.
3 Strain the mixture and return the liquid to the pot.
4 Stir in honey and simmer until thickened.
5 Pour into a jar and preserve in the refrigerator.

Usage Tips: Take 1 tbsp of this syrup daily during autumn to boost your immune system. Elderberries and echinacea are powerful immune boosters that help to prevent colds and flu.

38. DRY SKIN WINTER SALVE WITH CALENDULA AND SHEA BUTTER

Ingredients:

- 1/3 cup dried calendula flowers
- 1/2 cup shea butter
- 1/3 cup coconut oil
- 1/3 cup beeswax

- 12 drops lavender essential oil

Steps:

1 Infuse the calendula flowers in coconut oil over low heat for about1 hour.
2 Strain the oil and combine with shea butter and beeswax in a double boiler.
3 Heat until melted, then stir in lavender essential oil.
4 Pour into a jar and let cool.

Usage Tips: Apply this salve to dry skin areas during winter to keep your skin moisturized and protected. Calendula is known for its healing properties, while shea butter provides deep hydration.

39. SUMMER HEAT COOLING HIBISCUS AND MINT ICED TEA

Ingredients:

- 1 tbsp dried hibiscus flowers
- 1 tbsp dried mint leaves
- 4 cups boiling water
- 1 tbsp honey
- Ice cubes

Steps:

1 Transfer dried hibiscus flowers and dried mint leaves in your teapot.
2 Pour boiling water into the teapot.
3 Let steep for 8-9 min.
4 Strain the tea into a pitcher.
5 Stir in honey and let cool.
6 Serve over ice.

Usage Tips: Enjoy this refreshing iced tea on hot summer days. Hibiscus is known for its cooling properties and rich vitamin C content, while mint adds a refreshing flavor.

40. SPRING ALLERGY RELIEF NETTLE AND QUERCETIN TEA

Ingredients:

- 1 tsp dried nettle leaves
- 1 tsp quercetin powder
- 1 cup boiling water
- 1 tbsp honey

Steps:

1 Combine dried nettle leaves and quercetin powder in your teapot.
2 Pour boiling water over the mixture.
3 Let steep for 8-9 min.
4 Strain into a cup.
5 Stir in honey and serve.

Usage Tips: Drink this tea during allergy season to help alleviate symptoms. Nettle has natural antihistamine properties, and quercetin helps to stabilize mast cells and reduce inflammation.

41. SEASONAL DETOX DANDELION ROOT AND MILK THISTLE TEA

Ingredients:

- 1 tsp dried dandelion root
- 1 tsp dried milk thistle seeds
- 1 cup boiling water
- 1 tbsp honey

Steps:

1 Transfer dried dandelion root and dried milk thistle seeds in your teapot.
2 Pour boiling water into the teapot.
3 Let steep for 8-9 min.
4 Strain into a cup.
5 Stir in honey and serve.

Usage Tips: Use this tea periodically to detoxify and support your liver. Dandelion and milk thistle are both known for their liver-protective and detoxifying properties.

42. COLD PREVENTION ECHINACEA AND GINGER TONIC

Ingredients:

- 1 tsp dried echinacea root
- 1 tsp grated fresh ginger
- 1 cup boiling water
- 1 tbsp honey
- 1 tsp lemon juice

Steps:

1 Transfer dried echinacea root and grated fresh ginger in your teapot.
2 Pour boiling water over the mixture.
3 Let steep for 8-9 min.
4 Strain into a cup.

5 Stir in honey and lemon juice, then serve.

Usage Tips: Drink this tonic at the first sign of a cold to boost your immune system. Echinacea and ginger both have immune-boosting properties that help to fight off infections.

43. FLU RECOVERY THYME AND HONEY COUGH SYRUP

Ingredients:

- 1 cup water
- 1/2 cup dried thyme
- 1 cup honey

Steps:

1 Combine water and dried thyme in a pot.
2 Bring to a boil, then simmer for 15 min.
3 Strain the mixture and return the liquid to the pot.
4 Stir in honey and heat until thickened.
5 Pour into a jar and preserve in the refrigerator.

Usage Tips: Take 1 tbsp of this syrup as needed to soothe a cough. Thyme has antimicrobial properties that help to clear respiratory infections, while honey soothes the throat.

44. WINTER BLUES SAFFRON AND LEMON BALM TEA

Ingredients:

- 1/4 tsp saffron threads
- 1 tsp dried lemon balm leaves
- 1 cup boiling water
- 1 tbsp honey

Steps:

1 Combine saffron threads and dried lemon balm leaves in your teapot.
2 Pour boiling water over the mixture.
3 Let steep for 8-9 min.
4 Strain into a cup.
5 Stir in honey and serve.

Usage Tips: Drink this tea during winter to lift your mood and reduce anxiety. Saffron is known for its mood-enhancing properties, while lemon balm helps to calm the mind.

45. CALMING CHAMOMILE AND VANILLA BEDTIME TEA

Ingredients:

- 1 tsp dried chamomile flowers
- 1/2 vanilla bean, split
- 1 cup boiling water
- 1 tbsp honey

Steps:

1. Transfer dried chamomile flowers and split vanilla bean in your teapot.
2. Pour boiling water over the mixture.
3. Let steep for 8-9 min.
4. Strain into a cup.
5. Stir in honey and serve.

Usage Tips: Enjoy this tea before bedtime to promote restful sleep. Chamomile and vanilla both have calming properties that help to relax the mind and body, ensuring a peaceful night's rest.

46. SOOTHING LEMON BALM AND ROSE TEA

Ingredients:

- 1 tsp dried lemon balm leaves
- 1 tsp dried rose petals
- 1 cup boiling water
- 1 tbsp honey

Steps:

1. Transfer dried lemon balm leaves and dried rose petals in your teapot.
2. Pour boiling water over the mixture.
3. Let steep for 8-9 min.
4. Strain into a cup.
5. Stir in honey and serve.

Usage Tips: Sip this tea to soothe your nerves and uplift your spirits. Lemon balm and rose both have mood-enhancing and calming properties that help to reduce stress and anxiety.

47. STRESS RELIEF PASSIONFLOWER AND VALERIAN ROOT TEA

Ingredients:

- 1 tsp dried passionflower
- 1 tsp dried valerian root
- 1 cup boiling water
- 1 tbsp honey

Steps:

1. Transfer dried passionflower and dried valerian root in your teapot.
2. Pour boiling water into the teapot.
3. Let steep for 8-9 min.
4. Strain into a cup.
5. Stir in honey and serve.

Usage Tips: Drink this tea to reduce stress and promote relaxation. Passionflower and valerian root have natural sedative properties that help to calm the mind and body.

48. DIGESTIVE COMFORT PEPPERMINT AND LICORICE TEA

Ingredients:

- 1 tsp dried peppermint leaves
- 1 tsp dried licorice root
- 1 cup boiling water
- 1 tbsp honey

Steps:

1. Transfer dried peppermint leaves and dried licorice root in your teapot.
2. Pour boiling water into the teapot.
3. Let steep for 8-9 min.
4. Strain into a cup.
5. Stir in honey and serve.

Usage Tips: Enjoy this tea after meals to aid digestion and soothe your stomach. Peppermint and licorice both have digestive benefits that help to reduce bloating and discomfort.

49. DETOX GREEN TEA WITH BURDOCK AND NETTLE

Ingredients:

- 1 tsp green tea leaves
- 1 tsp dried burdock root
- 1 tsp dried nettle leaves
- 1 cup boiling water
- 1 tbsp honey

Steps:

1. Combine green tea leaves, dried burdock root, and dried nettle leaves in your teapot.
2. Pour boiling water into the teapot.
3. Let steep for 8-9 min.
4. Strain into a cup.
5. Stir in honey and serve.

Usage Tips: Drink this tea to support detoxification and overall health. Green tea, burdock, and nettle are all known for their cleansing and detoxifying properties.

50. HEARTWARMING CINNAMON AND APPLE SPICE TEA

Ingredients:

- 1 cinnamon stick
- 1/2 apple, sliced
- 1 cup boiling water
- 1 tbsp honey

Steps:

1. Combine cinnamon stick and sliced apple in your teapot.
2. Pour boiling water over the ingredients.
3. Let steep for 8-9 min.
4. Strain into a cup.
5. Stir in honey and serve.

Usage Tips: Enjoy this tea to warm your heart and soul on a chilly day. Cinnamon and apple provide a comforting and warming flavor that is perfect for cozy moments.

51. REJUVENATING WHITE TEA WITH JASMINE AND PEAR

Ingredients:

- 1 tsp white tea leaves
- 1 tsp dried jasmine flowers
- 1/2 pear, sliced
- 1 cup boiling water
- 1 tbsp honey

Steps:

1. Combine white tea leaves, dried jasmine flowers, and sliced pear in your teapot.
2. Pour boiling water over the mixture.
3. Let steep for about 6 min.
4. Strain into a cup.
5. Stir in honey and serve.

Usage Tips: Drink this tea for a rejuvenating and fragrant experience. White tea and jasmine flowers provide gentle stimulation, while pear adds a subtle sweetness.

52. RESTFUL SLEEP TEA WITH HOPS AND SKULLCAP

Ingredients:

- 1 tsp dried hops
- 1 tsp dried skullcap
- 1 cup boiling water
- 1 tbsp honey

Steps:

1. Transfer dried hops and dried skullcap in your teapot.
2. Pour boiling water into the teapot.
3. Let steep for 8-9 min.
4. Strain into a cup.
5. Stir in honey and serve.

Usage Tips: Drink this tea before bed to promote restful sleep. Hops and skullcap have calming and sedative properties that help to relax the mind and body, ensuring a good night's rest.

53. CLEAR MIND TEA WITH GINKGO AND GOTU KOLA

Ingredients:

- 1 tsp dried ginkgo biloba leaves
- 1 tsp dried gotu kola leaves
- 1 cup boiling water
- 1 tbsp honey

Steps:

1. Combine dried ginkgo biloba leaves and dried gotu kola leaves in your teapot.
2. Pour boiling water into the teapot.
3. Let steep for 8-9 min.
4. Strain into a cup.

5 Stir in honey and serve.

Usage Tips: Drink this tea to enhance mental clarity and focus. Ginkgo and gotu kola are important for their neuroprotective properties and capacity to improve cognitive function.

54.   UPLIFTING HIBISCUS AND CITRUS TEA

Ingredients:

- 1 tbsp dried hibiscus flowers
- 1 slice of orange
- 1 slice of lemon
- 1 cup boiling water
- 1 tbsp honey

Steps:

1 Combine dried hibiscus flowers, orange slice, and lemon slice in your teapot.
2 Pour boiling water over the mixture.
3 Let steep for 8-9 min.
4 Strain into a cup.
5 Stir in honey and serve.

Usage Tips: Enjoy this tea to uplift your spirits and energize your day. Hibiscus provides a tart and refreshing flavor, while citrus adds brightness and vitamin C.

55.   TRANQUILITY TEA WITH HOLY BASIL AND CACAO

Ingredients:

- 1 tsp dried holy basil leaves
- 1 tsp cacao nibs
- 1 cup boiling water
- 1 tbsp honey

Steps:

1 Transfer dried holy basil leaves and cacao nibs in your teapot.
2 Pour boiling water into the teapot.
3 Let steep for 8-9 min.
4 Strain into a cup.
5 Stir in honey and serve.

Usage Tips: Drink this tea to find tranquility and balance. Holy basil is an adaptogen that helps to reduce stress, while cacao provides a mood-enhancing boos.

2.3 The Benefits of Herbal Poultices

56.   ANTI-INFLAMMATORY TURMERIC AND GINGER POULTICE

Ingredients:

- 1 tsp ground turmeric
- 1 tsp grated fresh ginger
- 1 tbsp water
- Cheesecloth or muslin

Steps:

1 Combine ground turmeric, grated fresh ginger, and water to form a paste.
2 Spread the paste on cheesecloth or muslin.
3 Apply to the affected area for 15-18 min.

Usage Tips: Use this poultice to reduce inflammation and pain. Turmeric and ginger have natural anti-inflammatory properties that help to relieve swelling and discomfort.

57. PAIN RELIEF ARNICA AND WILLOW BARK COMPRESS

Ingredients:

- 1 tbsp dried arnica flowers
- 1 tbsp dried willow bark
- 1 cup boiling water
- Cheesecloth or muslin

Steps:

1 Transfer dried arnica flowers and dried willow bark in a bowl.
2 Pour boiling water into the teapot and let steep for 15 min.
3 Strain the mixture and soak the cheesecloth or muslin in the liquid.

4 Apply to the affected area for 20-30 minutes.

Usage Tips: Use this compress to relieve pain and inflammation. Arnica and willow bark are known for their pain-relieving properties, making this compress effective for sore muscles and joints.

58. WARMING MUSTARD AND EUCALYPTUS CHEST POULTICE

Ingredients:

- 1 tbsp mustard powder
- 1 tbsp eucalyptus oil
- 1 tbsp water
- Cheesecloth or muslin

Steps:

1 Combine mustard powder, eucalyptus oil, and water to form a paste.
2 Spread the paste on cheesecloth or muslin.
3 Apply to the chest area for 15-20 min.

Usage Tips: Use this poultice to relieve chest congestion and respiratory discomfort. Mustard and eucalyptus both have warming and decongestant properties that help to clear the airways.

59. SOOTHING ECZEMA CALENDULA AND OATMEAL POULTICE

Ingredients:

- 1 tbsp dried calendula flowers
- 1 tbsp ground oatmeal
- 1 cup boiling water
- Cheesecloth or muslin

Steps:

1 Transfer dried calendula flowers and ground oatmeal in a bowl.
2 Pour boiling water over the mixture and let steep for 8-9 min.
3 Strain the mixture and soak the cheesecloth or muslin in the liquid.
4 Apply to the affected area for 18-20 minu.

Usage Tips: Use this poultice to soothe eczema and reduce itching. Calendula and oatmeal have anti-inflammatory and moisturizing properties that help to calm irritated skin.

60. COOLING CUCUMBER AND ALOE VERA EYE COMPRESS

Ingredients:

- 1/2 cucumber, grated
- 2 tbsp fresh aloe vera gel
- Cheesecloth or muslin

Steps:

1 Combine grated cucumber and fresh aloe vera gel in a bowl.
2 Spread the mixture on cheesecloth or muslin.
3 Apply to the eye area for 15-20 minutes.

Usage Tips: Use this compress to reduce puffiness and soothe tired eyes. Cucumber and aloe vera both have cooling and anti-inflammatory properties that aid to refresh and rejuvenate the skin around the eyes.

61. BRUISE MINIMIZING PARSLEY AND WITCH HAZEL POULTICE

Ingredients:

- 1 tbsp chopped fresh parsley
- 1 tbsp witch hazel
- Cheesecloth or muslin

Steps:

1 Combine chopped fresh parsley and witch hazel in a bowl.
2 Spread the mixture on cheesecloth or muslin.
3 Apply to the affected area for 18-20 min.

Usage Tips: Use this poultice to minimize bruising and reduce inflammation. Parsley and witch hazel both have anti-inflammatory and astringent properties that help to speed up the healing process of bruises.

62. DETOXIFYING BENTONITE CLAY AND SEAWEED POULTICE

Ingredients:

- 1 tbsp bentonite clay
- 1 tbsp powdered seaweed
- 1 tbsp water
- Cheesecloth or muslin

Steps:

1. Combine bentonite clay, powdered seaweed, and water to form a paste.
2. Spread the paste on cheesecloth or muslin.
3. Apply to the affected area for 18-20 min.

Usage Tips: Use this poultice to detoxify and draw out impurities from the skin. Bentonite clay and seaweed are both known for their detoxifying properties, making this poultice effective for skin cleansing.

63. RELAXING LAVENDER AND CHAMOMILE NECK POULTICE

Ingredients:

- 1 tbsp dried lavender flowers
- 1 tbsp dried chamomile flowers
- 1 cup boiling water
- Cheesecloth or muslin

Steps:

1. Transfer dried lavender flowers and dried chamomile flowers in a bowl.
2. Pour boiling water into the teapot and let steep for 8-9 min.
3. Strain the mixture and soak the cheesecloth or muslin in the liquid.
4. Apply to the neck area for 18-20 min.

Usage Tips: Use this poultice to relax and soothe neck muscles. Lavender and chamomile both have calming and anti-inflammatory properties that help to reduce tension and promote relaxation.

64. REJUVENATING ROSE PETAL AND HONEY FACIAL POULTICE

Ingredients:

- 1 tbsp dried rose petals
- 1 tbsp honey
- 1 tbsp water
- Cheesecloth or muslin

Steps:

1. Combine dried rose petals, honey, and water to form a paste.
2. Spread the paste on cheesecloth or muslin.
3. Apply to the face for 15-20 minutes.

Usage Tips: Use this poultice to rejuvenate and hydrate the skin. Rose petals and honey both have moisturizing and anti-inflammatory properties that aid to nourish and rejuvenate the skin.

65. ANTIFUNGAL TEA TREE AND GARLIC FOOT WRAP

Ingredients:

- 12 drops tea tree essential oil
- 1 clove garlic, crushed
- 1 tbsp olive oil
- Cheesecloth or muslin

Steps:

1. Combine tea tree essential oil, crushed garlic, and olive oil in a bowl.
2. Spread the mixture on cheesecloth or muslin.
3. Apply to the affected area for 15-20 minutes.

Usage Tips: Use this foot wrap to treat fungal infections such as athlete's foot. Garlic and Tea tree oil have powerful antifungal properties that help to eliminate the fungus and promote healing.

66. SKIN HEALING COMFREY AND PLANTAIN LEAF POULTICE

Ingredients:

- 1 tbsp dried comfrey leaves
- 1 tbsp dried plantain leaves
- 1 cup boiling water

- Cheesecloth or muslin

Steps:

1 Transfer dried comfrey leaves and dried plantain leaves in a bowl.
2 Pour boiling water into the teapot and let steep for 8-9 min.
3 Strain the mixture and soak the cheesecloth or muslin in the liquid.

4 Apply to the affected area for 18-20 min.

Usage Tips: Use this poultice to promote skin healing and reduce inflammation. Comfrey and plantain are known for their skin-healing properties, making this poultice effective for cuts, scrapes, and minor wounds.

2.4 Herbal Infusions for Winter Wellness

67. IMMUNE-BOOSTING ELDERBERRY AND ASTRAGALUS TONIC

Ingredients:

- 1 tbsp dried elderberries
- 1 tbsp dried astragalus root
- 4 cups water
- 1 cup honey

Steps:

1 Combine dried elderberries, dried astragalus root, and water in a pot.
2 Bring to a boil, then simmer for about 45 min.
3 Strain the mixture and return the liquid to the pot.
4 Stir in honey and simmer until thickened.
5 Pour into a jar and preserve in the refrigerator.

Usage Tips: Take 1 tbsp of this tonic daily to boost your immune system during winter. Elderberries and astragalus both have powerful immune-boosting properties that help to prevent colds and flu.

68. WARMING GINGER AND CINNAMON TEA

Ingredients:

- 1 tsp grated fresh ginger
- 1 cinnamon stick
- 1 cup boiling water
- 1 tbsp honey

Steps:

1 Combine grated fresh ginger and cinnamon stick in your teapot.
2 Pour boiling water over the ingredients.
3 Let steep for 8-9 min.
4 Strain into a cup.
5 Stir in honey and serve.

Usage Tips: Enjoy this warming tea to boost circulation and stay warm during winter. Ginger and cinnamon both have warming properties that help to increase circulation and keep you cozy.

69. BONE STRENGTHENING HORSETAIL AND NETTLE INFUSION

Ingredients:

- 1 tsp dried horsetail
- 1 tsp dried nettle
- 2 cups water

Steps:

1 Combine dried horsetail and dried nettle in a pot.
2 Add water and bring to a boil.
3 Mix for 20 minutes.
4 Strain into cups and serve.

Usage Tips: Drink this infusion to support bone health. Horsetail and nettle are rich in minerals like silica and calcium, which are essential for strong bones.

70. SKIN NOURISHING SEA BUCKTHORN AND MINT TEA

Ingredients:

- 1 tsp dried sea buckthorn berries
- 1 tsp dried mint leaves

- 1 cup boiling water
- 1 tbsp honey

Steps:

1 Combine dried sea buckthorn berries and dried mint leaves in your teapot.
2 Pour boiling water into the teapot.
3 Let steep for 8-9 min.
4 Strain into a cup.
5 Stir in honey and serve.

Usage Tips: Enjoy this tea to nourish your skin. Sea buckthorn berries are rich in vitamins and antioxidants that promote skin health, while mint adds a refreshing flavor.

71. RESPIRATORY HEALTH MULLEIN AND EUCALYPTUS BREW

Ingredients:

- 1 tsp dried mullein leaves
- 1 tsp dried eucalyptus leaves
- 1 cup boiling water
- 1 tbsp honey

Steps:

1 Transfer dried mullein leaves and dried eucalyptus leaves in your teapot.
2 Pour boiling water into the teapot.
3 Let steep for 8-9 min.
4 Strain into a cup.
5 Stir in honey and serve.

Usage Tips: Drink this brew to support respiratory health and clear congestion. Mullein and eucalyptus both have expectorant properties that help to clear mucus and improve breathing.

72. DIGESTIVE AID FENNEL AND PEPPERMINT TEA

Ingredients:

- 1 tsp dried fennel seeds
- 1 tsp dried peppermint leaves
- 1 cup boiling water
- 1 tbsp honey

Steps:

1 Transfer dried fennel seeds and dried peppermint leaves in your teapot.
2 Pour boiling water into the teapot.
3 Let steep for 8-9 min.

4 Strain into a cup.
5 Stir in honey and serve.

Usage Tips: Drink this tea after meals to aid digestion and soothe your stomach. Fennel and peppermint both have digestive benefits that help to reduce bloating and discomfort.

73. SOOTHING THROAT LICORICE AND MARSHMALLOW ROOT TEA

Ingredients:

- 1 tsp dried licorice root
- 1 tsp dried marshmallow root
- 1 cup boiling water
- 1 tbsp honey

Steps:

1 Transfer dried licorice root and dried marshmallow root in your teapot.
2 Pour boiling water into the teapot.
3 Let steep for 8-9 min.
4 Strain into a cup.
5 Stir in honey and serve.

Usage Tips: Drink this tea to soothe a sore throat and reduce irritation. Licorice root and marshmallow root both have demulcent properties that help to coat and soothe the throat.

74. CIRCULATION BOOSTING GINKGO AND CAYENNE PEPPER TEA

Ingredients:

- 1 tsp dried ginkgo biloba leaves
- 1/4 tsp cayenne pepper
- 1 cup boiling water
- 1 tbsp honey

Steps:

1 Combine dried ginkgo biloba leaves and cayenne pepper in your teapot.
2 Pour boiling water over the mixture.
3 Let steep for 8-9 min.
4 Strain into a cup.
5 Stir in honey and serve.

Usage Tips: Drink this tea to boost circulation and stay warm. Ginkgo biloba and cayenne pepper both have circulatory-boosting properties that help to increase blood flow and keep you warm.

75. ANTI-COLD LEMON, HONEY, AND THYME INFUSION

Ingredients:

- 1 slice of lemon
- 1 tbsp honey
- 1 tsp dried thyme
- 1 cup boiling water

Steps:

1 Combine lemon slice, honey, and dried thyme in your teapot.
2 Pour boiling water over the ingredients.
3 Let steep for 8-9 min.
4 Strain into a cup and serve.

Usage Tips: Drink this infusion at the first sign of a cold to boost your immune system. Lemon and honey provide vitamin C and soothing properties, while thyme has antimicrobial properties.

76. SLEEP-ENHANCING CHAMOMILE AND LAVENDER TEA

Ingredients:

- 1 tsp dried chamomile flowers
- 1 tsp dried lavender flowers
- 1 cup boiling water
- 1 tbsp honey

Steps:

1 Transfer dried chamomile flowers and dried lavender flowers in your teapot.
2 Pour boiling water into the teapot.
3 Let steep for 8-9 min.
4 Strain into a cup.
5 Stir in honey and serve.

Usage Tips: Drink this tea before bed to promote restful sleep. Chamomile and lavender both have calming and sedative properties that help to relax the mind and body, ensuring a good night's rest.

77. MOOD-LIFTING ST. JOHN'S WORT AND ROSEHIP TEA

Ingredients:

- 1 tsp dried St. John's wort
- 1 tsp dried rosehips
- 1 cup boiling water
- 1 tbsp honey

Steps:

1 Combine dried St. John's wort and dried rosehips in your teapot.
2 Pour boiling water into the teapot.
3 Let steep for 8-9 min.
4 Strain into a cup.
5 Stir in honey and serve.

Usage Tips: Drink this tea to uplift your mood and reduce symptoms of depression. St. John's wort is known for its natural antidepressant properties, while rosehips provide a boost of vitamin C.

2.5 Wellness Routines for Seniors

78. MEMORY-ENHANCING BACOPA AND GINKGO TEA

Ingredients:

- 1 tsp dried bacopa leaves
- 1 tsp dried ginkgo biloba leaves
- 1 cup boiling water
- 1 tbsp honey

Steps:

1 Combine dried bacopa leaves and dried ginkgo biloba leaves in your teapot.
2 Pour boiling water into the teapot.
3 Let steep for 8-9 min.
4 Strain into a cup.
5 Stir in honey and serve.

Usage Tips: Drink this tea to enhance memory and cognitive function. Bacopa and ginkgo biloba are both known for their neuroprotective properties and ability to improve brain health.

79. JOINT HEALTH TURMERIC AND BLACK PEPPER CAPSULES

Ingredients:

- 1/2 cup ground turmeric
- 1/3 cup ground black pepper
- Empty gelatin capsules

Steps:

1 Combine ground turmeric and ground black pepper in a bowl.
2 Fill empty gelatin capsules with the mixture.
3 Store the capsules in an airtight container.

Usage Tips: Take 1-2 capsules daily to support joint health and reduce inflammation. Turmeric and black pepper have anti-inflammatory properties that help to relieve joint pain and stiffness.

80. HEART HEALTHY HAWTHORN AND GARLIC TONIC

Ingredients:

- 1 tsp dried hawthorn berries
- 1 clove garlic, crushed
- 1 cup boiling water
- 1 tbsp honey

Steps:

1 Combine dried hawthorn berries and crushed garlic in your teapot.
2 Pour boiling water into the teapot.
3 Let steep for 8-9 min.
4 Strain into a cup.
5 Stir in honey and serve.

Usage Tips: Drink this tonic to support heart health and improve circulation. Hawthorn berries and garlic both have cardiovascular benefits that help to maintain a healthy heart.

81. VISION SUPPORT LUTEIN AND BILBERRY SMOOTHIE

Ingredients:

- 1 cup fresh or frozen bilberries
- 1 tsp lutein powder
- 1 banana
- 1 cup almond milk
- 1 tbsp honey

Steps:

1 Combine fresh or frozen bilberries, lutein powder, banana, almond milk, and honey in a blender.
2 Mix until smooth.
3 Pour into a glass and drink.

Usage Tips: Enjoy this smoothie to support vision health and protect your eyes. Bilberries are rich in antioxidants, while lutein is known for its protective effects on the eyes.

82. IMMUNE SUPPORT SHIITAKE AND REISHI MUSHROOM SOUP

Ingredients:

- 1 cup sliced shiitake mushrooms
- 1 cup sliced reishi mushrooms
- 4 cups vegetable broth
- 1 onion, chopped
- 2 cloves garlic, minced
- 1 tbsp olive oil
- Salt and pepper to taste

Steps:

1 Heat olive oil in a pot and sauté chopped onion and minced garlic until fragrant.
2 Add sliced shiitake mushrooms and sliced reishi mushrooms and cook until softened.
3 Pour in vegetable broth and bring to a boil.
4 Diminish heat and simmer for about 30 min.
5 Add salt and pepper.

Usage Tips: Enjoy this soup to boost your immune system and support overall health. Shiitake and reishi mushrooms are both known for their immune-boosting properties.

83. DIGESTIVE COMFORT GINGER AND CHAMOMILE TEA

Ingredients:

- 1 tsp grated fresh ginger
- 1 tsp dried chamomile flowers
- 1 cup boiling water
- 1 tbsp honey

Steps:

1. Combine grated fresh ginger and dried chamomile flowers in your teapot.
2. Pour boiling water into the teapot.
3. Let steep for 8-9 min.
4. Strain into a cup.
5. Stir in honey and serve.

Usage Tips: Drink this tea after meals to aid digestion and reduce bloating. Ginger and chamomile both have digestive benefits that help to soothe the stomach and improve digestion.

84. BONE DENSITY SAGE AND SILICA TEA

Ingredients:

- 1 tsp dried sage leaves
- 1 tsp dried horsetail
- 1 cup boiling water
- 1 tbsp honey

Steps:

1. Transfer dried sage leaves and dried horsetail in your teapot.
2. Pour boiling water into the teapot.
3. Let steep for 8-9 min.
4. Strain into a cup.
5. Stir in honey and serve.

Usage Tips: Drink this tea to support bone density and strength. Sage and horsetail are both rich in minerals that help to maintain healthy bones.

85. ENERGY BOOSTING MACA AND SIBERIAN GINSENG DRINK

Ingredients:

- 1 tsp maca powder
- 1 tsp Siberian ginseng powder
- 1 cup almond milk
- 1 tbsp honey

Steps:

1. Combine maca powder, Siberian ginseng powder, almond milk, and honey in a blender.
2. Mix until smooth.
3. Pour into a glass and drink.

Usage Tips: Enjoy this drink in the morning to boost energy levels and reduce fatigue. Maca and Siberian ginseng are both adaptogens that help to increase stamina and improve resilience.

86. STRESS RELIEF ASHWAGANDHA AND LEMON BALM ELIXIR

Ingredients:

- 1 tsp dried ashwagandha root
- 1 tsp dried lemon balm leaves
- 1 cup boiling water
- 1 tbsp honey

Steps:

1. Transfer dried ashwagandha root and dried lemon balm leaves in your teapot.
2. Pour boiling water into the teapot.
3. Let steep for 8-9 min.
4. Strain into a cup.
5. Stir in honey and serve.

Usage Tips: Drink this elixir to reduce stress and promote relaxation. Ashwagandha and lemon balm both have calming properties that help to balance stress hormones and support overall well-being.

87. SLEEP INDUCING VALERIAN AND PASSIONFLOWER TEA

Ingredients:

- 1 tsp dried valerian root
- 1 tsp dried passionflower
- 1 cup boiling water
- 1 tbsp honey

Steps:

1. Transfer dried valerian root and dried passionflower in your teapot.
2. Pour boiling water into the teapot.

3 Let steep for 8-9 min.
4 Strain into a cup.
5 Stir in honey and serve.

Usage Tips: Drink this tea before bed to promote restful sleep. Valerian and passionflower both have calming and sedative properties that help to relax the mind and body.

---

88. MUSCLE RECOVERY COMFREY AND ARNICA SALVE

Ingredients:

- 1/3 cup dried comfrey leaves
- 1/3 cup dried arnica flowers
- 1/2 cup coconut oil
- 1/3 cup beeswax
- 12 drops peppermint essential oil

Steps:

1 Infuse the dried comfrey leaves and dried arnica flowers in coconut oil over low heat for 1 hour.
2 Strain the oil and combine with beeswax in a double boiler.
3 Heat until melted, then stir in peppermint essential oil.
4 Pour into a jar and let cool.

Usage Tips: Apply this salve to sore muscles to promote recovery and reduce inflammation. Comfrey and arnica both have healing properties that help to soothe and repair muscles.

2.6 Herbs for Holistic Recovery and Rejuvenation

89. RECOVERY BOOST ADAPTOGEN BLEND WITH RHODIOLA AND HOLY BASIL

Ingredients:

- 1 tsp dried rhodiola root
- 1 tsp dried holy basil leaves
- 1 cup boiling water
- 1 tbsp honey

Steps:

1 Combine dried rhodiola root and dried holy basil leaves in your teapot.
2 Pour boiling water into the teapot.
3 Let steep for 8-9 min.
4 Strain into a cup.
5 Stir in honey and serve.

Usage Tips: Drink this blend to boost recovery and reduce stress. Rhodiola and holy basil are adaptogens that help to balance stress hormones and improve resilience.

90. REJUVENATING SKIN TONIC WITH GOTU KOLA AND POMEGRANATE

Ingredients:

- 1 tsp dried gotu kola leaves
- 1/3 cup pomegranate juice
- 1 cup boiling water
- 1 tbsp honey

Steps:

1 Transfer dried gotu kola leaves and boiling water in your teapot.
2 Let steep for 8-9 min, then strain into a cup.
3 Stir in pomegranate juice and honey.

Usage Tips: Enjoy this tonic to rejuvenate your skin from within. Gotu kola is known for its skin-healing properties, while pomegranate is rich in antioxidants that promote skin health.

91. ENERGY RESTORATION SCHISANDRA AND BEETROOT JUICE

Ingredients:

- 1 tsp dried schisandra berries
- 1/3 cup beetroot juice
- 1 cup boiling water
- 1 tbsp honey

Steps:

1 Combine dried schisandra berries and boiling water in your teapot.
2 Let steep for 8-9 min, then strain into a cup.
3 Stir in beetroot juice and honey, then serve.

Usage Tips: Drink this juice to restore energy and vitality. Schisandra is an adaptogen that helps to reduce fatigue, while beetroot juice provides a natural energy boost.

92. REVITALIZING ROSEMARY AND SAGE SCALP TONIC

Ingredients:

- 1 tbsp dried rosemary leaves
- 1 tbsp dried sage leaves
- 1 cup boiling water

Steps:

1 Transfer dried rosemary leaves and dried sage leaves in your teapot.
2 Pour boiling water into the teapot.
3 Let steep for 8-9 min.
4 Strain into a cup and let cool.

Usage Tips: Use this tonic to revitalize your scalp and promote hair health. Rosemary and sage both have stimulating properties that help to improve scalp circulation and strengthen hair.

93. HEALING ALOE VERA AND WHEATGRASS SHOT

Ingredients:

- 1 tbsp fresh aloe vera gel
- 1 tbsp wheatgrass juice

Steps:

1 Combine fresh aloe vera gel and wheatgrass juice in a small glass.
2 Stir well and serve.

Usage Tips: Take this shot daily to support healing and detoxification. Aloe vera and wheatgrass are both known for their healing and cleansing properties.

94. DETOXIFYING DANDELION AND MILK THISTLE TEA

Ingredients:

- 1 tsp dried dandelion root
- 1 tsp dried milk thistle seeds
- 1 cup boiling water
- 1 tbsp honey

Steps:

1 Transfer dried dandelion root and dried seeds in your teapot.
2 Pour boiling water into the teapot.
3 Let steep for 8-9 min.
4 Strain into a cup.
5 Stir in honey and serve.

Usage Tips: Drink this tea to support liver detoxification. Dandelion and milk thistle are both known for their liver-protective and detoxifying properties.

95. ANTI-AGING ACAI AND GOJI BERRY SMOOTHIE

Ingredients:

- 1/3 cup acai berries
- 1/3 cup goji berries
- 1 banana
- 1 cup almond milk
- 1 tbsp honey

Steps:

1 Combine acai berries, goji berries, banana, almond milk, and honey in a blender.
2 Mix until smooth.
3 Pour into a glass and drink.

Usage Tips: Enjoy this smoothie for its anti-aging benefits. Acai and goji berries are rich in antioxidants that help to fight free radicals and promote youthful skin.

96. STRESS RECOVERY LEMON BALM AND CATNIP TEA

Ingredients:

- 1 tsp dried lemon balm leaves
- 1 tsp dried catnip leaves
- 1 cup boiling water
- 1 tbsp honey

Steps:

1 Combine dried lemon balm leaves and dried catnip leaves in your teapot.
2 Pour boiling water into the teapot.
3 Let steep for 8-9 min.
4 Strain into a cup.
5 Stir in honey and serve.

Usage Tips: Drink this tea to support stress recovery and relaxation. Lemon balm and catnip both have calming properties that help to reduce stress and promote relaxation.

97. HORMONAL BALANCE CHASTE TREE AND RASPBERRY LEAF TINCTURE

Ingredients:

- 1/2 cup dried chaste tree berries
- 1/2 cup dried raspberry leaves
- 1 cup vodka or brandy

Steps:

1. Combine dried chaste tree berries, dried raspberry leaves, and vodka or brandy in a jar.
2. Seal the jar and let sit for about 1 month, shaking daily.
3. Strain the mixture and store the liquid in a glass bottle.

Usage Tips: Take 1 tsp of this tincture daily to support hormonal balance. Chaste tree and raspberry leaf are both known for their hormone-balancing properties.

98. MUSCLE SOOTHE ARNICA AND LAVENDER MASSAGE OIL

Ingredients:

- 1/3 cup dried arnica flowers
- 1/3 cup dried lavender flowers
- 1 cup carrier oil (such as almond or olive oil)

Steps:

1. Infuse the dried arnica flowers and dried lavender flowers in the carrier oil over low heat for about 50-60 min..
2. Strain the oil and pour into a glass bottle.

Usage Tips: Use this massage oil to soothe sore muscles and reduce inflammation. Arnica and lavender both have anti-inflammatory and relaxing properties that help to relieve muscle pain.

99. MENTAL CLARITY BRAHMI AND PEPPERMINT INFUSION

Ingredients:

- 1 tsp dried brahmi leaves
- 1 tsp dried peppermint leaves
- 1 cup boiling water
- 1 tbsp honey

Steps:

1. Transfer dried brahmi leaves and dried peppermint leaves in your teapot.
2. Pour boiling water into the teapot.
3. Let steep for 8-9 min.
4. Strain into a cup.
5. Stir in honey and serve.

Usage Tips: Drink this infusion to enhance mental clarity and focus. Brahmi and peppermint are both known for their cognitive-enhancing properties.

Chapter 3: Herbal Wellness Practices for Families

3.1 Daily Wellness Routines.

Morning Herbal Rituals

Morning herbal rituals are a wonderful way to start the day with intention and mindfulness, incorporating the natural benefits of herbs into your daily routine. Beginning the day with a cup of herbal tea sets a calming tone and provides gentle energy without the jitters associated with caffeine. Herbs such as peppermint, lemon balm, and holy basil are excellent choices. Peppermint invigorates the senses and aids digestion, lemon balm offers a mild calming effect while enhancing mood, and holy basil, known as tulsi, is revered for its adaptogenic properties, helping to balance stress levels.

Incorporating herbal tinctures or supplements into your morning routine can also be highly beneficial. A few drops of a high-quality herbal tincture in a glass of water can provide a concentrated dose of herbal goodness. For instance, ginseng can boost energy levels, echinacea can support the immune system, and ashwagandha can help manage stress. These tinctures are easily absorbed by the body, making them an efficient way to reap the benefits of herbs.

Starting the day with a facial steam using herbs can also rejuvenate the skin and mind. Boiling water with herbs like chamomile, lavender, and rosemary, then allowing the steam to open your pores while inhaling the aromatic vapors can be both invigorating and relaxing. Chamomile soothes the skin, lavender provides a calming effect, and rosemary can enhance focus and mental clarity.

Another beneficial practice is to create an herbal-infused oil to use in a self-massage or as part of your skincare routine. Infusing oils with herbs such as calendula, rose, or lavender can create nourishing and healing treatments for the skin. Massaging your face and body with these oils not only hydrates the skin but also promotes circulation and reduces tension. This practice can be particularly grounding, providing a moment of calm before the busyness of the day begins.

Incorporating herbs into your morning smoothie is another excellent way to start the day with a nutritional boost. Adding herbs like fresh mint, basil, or cilantro not only enhances the flavor but also adds a range of health benefits. Mint can soothe the digestive tract, basil offers anti-inflammatory properties, and cilantro can help detoxify the body. Combining these herbs with fruits, vegetables, and a source of protein creates a balanced and nourishing breakfast.

Practicing mindfulness or meditation with the aid of herbs can also be a powerful morning ritual. Burning sage or using essential oils like frankincense or sandalwood can create a serene environment, enhancing your meditation practice. These herbs have been traditionally used to clear negative energy, promote mental clarity, and connect with deeper spiritual practices.

Starting your day with these herbal rituals can transform your morning into a time of self-care and wellness, setting a positive and nurturing tone for the rest of the day. Integrating the healing properties of herbs into your morning routine helps you to connect with nature, support your health, and embrace a holistic approach to daily living.

Herbal Supplements for Daily Health

Herbal supplements for daily health are a convenient and effective way to integrate the powerful benefits of herbs into your wellness routine. These supplements come in various forms, including capsules, tinctures, powders, and teas, making it easy to find a method that fits seamlessly into your lifestyle. They offer targeted support for various aspects of health, from boosting the immune system to enhancing mental clarity and managing stress.

One of the most popular herbal supplements is echinacea, well-known for its immune-boosting properties. Regular intake of echinacea, particularly during the cold and flu season, can help reduce the severity and duration of symptoms. This herb is often taken in capsule form or as a tincture, providing an easy way to support your immune health daily.

Ashwagandha, another widely used herb, is prized for its adaptogenic properties. Adaptogens help the body adapt to stress and maintain balance. Taking ashwagandha supplements can improve energy levels, reduce stress, and enhance overall well-being. This herb is available in capsules, powders, and tinctures, offering flexibility in how you choose to incorporate it into your routine.

Turmeric is renowned for its potent anti-inflammatory and antioxidant properties. Regular consumption of turmeric supplements can help manage inflammation, support joint health, and enhance cognitive function. Turmeric is often combined with black pepper in supplements to increase its bioavailability, ensuring you receive the maximum benefit from this powerful herb.

Ginkgo biloba is another herb commonly used to enhance cognitive function and support mental clarity. It improves blood circulation to the brain, which can enhance memory, focus, and overall cognitive performance. Ginkgo biloba supplements are available in various forms, including capsules and liquid extracts, making it easy to add to your daily regimen.

For digestive health, supplements like ginger and peppermint are highly effective. Ginger is known for its ability to soothe the digestive tract and alleviate nausea, while peppermint can help relieve symptoms of irritable bowel syndrome (IBS) and promote overall digestive comfort. These herbs can be taken in capsule form or as tinctures, providing convenient options for daily use.

Adaptogens like rhodiola and holy basil are also excellent choices for daily supplementation, particularly for their stress-relieving and energy-boosting properties. Rhodiola helps improve physical and mental stamina, while holy basil, also known as tulsi, is revered for its ability to balance the body and mind, reduce stress, and support the immune system.

Incorporating herbal supplements into your daily health routine can provide a natural and effective way to support your body's functions and enhance overall well-being. It's essential to choose high-quality supplements from reputable sources to ensure you are getting the most benefit from these potent natural remedies. Whether you're looking to boost your immune system, manage stress, improve cognitive function, or support digestive health, there's an herbal supplement that can help you achieve your health goals naturally and holistically.

Midday Stress Relief Practices

Midday stress relief practices are essential for maintaining balance and productivity throughout the day. Incorporating herbal remedies and mindful activities into your routine can significantly reduce stress levels, enhance focus, and rejuvenate your mind and body. Here are some effective practices to help you find calm and restore energy during the midday slump.

One of the simplest and most effective midday stress relief practices is enjoying a calming herbal tea. Herbal teas such as chamomile, lavender, and lemon balm are well-known for their soothing properties. Taking a break to brew and sip on a cup of these herbal teas can help you unwind and reset your mind. Chamomile tea is particularly effective for reducing anxiety and promoting relaxation, while lavender and lemon balm can uplift your mood and provide a sense of tranquility.

Incorporating aromatherapy into your midday routine is another powerful way to combat stress. Essential oils like lavender, bergamot, and ylang-ylang have calming and stress-relieving effects. Using a diffuser with these essential oils in your workspace can create a peaceful environment that promotes relaxation and mental clarity. Alternatively, you can apply a few drops of essential oil to a tissue or cotton ball and inhale deeply to experience immediate calming effects.

Taking a brief walk outside, especially in a natural setting, can do wonders for your mental health. Nature has a restorative effect, and walking in a park or garden can help reduce stress and improve your mood. If you can't get outside, try a few minutes of gentle stretching or yoga at your desk. Poses like the forward fold, seated twist, and cat-cow stretch can relieve tension in your muscles and promote a sense of calm.

Mindful breathing exercises are another excellent midday stress relief practice. Taking just five minutes to focus on your breath can significantly reduce stress levels and enhance your ability to concentrate. A simple technique is the 4-7-8 breathing exercise: inhale through your nose for a count of four, hold your breath for a count of seven, and exhale slowly through your mouth for a count of eight. Repeat this cycle several times to calm your nervous system and clear your mind.

Midday meditation is also highly effective for managing stress. Even a short, five-minute meditation session can help you reset and regain focus. Find a quiet space, close your eyes, and focus on your breath. Allow your thoughts to come and go without judgment, bringing your attention back to your breath whenever your mind starts to wander. Guided meditation apps can be particularly helpful if you are new to meditation or need a little extra support.

Additionally, herbal supplements like ashwagandha and rhodiola can be taken midday to help manage stress and improve energy levels. Ashwagandha is an adaptogen known for its ability to reduce cortisol levels and promote a sense of calm, while rhodiola helps enhance mental clarity and combat fatigue. These supplements can be taken in capsule form or as tinctures, providing a convenient way to support your stress relief efforts.

Incorporating these midday stress relief practices into your routine can significantly enhance your well-being and productivity. By taking the time to care for your mind and body, you can navigate the rest of your day with greater ease and focus. Remember that small, consistent actions can make a big difference in managing stress and maintaining a balanced lifestyle.

Evening Relaxation and Sleep Enhancement

Evening relaxation and sleep enhancement are crucial components of a holistic approach to wellness. The transition from a busy day to a peaceful night can significantly impact the quality of your sleep and overall health. Incorporating herbal remedies and calming practices into your evening routine can promote deep relaxation, reduce stress, and prepare your mind and body for restorative sleep.

Begin your evening relaxation with a soothing herbal tea. Chamomile, valerian root, and passionflower teas are well-known for their sedative properties and can help you unwind after a long day. Chamomile is particularly effective for its mild tranquilizing effects, making it an excellent choice for easing anxiety and promoting calmness. Valerian root acts as a natural sedative, helping to reduce the time it takes to fall asleep and improve sleep quality. Passionflower, known for its calming effects, can help alleviate nervousness and encourage a restful night's sleep. Sipping on a warm cup of herbal tea about an hour before bedtime can create a calming ritual that signals your body it's time to relax.

A warm herbal bath can also be incredibly beneficial for evening relaxation. Adding a handful of dried lavender flowers, rose petals, or chamomile blossoms to your bathwater can create a fragrant and soothing soak. The warm water helps to relax tense muscles and the aromatic herbs provide additional calming benefits. Lavender, in particular, is renowned for its ability to reduce stress and promote relaxation. As you soak, focus on deep, slow breathing to enhance the calming effects and prepare your body for sleep.

Incorporating aromatherapy into your evening routine can further enhance relaxation. Essential oils like lavender, sandalwood, and ylang-ylang are known for their relaxing and sedative properties. Use an essential oil diffuser in your bedroom to fill the air with these calming scents. You can also create a pillow spray by diluting a few drops of essential oil in water and lightly misting your pillow before bed. The soothing aroma will help to calm your mind and promote a peaceful sleep environment.

Practicing gentle yoga or stretching before bed can help release physical tension and quiet your mind. Focus on poses that promote relaxation and stress relief, such as child's pose, legs up the wall, and seated forward bend. These poses can help to release tension in your back, shoulders, and hips, areas where stress often accumulates. Combining these stretches with mindful breathing can further enhance the calming effects and prepare your body for sleep.

Engaging in a mindfulness or meditation practice before bed can also significantly improve sleep quality. Guided meditation, progressive muscle relaxation, or simple deep breathing exercises can help to calm your mind and reduce anxiety. Find a quiet, comfortable place to sit or lie down, close your eyes, and focus on your breath. Allow your thoughts to pass without judgment and bring your attention back to your breath whenever your mind starts to wander. Even just a few minutes of meditation can create a sense of inner peace and readiness for sleep.

Herbal supplements such as melatonin, magnesium, and L-theanine can also be beneficial for enhancing sleep. Melatonin is a natural hormone that regulates sleep-wake cycles, and taking a melatonin supplement can help to improve sleep onset and quality. Magnesium helps to relax muscles and calm the nervous system, making it easier to fall asleep. L-theanine, an amino acid found in green tea, promotes relaxation and can help to reduce the symptoms of anxiety. These supplements can be taken in capsule form or as part of a calming bedtime drink.

Creating a bedtime routine that includes these herbal remedies and relaxation practices can significantly enhance your sleep quality and overall well-being. By dedicating time to unwind and prepare for sleep, you can promote a deeper, more restorative rest and wake up feeling refreshed and rejuvenated. Remember that consistency is key, and establishing a regular evening routine will help to reinforce these healthy habits.

Weekly Detox and Rejuvenation

Weekly detox and rejuvenation practices can play a vital role in maintaining overall health and wellness. These practices help to cleanse the body of toxins, rejuvenate the mind and spirit, and provide a reset that can enhance your well-being. Incorporating herbal remedies into your weekly detox routine can amplify these benefits, as many herbs have natural detoxifying and revitalizing properties.

Begin your weekly detox with a focus on hydration. Drinking plenty of water is essential for flushing out toxins from the body. Enhance your hydration with a detoxifying herbal water infusion. Add slices of cucumber, lemon, and a few sprigs of fresh mint to a pitcher of water. Cucumber is known for its hydrating and anti-inflammatory properties, while lemon aids digestion and detoxification. Mint adds a refreshing taste and can help soothe the digestive tract. Drink this infusion throughout the day to stay hydrated and support your body's natural detox processes.

Incorporate a detoxifying herbal tea into your weekly routine. Dandelion root tea is an excellent choice, as it supports liver function and acts as a gentle diuretic, helping to flush out toxins. Burdock root tea is another effective option, known for its blood-purifying properties. These teas can be consumed daily or several times a week during your detox period. Preparing a blend of these detoxifying herbs can provide a powerful boost to your detox efforts.

A weekly herbal bath can also be an integral part of your detox routine. Prepare a detox bath with Epsom salts and a blend of detoxifying herbs such as rosemary, thyme, and sage. Epsom salts help to draw out impurities through the skin and relieve muscle tension, while the herbs provide additional detoxifying benefits. Rosemary stimulates circulation and aids in the removal of toxins, thyme has antiseptic and cleansing properties, and sage helps to reduce inflammation. Soaking in this herbal bath for 20-30 minutes can help to cleanse your body and leave you feeling rejuvenated.

Incorporate dry brushing into your weekly detox practices. Dry brushing involves using a natural bristle brush to gently exfoliate the skin and stimulate lymphatic drainage, which helps to remove toxins from the body. Start at your feet and brush upwards in long, sweeping motions towards your heart. This technique not only supports detoxification but also improves circulation and promotes smoother, healthier skin.

Consider adding a weekly herbal steam to your routine. Herbal steams can open up your pores, allowing toxins to be released from your skin. Boil a pot of water and add detoxifying herbs such as eucalyptus, chamomile, and peppermint. Eucalyptus has powerful antibacterial properties and helps to clear respiratory passages, chamomile soothes the skin and reduces inflammation, and peppermint invigorates the senses and aids in cleansing. Lean over the pot with a towel draped over your head to create a tent, and breathe deeply for about 10-15 minutes. This herbal steam can help to clear your skin and respiratory system while providing a calming and rejuvenating experience.

Support your detox efforts with a nutrient-dense diet rich in whole foods. Incorporate plenty of fruits, vegetables, whole grains, and lean proteins into your meals. Focus on foods that are known for their detoxifying properties, such as leafy greens, garlic, and berries. Leafy greens like kale and spinach are packed with chlorophyll, which helps to cleanse the blood. Garlic contains sulfur compounds that activate liver enzymes responsible for detoxification. Berries are rich in antioxidants, which help to neutralize toxins and protect your cells.

End your weekly detox with a period of rest and relaxation. Allow your body and mind to fully unwind by engaging in activities that promote relaxation and stress relief. This could include practices such as yoga, meditation, or simply spending time in nature. Giving yourself this time to relax and rejuvenate can enhance the benefits of your detox routine and leave you feeling refreshed and revitalized for the week ahead.

By incorporating these weekly detox and rejuvenation practices into your routine, you can support your body's natural detoxification processes, improve your overall health, and enhance your sense of well-being. Consistency is key, and making these practices a regular part of your life can lead to long-term benefits and a greater sense of vitality.

3.2 Herbal Activities for Families

3.2.1 Making Herbal Soaps Together

Creating herbal soaps at home is a wonderful way to introduce your family to the world of natural skincare. The process is straightforward and allows for creativity in choosing herbs, scents, and shapes. Making soap from scratch can also help children and adults alike understand the importance of natural ingredients and the benefits they bring to our skin. Below is a step-by-step guide to making herbal soaps together as a family.

Steps for Making Herbal Soaps:

1. Gather Materials and Ingredients:

- Soap base (such as glycerin or goat's milk)
- Dried herbs (like lavender, calendula, chamomile)
- Essential oils (optional, for fragrance)
- Soap molds
- Microwave-safe container or double boiler
- Mixing utensils (spoon, whisk)
- Knife or grater (if using a solid soap base)

2. Prepare Your Workspace:

- Clean and sanitize your workspace to ensure all equipment and surfaces are free of contaminants.
- Lay out all your materials and ingredients to ensure everything is within reach.

3. Melt the Soap Base:

- Cut the soap base into small, uniform pieces to ensure even melting.
- Place the pieces in a microwave-safe container or double boiler.
- If using a microwave, heat the soap base in short intervals (20-30 seconds), stirring in between until fully melted.
- If using a double boiler, heat the soap base over low to medium heat, stirring occasionally until melted.

4. Add Herbs and Essential Oils:

- Once the soap base is fully melted, remove it from the heat source.

- Add a small handful of dried herbs to the melted soap. Stir gently to distribute the herbs evenly.
- If desired, add a few drops of essential oils for fragrance. Common choices include lavender, peppermint, and chamomile essential oils.

5. Pour into Molds:

- Carefully pour the mixture into soap molds. Fill each mold to the top to ensure a full-sized soap bar.
- Tap the molds gently on the countertop to release any air bubbles that may have formed.

6. Allow to Set:

- Let the soap cool and harden at room temperature for several hours. Alternatively, you can place the molds in the refrigerator to speed up the process.
- Ensure the soap is completely set before attempting to remove it from the molds.

7. Remove from Molds:

- Once the soap is fully hardened, carefully remove each bar from its mold. If the soap is difficult to remove, gently press on the bottom of the mold or use a small knife to loosen the edges.

8. Cure and Store:

- Allow the soap bars to cure for at least 24 hours in a cool, dry place. This helps the soap to firm up and ensures it lasts longer when used.
- Store the finished soap bars in an airtight container or wrap them individually in plastic wrap or wax paper to keep them fresh.

Tips for Family Soap-Making:

- Let children choose the herbs and essential oils they want to use. This makes the activity more engaging and personalized.
- Use different shapes and sizes of molds to create a variety of soap bars.
- Label the soaps with the names of the herbs and oils used, and include the date they were made.

Making herbal soaps together is a rewarding activity that not only produces a useful end product but also fosters family bonding and creativity. Enjoy the process, experiment with different combinations, and have fun creating your own herbal soaps at home!

3.2.2 Creating a Family Herb Garden

Starting a family herb garden is an excellent project that can involve everyone, from young children to adults. It's a hands-on way to learn about plant life cycles, the importance of sustainable gardening, and the specific uses of different herbs. Whether you have a large backyard or a small balcony, you can create a thriving herb garden that brings both joy and practical benefits to your family.

Steps for Creating a Family Herb Garden:

1. Choose the Location:

- Select a sunny spot for your herb garden, as most herbs thrive with at least 6-8 hours of sunlight daily. This could be a section of your yard, a raised garden bed, or even containers on a patio or windowsill.
- Ensure the location has good drainage to prevent waterlogging, which can harm the herbs.

2. Plan Your Garden:

- Decide which herbs you want to grow. Consider the culinary, medicinal, and aromatic uses of each herb. Common choices include basil, parsley, thyme, rosemary, mint, and lavender.
- Draw a simple layout of your garden, considering the space each herb will need to grow. Taller herbs like rosemary should be placed at the back or center, while shorter herbs like thyme and basil can be placed at the front or edges.

3. Prepare the Soil:

- Test the soil in your chosen location to ensure it's suitable for growing herbs. Herbs prefer well-drained soil with a pH between 6.0 and 7.5.
- If needed, amend the soil with organic matter such as compost or aged manure to improve fertility and drainage.
- For container gardening, use a high-quality potting mix that provides good drainage and nutrients.

4. Plant the Herbs:

- Purchase herb seedlings from a nursery or start your own from seeds. Starting from seedlings is often easier and faster, especially for beginners.
- Dig holes in the soil according to the size of the root ball of each plant. Space the plants according to their growth habits—typically 12-18 inches apart for most herbs.

- Gently remove the seedlings from their pots and loosen the roots before placing them in the holes. Cover the roots with soil and press down gently to remove air pockets.

5. Water and Mulch:

- Water the newly planted herbs thoroughly to help them establish. Keep the soil consistently moist but not waterlogged.
- Apply a layer of mulch around the plants to retain moisture, suppress weeds, and regulate soil temperature. Organic mulch such as straw, bark chips, or compost works well.

6. Care and Maintenance:

- Regularly water the herbs, especially during dry spells. Herbs in containers may need more frequent watering than those planted in the ground.
- Fertilize sparingly with a balanced organic fertilizer if necessary. Over-fertilizing can reduce the flavor and aroma of herbs.
- Prune the herbs regularly to encourage bushy growth and prevent flowering, which can reduce the potency of the leaves. Use the pruned leaves in your cooking or drying projects.

7. Harvesting:

- Harvest herbs in the morning after the dew has dried but before the sun is too hot. This is when the essential oils, which give herbs their flavor and aroma, are at their peak.
- Use sharp scissors or pruning shears to cut the herbs. Avoid stripping more than one-third of the plant at a time to ensure continued healthy growth.
- Store fresh herbs in a cool, dry place or use them immediately. You can also dry or freeze excess herbs for later use.

8. Engage the Family:

- Involve children in all stages of the gardening process, from planning and planting to watering and harvesting. This teaches them valuable skills and creates a sense of ownership and pride in the garden.
- Create garden markers together to label each herb. This can be a fun craft activity using stones, sticks, or recycled materials.
- Encourage family members to use the herbs in cooking, teas, and homemade remedies, fostering an appreciation for fresh, natural ingredients.

Creating a family herb garden is a rewarding activity that provides fresh herbs and valuable life lessons. Enjoy the process of nurturing your garden and reaping the benefits of your hard work. With care and attention, your family herb garden will thrive, offering an ongoing source of joy and health.

3.2.3 DIY Herbal Bath Bombs

Herbal bath bombs are a delightful way to combine the benefits of aromatherapy and herbal skincare. By incorporating dried herbs, essential oils, and natural ingredients, you can create bath bombs that are both beautiful and beneficial. Whether you want to relax, rejuvenate, or relieve stress, these DIY bath bombs can be tailored to your needs and preferences.

Steps for Making DIY Herbal Bath Bombs:

1. Gather Ingredients and Supplies:

- Dry Ingredients:
    - 1 cup baking soda
    - 1/2 cup citric acid
    - 1/2 cup Epsom salts
    - 1/2 cup cornstarch
    - Dried herbs (such as lavender, chamomile, or rose petals)
- Wet Ingredients:
    - 2 1/2 tablespoons coconut oil (melted)
    - 1 tablespoon water
    - 15-20 drops of essential oils (such as lavender, eucalyptus, or peppermint)
- Supplies:
    - Mixing bowls
    - Whisk
    - Spray bottle filled with water
    - Silicone molds or bath bomb molds
    - Gloves (optional for mixing)

2. Prepare the Dry Ingredients:

- In a large mixing bowl, combine the baking soda, citric acid, Epsom salts, and cornstarch. Use a whisk to mix thoroughly, breaking up any clumps.
- Add a handful of dried herbs to the dry mixture. Ensure they are finely chopped or crushed to evenly distribute throughout the bath bombs.

3. Mix the Wet Ingredients:

- In a separate bowl, mix the melted coconut oil, water, and essential oils. Stir well to combine.

- The choice of essential oils can be based on the desired effect: lavender for relaxation, eucalyptus for respiratory relief, or peppermint for invigoration.

4. Combine Wet and Dry Ingredients:

- Slowly pour the wet ingredients into the dry mixture, whisking continuously. It's important to add the wet mixture gradually to prevent the citric acid from reacting prematurely.
- If the mixture starts to fizz, slow down the addition of the wet ingredients and continue whisking.

5. Achieve the Right Consistency:

- Once the wet and dry ingredients are combined, the mixture should hold together when squeezed. If it's too dry and crumbly, use the spray bottle to add a few spritzes of water, mixing well after each spritz until the right consistency is achieved.
- Be cautious not to add too much water, as this can activate the citric acid and ruin the mixture.

6. Mold the Bath Bombs:

- Firmly pack the mixture into the molds, pressing down to ensure there are no air pockets. Overfill the molds slightly and press the two halves together if using spherical molds.
- Allow the bath bombs to sit in the molds for at least 24 hours to harden. If using silicone molds, they may harden more quickly and can be removed after a few hours.

7. Dry and Store the Bath Bombs:

- Once the bath bombs are fully hardened, gently remove them from the molds. Place them on a parchment-lined baking sheet to dry for an additional 24-48 hours.
- Store the finished bath bombs in an airtight container to protect them from moisture. They can be wrapped individually in tissue paper or plastic wrap for gifting.

8. Tips for Customizing Your Bath Bombs:

- **Colors:** Add natural colorants such as beetroot powder for pink, spirulina for green, or turmeric for yellow. Mix these with the dry ingredients before adding the wet mixture.
- **Shapes:** Experiment with different mold shapes, such as hearts, stars, or flowers, to make the bath bombs more visually appealing.
- **Decorations:** Sprinkle extra dried herbs or flower petals on top of the bath bombs before they harden for a decorative touch.

Creating DIY herbal bath bombs is a rewarding and enjoyable project that the whole family can participate in. Not only do you get to enjoy the soothing effects of a luxurious bath, but you also gain the satisfaction of crafting something beautiful and beneficial from natural ingredients.

3.2.4 Herbal Crafting: Making Sachets and Potpourri

Herbal sachets and potpourri are traditional ways to use dried herbs and flowers to freshen up closets, drawers, and rooms. These aromatic creations not only add a pleasant scent to your home but also offer various benefits, such as repelling insects, promoting relaxation, and enhancing mood. By combining different herbs and essential oils, you can customize the aroma to suit your preferences and needs.

Making Herbal Sachets:

1. Gather Ingredients and Supplies:

- Herbs and Flowers:
    - Lavender
    - Rose petals
    - Chamomile
    - Mint
    - Lemon balm
- Essential Oils (optional):
    - Lavender oil
    - Rose oil
    - Peppermint oil
- Supplies:
    - Small fabric bags (muslin, cotton, or organza)
    - Ribbon or string
    - Scissors
    - Mixing bowl

2. Prepare the Herbs:

- Select dried herbs and flowers based on their fragrance and properties. Lavender is calming, rose petals are uplifting, and mint is invigorating.
- If desired, mix different herbs to create a blend. For example, a relaxing blend might include lavender, chamomile, and lemon balm.

3. Add Essential Oils:

- To enhance the scent, add a few drops of essential oils to the dried herb mixture. Essential oils can intensify the fragrance and add therapeutic benefits.
- Mix the herbs and oils thoroughly in a bowl to ensure even distribution.

4. Fill the Sachets:

- Spoon the herb mixture into the small fabric bags. Fill each bag about three-quarters full to allow the aroma to circulate.
- Tie the top of the bag tightly with ribbon or string to secure the contents.

5. Decorate the Sachets:

- For a decorative touch, add small charms, dried flowers, or labels to the sachets. This can make them more attractive if you're giving them as gifts.
- You can also sew or embroider designs onto the fabric bags for a personalized touch.

6. Usage Tips:

- Place herbal sachets in drawers, closets, or under pillows to enjoy their fragrance. Lavender sachets are particularly nice for promoting restful sleep when placed near your bed.
- Replace the contents of the sachets every few months to maintain their potency.

Making Potpourri:
1. Gather Ingredients and Supplies:

- Herbs and Flowers:
  - Rose petals
  - Lavender
  - Orange or lemon peel
  - Cinnamon sticks
  - Cloves
- Essential Oils (optional):
  - Rose oil
  - Citrus oil
  - Clove oil
- Supplies:
  - Large mixing bowl
  - Wooden spoon
  - Airtight containers (for storage)
  - Decorative bowls or jars (for display)

2. Prepare the Ingredients:

- Collect dried herbs, flowers, and spices. Ensure they are completely dry to prevent mold and spoilage.

- For added color and texture, include small pine cones, star anise, or dried fruit slices.

3. Mix the Potpourri:

- In a large mixing bowl, combine the dried ingredients. Use a wooden spoon to mix them gently.
- Add a few drops of essential oils to the mixture. Essential oils will boost the fragrance and can be chosen based on your desired effect (e.g., rose oil for romance, citrus oil for freshness).

4. Cure the Potpourri:

- Transfer the mixture to an airtight container and let it sit for 4-6 weeks. This allows the fragrances to blend and intensify.
- Shake the container occasionally to redistribute the essential oils.

5. Display the Potpourri:

- Once cured, transfer the potpourri to decorative bowls or jars. Place them around your home to add a pleasant aroma and a touch of natural beauty.
- Potpourri can also be refreshed with a few additional drops of essential oil if the scent starts to fade.

6. Usage Tips:

- Use potpourri in living rooms, bathrooms, or any space where you want to enjoy a natural fragrance.
- Consider creating seasonal potpourri blends. For example, use cinnamon and cloves for a winter scent, or lavender and lemon for a refreshing summer aroma.

Herbal crafting with sachets and potpourri is a creative way to harness the natural fragrances of herbs and flowers. These crafts not only enhance the ambiance of your home but also offer therapeutic benefits, making them a delightful addition to your herbal repertoire.

BOOK 7: SPIRITUAL AND HOLISTIC HERBAL PRACTICES

In our fast-paced, modern world, many seek solace and balance through spiritual and holistic practices. This section delves into the profound ways herbs can support mental wellness, spiritual growth, and holistic healing. This book explores how herbs can be seamlessly integrated into practices such as meditation, mindfulness, and rituals, offering a pathway to inner peace and deeper connection with nature.

Herbs have long been revered for their spiritual properties. Ancient cultures around the world have used herbs in various spiritual practices, from incense burning to creating sacred smudge sticks. These practices are not merely rituals of the past; they continue to offer significant benefits for mental and emotional health today. By incorporating herbs into your spiritual routines, you can enhance your mental clarity, emotional stability, and overall sense of well-being.

This book offers a comprehensive guide to using herbs for mental wellness and spiritual growth. We explore herbs known for their calming, uplifting, and grounding properties, such as lavender, sage, and frankincense. These herbs can help ease anxiety, improve focus, and foster a sense of tranquility. By understanding the properties of these herbs, you can create personalized blends that support your spiritual and mental health needs.

Meditation and mindfulness are powerful tools for achieving mental clarity and emotional balance. Integrating herbs into these practices can deepen your experience, making it more enriching and effective. This book provides detailed guidance on how to use herbs in various forms—such as teas, tinctures, and essential oils—to enhance your meditation and mindfulness routines. Whether you are seeking to calm a busy mind or cultivate a deeper sense of presence, herbs can be valuable allies in your journey.

Rituals are another important aspect of spiritual practice, and herbs play a significant role in creating meaningful and transformative experiences. This book offers step-by-step instructions for creating herbal incense, smudge sticks, and spiritual baths. These practices can purify your space, cleanse your aura, and help you connect with your inner self on a profound level. By incorporating these rituals into your daily life, you can create a sanctuary of peace and harmony, fostering spiritual growth and emotional healing.

Here you will find a wealth of knowledge and practical advice on harnessing the power of herbs for mental wellness and spiritual enrichment. Whether you are new to these practices or looking to deepen your existing knowledge, this book provides the tools and insights needed to integrate herbs into your spiritual and holistic routines. Embrace the wisdom of nature and discover how herbs can transform your mental and spiritual well-being, leading you towards a more balanced and fulfilling life.

Chapter 1: Herbs for Mental Wellness and Spiritual Growth

1.1 Natural Stress Management

1. LAVENDER AND CHAMOMILE CALM TEA

Ingredients:

- 1 tsp dried lavender flowers
- 1 tsp dried chamomile flowers
- 2 cups boiling water
- Honey to taste

Steps:

1 Combine lavender and chamomile flowers in your teapot.
2 Put boiling water into the teapot.
3 Let steep for 7-8 min.
4 Strain into a cup.
5 Add honey to taste, if desired.

Usage Tips: Enjoy this tea in the evening to help relax and unwind before bedtime.

2. ASHWAGANDHA ROOT TONIC

Ingredients:

- 1 tsp ashwagandha root powder
- 1 cup warm milk
- 1/2 tsp honey
- 1/4 tsp cinnamon

Steps:

1 Warm the milk in a small saucepan over low heat.

2 Put in ashwagandha root powder, honey, and cinnamon.
3 Whisk until well combined and smooth.
4 Pour into a cup and serve warm.

Usage Tips: Drink this tonic in the evening to promote relaxation and reduce stress.

3. HOLY BASIL NIGHTCAP

Ingredients:

- 1 tsp dried holy basil leaves
- 1 cup boiling water
- Honey to taste

Steps:

1 Place holy basil leaves in a cup.
2 Put boiling water over the leaves.
3 Let steep for 7-8 min.
4 Transfer into a cup.
5 Add honey to taste, if desired.

Usage Tips: Drink this calming tea before bed to help ease anxiety and promote restful sleep.

4. STRESS RELIEF HERBAL BATH SOAK

Ingredients:

- 1 cup Epsom salts
- 1/2 cup baking soda
- 1/3 cup dried lavender flowers
- 1/3 cup dried chamomile flowers

- 8 drops lavender essential oil

Steps:

1 Mix Epsom salts, baking soda, dried lavender, and chamomile flowers in a bowl.
2 Add lavender essential oil and mix.
3 Store the mixture in an airtight container.
4 When ready to use, add 1/2 cup of the mixture to a warm bath and soak for about 25 min.

Usage Tips: Use this bath soak to relieve stress and relax muscles after a long day.

---

5. VALERIAN HOP SLEEP POTION

Ingredients:

- 1 tsp dried valerian root
- 1 tsp dried hop flowers
- 1 cup boiling water
- Honey to taste

Steps:

1 Place valerian root and hop flowers in your teapot.
2 Put boiling water into the teapot.
3 Let steep for 12-14 min.
4 Strain into a cup.
5 Add honey to taste, if desired.

Usage Tips: Drink this potion 30 minutes before bedtime to help improve sleep quality.

---

6. SOOTHING LEMON BALM ELIXIR

Ingredients:

- 1 tsp dried lemon balm leaves
- 1 cup hot water
- 1 tsp honey
- 1 tsp lemon juice

Steps:

1 Transfer the dried lemon balm leaves in a cup.
2 Put hot water over the leaves.
3 Let steep for 7-8 min.
4 Strain into a glass.
5 Add honey and lemon juice.

Usage Tips: Enjoy this elixir in the afternoon to soothe nerves and uplift your mood.

---

7. PASSIONFLOWER RELAXATION DROPS

Ingredients:

- 1 cup boiling water
- 1 tsp dried passionflower
- 1 tsp dried lemon balm
- 12 drops valerian tincture

Steps:

1 Combine passionflower and lemon balm in a cup.
2 Put boiling water into the cup.
3 Let steep for 8-9 min.
4 Strain into a dropper bottle.
5 Add valerian tincture drops.

Usage Tips: Take a few drops under the tongue as needed for relaxation and stress relief.

---

8. GINGER-MINT ANTI-STRESS DRINK

Ingredients:

- 1-inch piece fresh ginger, sliced
- 1 tsp dried peppermint leaves
- 2 cups boiling water
- Honey to taste

Steps:

1 Combine ginger slices and peppermint leaves in your teapot.
2 Put boiling water into the teapot.
3 Let steep for 12-14 min.
4 Strain into a cup.
5 Add honey to taste.

Usage Tips: This refreshing drink can be enjoyed hot or cold to reduce stress and improve digestion.

---

9. ROSEMARY CITRUS REFRESHER

Ingredients:

- 1 sprig fresh rosemary
- 1/2 lemon, sliced
- 1/2 orange, sliced
- 4 cups cold water

Steps:

1 Place rosemary sprig, lemon slices, and orange slices in a pitcher.
2 Add cold water and stir.
3 Let infuse in the refrigerator for about 180-200 min.
4 Serve chilled.

Usage Tips: Enjoy this refreshing drink throughout the day to stay hydrated and invigorated.

10. HERBAL NECK PILLOW BLEND

Ingredients:

- 1/2 cup dried lavender flowers
- 1/2 cup dried chamomile flowers
- 1/3 cup dried rosemary
- 1/3 cup dried peppermint leaves

Steps:

1 Mix all dried herbs in a bowl and stir well.

2 Fill a small fabric pouch or neck pillow with the herb blend.
3 Sew or tie the pouch closed.

Usage Tips: Heat the neck pillow in the microwave for 30 seconds and place it around your neck to relieve stress and tension.

11. ADAPTOGEN POWER SMOOTHIE

Steps: 1/2 cup spinach

- 1/2 cup almond milk
- 1 tbsp almond butter
- 1 tsp maca powder
- 1/2 tsp ashwagandha powder
- 1 tsp honey
- 1 banana

1 Mix all ingredients in a blender.
2 Mix until smooth.
3 Transfer into a glass and drink immediately.

Usage Tips: This smoothie is perfect for a morning energy boost and stress management.

1.2 Herbs for Relaxation and Meditation

12. CENTRING SAGE SMUDGE STICK

Ingredients:

- Fresh sage leaves
- Cotton string

Steps:

1 Gather a bundle of fresh sage leaves.
2 Tightly wrap the cotton string around the bundle, starting at the base and working your way up.
3 Allow the smudge stick to dry in a cool, dry place for a couple of weeks.

Usage Tips: Light the end of the smudge stick and blow out the flame, allowing the smoke to cleanse and center your space.

13. MINDFUL BREATHING HERBAL SACHET

Ingredients:

- 1/3 cup dried lavender flowers
- 1/3 cup dried chamomile flowers
- 1/3 cup dried mint leaves
- 1 small fabric sachet

Steps:

1 Mix all dried herbs in a bowl and blend.
2 Fill the fabric sachet with the herb blend.
3 Tie or sew the sachet closed.

Usage Tips: Hold the sachet close to your nose and breathe deeply during meditation or mindful breathing exercises.

14. TRANQUIL LOTUS TEA

Ingredients:

- 1 tsp dried lotus flowers
- 1 tsp dried chamomile flowers
- 1 cup boiling water
- Honey to taste

Steps:

1. Combine dried lotus and chamomile flowers in your teapot.
2. Pour boiling water into the teapot.
3. Let steep for 7-8 min.
4. Strain into a glass.
5. Add honey to taste, if desired.

Usage Tips: Drink this tea during or after meditation to promote tranquility and relaxation.

15. ZEN GARDEN HERBAL INFUSION

Ingredients:

- 1 tsp dried green tea leaves
- 1 tsp dried peppermint leaves
- 1/2 tsp dried lavender flowers
- 1 cup hot water

Steps:

1. Combine all dried herbs in your teapot.
2. Put hot water into the teapot.
3. Let steep for 5-7 minutes.
4. Strain into a glass.

Usage Tips: Enjoy this infusion in a peaceful setting to create a Zen-like atmosphere and enhance your meditation practice.

16. FRANKINCENSE MEDITATION BALM

Ingredients:

- 1/3 cup coconut oil
- 1/3 cup beeswax pellets
- 8 drops frankincense essential oil
- 5 drops lavender essential oil

Steps:

1. Melt coconut oil and beeswax pellets together in a double boiler.
2. Take off from heat and add essential oils.
3. Transfer the mixture into a small jar or tin and let it cool and solidify.

Usage Tips: Apply a small amount to your temples and pulse points before meditation to promote calm and focus.

17. SANDALWOOD SERENITY SALVE

Ingredients:

- 1/3 cup shea butter
- 1/3 cup coconut oil
- 12 drops sandalwood essential oil
- 12 drops chamomile essential oil

Steps:

1. Melt shea butter and coconut oil together in a double boiler.
2. Take off from heat and add essential oils.
3. Transfer the mixture into a small jar or tin and let it cool and solidify.

Usage Tips: Massage this salve onto your wrists and neck before meditation to create a serene and calming effect.

18. CHAKRA BALANCING TINCTURE

Ingredients:

- 1/3 cup dried holy basil
- 1/3 cup dried ashwagandha root
- 1/3 cup dried gotu kola
- 1 cup vodka or glycerin (for alcohol-free version)

Steps:

1. Mix all dried herbs in a jar.
2. Put vodka or glycerin into the jar, until they are fully submerged.
3. Seal the jar and let it sit in a cool, dark place for about 30 days, stirring occasionally.
4. Strain the tincture into a dropper bottle.

Usage Tips: Take a few drops under the tongue or in water daily to help balance your chakras and promote overall well-being.

19. QUIET MIND HERBAL CAPSULES

Ingredients:

- 1/3 cup dried lavender flowers
- 1/3 cup dried chamomile flowers

- 1/3 cup dried lemon balm
- Empty gelatin or vegetarian capsules

Steps:

1 Grind all dried herbs into a fine powder using a mortar and pestle or coffee grinder.
2 Fill the empty capsules with the powdered herbs using a capsule machine or by hand.
3 Store the filled capsules in an airtight container.

Usage Tips: Take one capsule before meditation or as needed to calm the mind and promote relaxation.

20. REFLECTIVE MYRRH MIST

Ingredients:

- 1 cup distilled water
- 8 drops myrrh essential oil
- 6 drops lavender essential oil
- 1 tbsp witch hazel

Steps:

1 Mix all ingredients in a spray bottle.
2 Stir well to combine.

Usage Tips: Spray this mist in your meditation space or around your body to create a reflective and calming atmosphere.

21. CALMING HERBAL INCENSE BLEND

Ingredients:

- dried lavender flowers (1 part)
- dried chamomile flowers (1 part)
- dried rosemary (1 part)
- dried sage (1 part)

Steps:

1 Mix all dried herbs in a bowl.
2 Blend well to ensure an even blend.
3 Preserve the blend in an airtight container.
4 To use, place a small amount on a charcoal disc or in an incense burner.

Usage Tips: Use this incense blend during meditation or relaxation sessions to create a calming atmosphere.

22. REFLECTIVE MYRRH MIST

Ingredients:

- 1 cup distilled water
- 8 drops myrrh essential oil
- 6 drops lavender essential oil
- 1 tbsp witch hazel

Steps:

1 Mix all ingredients in a spray bottle.
2 Stir well to combine.

Usage Tips: Spray this mist in your meditation space or around your body to create a reflective and calming atmosphere.

1.3 Non-Medicinal Fatigue Management

23. ENERGY BOOSTING MACA SMOOTHIE

Ingredients:

- 1 banana
- 1 cup almond milk
- 1 tbsp maca powder
- 1 tbsp almond butter
- 1 tsp honey
- 1/2 cup ice

Steps:

1 Put all ingredients in a blender.
2 Mix until smooth.
3 Transfer into a glass and serve immediately.

Usage Tips: Drink this smoothie in the morning or as a midday snack for a natural energy boost.

24.   SIBERIAN GINSENG ENERGY BALLS

Ingredients:

- 1 cup rolled oats
- 1/2 cup almond butter
- 1/3 cup honey
- 1/3 cup dried cranberries
- 1 tbsp Siberian Ginseng powder
- 1 tsp vanilla extract

Steps:

1 Transfer all ingredients in a bowl.
2 Blend well until a dough forms.
3 Roll into small balls.
4 Place on a baking sheet.
5 Refrigerate for about 60-70 min before serving.

Usage Tips: These energy balls make a perfect snack to combat fatigue and boost stamina.

25.   CAFFEINE-FREE GREEN WAKE-UP BREW

Ingredients:

- 1 tsp dried green tea leaves
- 1 tsp dried peppermint leaves
- 1 tsp dried lemon balm
- 2 cups boiling water

Steps:

1 Combine all dried herbs in your teapot.
2 Put boiling water into the teapot.
3 Let steep for 5-7 minutes.
4 Strain into a glass.

Usage Tips: Enjoy this brew in the morning to gently wake up your body and mind without caffeine.

26.   QUICK ENERGY HERBAL DROPS

Ingredients:

- 1/3 cup dried ginseng root
- 1/3 cup dried rhodiola root
- 1/3 cup dried eleuthero root
- 1 cup vodka or glycerin (for alcohol-free version)

Steps:

1 Mix all dried herbs in a jar.

2 Flow vodka or glycerin into the jar, so they'll be fully submerged.
3 Seal the jar and let it sit in a cool, dark place for about 30 days, mixing occasionally.
4 Strain the tincture into a dropper bottle.

Usage Tips: Take a few drops under the tongue or in water for a quick energy boost.

27.   RHODIOLA ROSEA REVITALIZER

Ingredients:

- 1 tsp dried Rhodiola Rosea root
- 1 cup hot water
- Honey to taste

Steps:

1 Transfer dried Rhodiola root in a cup.
2 Put hot water over the root.
3 Let steep for 12-14 min.
4 Strain into a cup.
5 Add honey to taste, if desired.

Usage Tips: Drink this revitalizing tea in the morning or early afternoon for a natural energy lift.

28.   SCHISANDRA CHINENSIS BERRY DRINK

Ingredients:

- 1 tbsp dried Schisandra berries
- 2 cups boiling water
- 1 tsp honey

Steps:

1 Place dried Schisandra berries in your teapot.
2 Put boiling water over the berries.
3 Let steep for 15-20 minutes.
4 Strain into a glass.
5 Stir in honey.

Usage Tips: Enjoy this drink to enhance energy levels and improve mental clarity.

29. CORDYCEPS POWER SHAKE

Ingredients:

- 1 cup almond milk
- 1 tbsp Cordyceps powder
- 1 banana
- 1 tbsp cocoa powder
- 1 tsp honey

Steps:

1 Mix all ingredients in a blender.
2 Mix until smooth.
3 Pour into a glass and drink immediately.

Usage Tips: Drink this power shake in the morning or after a workout for sustained energy.

30. INVIGORATING PEPPERMINT INFUSION

Ingredients:

- 1 tsp dried peppermint leaves
- 1 cup boiling water
- Lemon slice for garnish

Steps:

1 Place dried peppermint leaves in a cup.
2 Pour boiling water over the leaves.
3 Let steep for 68 min.
4 Strain into a cup.
5 Garnish with a lemon slice.

Usage Tips: Enjoy this refreshing infusion whenever you need a quick pick-me-up.

31. NETTLE AND HONEY VITALITY ELIXIR

Ingredients:

- 1 tsp dried nettle leaves
- 1 cup hot water
- 1 tsp honey
- 1 tsp lemon juice

Steps:

1 Place dried nettle leaves in a cup.
2 Put hot water into the leaves.
3 Let steep for 8-9 min.
4 Strain into a cup.
5 Stir in honey and lemon juice.

Usage Tips: Drink this elixir daily to support energy levels and overall vitality.

32. GUARANA SEED ENERGY FIZZ

Ingredients:

- 1 tsp guarana seed powder
- 1 cup sparkling water
- 1/2 lemon (juice)
- 1 tsp honey

Steps:

1 Combine guarana seed powder, lemon juice, and honey in a glass.
2 Stir well to mix.
3 Add sparkling water and stir gently.

Usage Tips: Enjoy this fizzy drink in the morning or early afternoon for a natural energy boost.

33. REFRESHING SPEARMINT ICED TEA

Ingredients:

- 1/3 cup dried spearmint leaves
- 4 cups boiling water
- Ice
- Lemon slices for garnish

Steps:

1 Put dried spearmint leaves into a teapot.
2 Pour hot water over the leaves.
3 Allow the tea to steep for 8-9 minutes.
4 Strain the tea into a pitcher.
5 Cool it down, then refrigerate until chilled.
6 Serve it over ice with lemon slices for garnish.

Usage Tips: This iced tea is perfect for a refreshing and invigorating drink on a hot day.

34. GINSENG AND JUJUBE RECHARGE TEA

Ingredients:

- 1 tsp dried ginseng root
- 3 dried jujube fruits
- 2 cups boiling water
- Honey to taste

Steps:

1 Put dried ginseng root and jujube fruits in your teapot.
2 Pour hot water into the teapot.
3 Allow the mixture to steep for 15-20 minutes.
4 Strain the tea into a cup.
5 Sweeten with honey, if desired.

Usage Tips: Drink this tea in the morning or afternoon to help recharge your energy levels.

35. ENERGIZING CITRUS HERB WATER

Ingredients:

- 1 lemon, sliced
- 1 orange, sliced
- 1 lime, sliced
- 1/3 cup fresh mint leaves
- 4 cups cold water

Steps:

1 Place lemon, orange, and lime slices in a pitcher.
2 Add fresh mint leaves and cold water.
3 Stir well and refrigerate for about a couple of hours before drinking.

Usage Tips: Drink this citrus-infused water throughout the day to stay hydrated and energized.

36. LEMON BALM AND HAWTHORN HEART TONIC

Ingredients:

- 1 tsp dried lemon balm leaves
- 1 tsp dried hawthorn berries
- 1 cup boiling water
- Honey to taste

Steps:

1 Put dried lemon balm leaves and hawthorn berries into a teapot.
2 Pour hot water into the teapot.
3 Allow it to steep for 12-14 minutes.
4 Strain the mixture into a cup.
5 Sweeten with honey, if you like.

Usage Tips: This tonic is great for supporting heart health and calming the mind.

37. CHAKRA ALIGNING ESSENTIAL OIL BLEND

Ingredients:

- 5 drops lavender essential oil
- 5 drops frankincense essential oil
- 5 drops sandalwood essential oil
- 2 tbsp carrier oil (e.g., jojoba or almond oil)

Steps:

1 Combine all essential oils in a small bottle.
2 Add the carrier oil and mix well.
3 Secure the bottle with a cap and shake gently to blend.

Usage Tips: Apply a few drops to your pulse points or use in a diffuser during meditation to help align your chakras.

38. BALANCING ADAPTOGEN BLEND

Ingredients:

- 1 tsp ashwagandha powder
- 1 tsp reishi mushroom powder
- 1 tsp maca powder
- 1 cup warm almond milk
- Honey to taste

Steps:

1 Combine ashwagandha, reishi, and maca powders in a cup.
2 Pour warm almond milk over the powders and stir well.
3 Add honey to taste, if desired.

Usage Tips: Drink this blend in the morning or evening to help balance stress and support energy levels.

---

39.   ELECTRIFYING GINGER LEMONADE

Ingredients:

- 1-inch piece fresh ginger, sliced
- 1 lemon, juiced
- 2 cups cold water
- 1 tbsp honey
- Ice

Steps:

1 Place ginger slices in a pitcher.
2 Add lemon juice, cold water, and honey.
3 Stir well to combine.
4 Serve over ice.

Usage Tips: Enjoy this refreshing lemonade to boost energy and improve digestion.

---

40.   GOLDEN TURMERIC AND BLACK PEPPER SHOT

Ingredients:

- 1/2 tsp turmeric powder
- 1/4 tsp black pepper
- 1 tbsp lemon juice
- 1/3 cup warm water

Steps:

1 Combine turmeric powder, black pepper, and lemon juice in a small glass.
2 Add warm water and stir well.

Usage Tips: Take this shot in the morning to kickstart your metabolism and reduce inflammation.

41.REJUVENATING ASTRAGALUS BROTH

Ingredients:

- 1 tbsp dried astragalus root
- 4 cups water
- 1 garlic clove, minced
- 1 small piece of ginger, sliced
- Salt to taste

Steps:

1 Mix all ingredients in a pot.
2 Bring to a boil, then reduce heat and simmer for 35-40 min.
3 Strain into a bowl and season with salt to taste.

Usage Tips: Drink this broth as a nourishing tonic to support overall vitality.

---

42.   ROSE HIP RENEWAL DRINK

Ingredients:

- 1 tbsp dried rose hips
- 1 cup boiling water
- Honey to taste

Steps:

1 Add dried rose hips to a teapot.
2 Pour hot water over the rose hips.
3 Steep for 12-14 minutes.
4 Strain the tea into a cup.
5 Sweeten with honey, if preferred.

Usage Tips: Enjoy this drink daily to boost your immune system and support skin health.

---

43.   POMEGRANATE AND MINT VITALITY BOOSTER

Ingredients:

- 1 cup pomegranate juice
- 1/3 cup fresh mint leaves
- 1 cup sparkling water
- Ice

Steps:

1 Combine pomegranate juice and fresh mint leaves in a pitcher.
2 Stir well and let sit for 8-9 min.
3 Add sparkling water and ice, then stir gently.

Usage Tips: This vibrant drink is perfect for boosting energy and refreshing your mind.

44. REVITALIZING HERBAL COMPRESSION MIX

Ingredients:

- 1/3 cup dried rosemary
- 1/3 cup dried lavender
- 1/3 cup dried peppermint
- 1 quart hot water

Steps:

1 Mix all dried herbs in a bowl.
2 Pour hot water into the bowl and let them steep for 8-9 minutes.
3 Strain the liquid.
4 Soak a cloth in the herbal infusion and wring out the excess.

Usage Tips: Apply the herbal compress to your forehead or neck to relieve fatigue and invigorate your senses.

1.5 Natural Management of Strong Emotions

45. CALMING KAVA COCKTAIL

Ingredients:

- 1 tbsp kava root powder
- 1 cup coconut milk
- 1 tsp honey
- 1/2 tsp cinnamon

Steps:

1 Combine kava root powder and coconut milk in a blender.
2 Blend until smooth.
3 Strain the mixture into a cup to remove any solids.
4 Stir in honey and cinnamon.
5 Serve chilled.

Usage Tips: Enjoy this calming cocktail in the evening to help reduce anxiety and promote relaxation.

46. EMOTIONAL BALANCE HERBAL TONIC

Ingredients:

- 1 tsp dried lemon balm
- 1 tsp dried chamomile
- 1 tsp dried lavender
- 1 cup boiling water
- Honey to taste

Steps:

1 Place dried lemon balm, chamomile, and lavender in your teapot.
2 Pour hot water into the teapot.
3 Steep for 8-9 minutes.
4 Strain the tea into a cup.

5 Sweeten with honey, if preferred.

Usage Tips: Drink this tonic daily to help maintain emotional balance and calmness.

47. PASSIONFLOWER PEACE TEA

Ingredients:

- 1 tsp dried passionflower
- 1 tsp dried peppermint
- 1 cup boiling water
- Honey to taste

Steps:

1 Put dried passionflower and peppermint in your teapot.
2 Pour hot water into the teapot.
3 Steep for 8-9 minutes.
4 Strain the tea into a cup.
5 Add honey for sweetness, if desired.

Usage Tips: Enjoy this tea in the evening to promote peace and relaxation.

48. BLUE VERVAIN TRANQUILITY TINCTURE

Ingredients:

- 1/3 cup dried blue vervain
- 1 cup vodka or glycerin (for alcohol-free version)

Steps:

1 Place dried blue vervain in a jar.
2 2   Pour vodka or glycerin over the herbs, ensuring they are fully submerged.

3 Close the jar tightly and keep it in a cool, dark place for about 30 days, shaking it now and then.

4 Filter the tincture into a dropper bottle.

Usage Tips: Take a few drops under the tongue or in water to promote tranquility and reduce stress.

49. CBD HERBAL CALM DROPS

Ingredients:

- 1/3 cup dried lavender
- 1/3 cup dried chamomile
- 1 cup carrier oil (e.g., MCT oil or olive oil)
- 1 tsp CBD oil

Steps:

1 Put dried lavender and chamomile in a jar.

2 Pour carrier oil into the jar, making sure they are fully covered.

3 Seal the jar and let it sit in a cool, dark place for about 30 days, shaking occasionally.

4 Strain the oil into a dropper bottle and add CBD oil.

Usage Tips: Take a few drops under the tongue or in water as needed for calming effects.

50. SOOTHING CHAMOMILE LAVENDER SPRAY

Ingredients:

- 1 cup distilled water
- 12 drops chamomile essential oil
- 12 drops lavender essential oil
- 1 tbsp witch hazel

Steps:

1 Put all ingredients into a spray bottle.

2 Shake thoroughly to combine.

Usage Tips: Spray this soothing mist on your pillow, bedding, or around your room to create a calming environment.

51. AROMATIC STRESS RELIEF ROLLER

Ingredients:

- 8 drops lavender essential oil
- 4 drops chamomile essential oil
- 4 drops bergamot essential oil
- 1 tbsp carrier oil (e.g., jojoba or almond oil)

Steps:

1 Combine all essential oils in a small bottle.

2 Add the carrier oil and mix thoroughly.

3 Secure the bottle with a roller cap.

Usage Tips: Apply to wrists, temples, or neck during stressful moments to help alleviate tension.

52. SERENITY NOW HERBAL INHALER

Ingredients:

- 4 drops frankincense essential oil
- 4 drops lavender essential oil
- 5 drops sandalwood essential oil
- Cotton wick
- Inhaler tube

Steps:

1 Place the cotton wick in a small dish.

2 Add the essential oils to the wick.

3 Insert the wick into the inhaler tube and secure it.

Usage Tips: Inhale deeply whenever you need a moment of calm and serenity.

53. HAWTHORN HEART SOOTHE SYRUP

Ingredients:

- 1 cup dried hawthorn berries
- 4 cups water
- 1 cup honey

Steps:

1 Place dried hawthorn berries and water in a saucepan.

2 Bring to a boil, then reduce heat and let it simmer for 30 minutes.

3   Strain the mixture and return the liquid to the saucepan.
4   Mix in honey until it is fully dissolved.
5   Transfer the syrup to a bottle and refrigerate.

Usage Tips: Take 1-2 tbsp daily to support heart health and emotional well-being.

54.   ST. JOHN'S WORT STABILITY SMOOTHIE

Ingredients:

- 1 banana
- 1 cup almond milk
- 1 tbsp St. John's Wort tincture
- 1 tbsp almond butter
- 1 tsp honey

Steps:

1   Combine all ingredients in a blender.
2   Blend until smooth.
3   Pour into a glass and serve right away.

Usage Tips: Drink this smoothie in the morning to help stabilize mood and boost emotional resilience.

55.   EMOTIONAL RESCUE BATH SALTS

Ingredients:

- 1 cup Epsom salts
- 1/2 cup sea salt
- 12 drops lavender essential oil
- 4 drops ylang-ylang essential oil
- 4 drops geranium essential oil

Steps:

1   Combine all ingredients in a bowl and mix thoroughly.
2   Transfer the mixture to an airtight container.
3   When you're ready to use, add 1/2 cup of the bath salts to warm bathwater and soak for at least 20 minutes.

Usage Tips: Use these bath salts to relax your body and mind during stressful times.

1.6 Mindfulness and Herbs for a Serene Mind

56.   MINDFUL MORNING HERBAL TEA

Ingredients:

- 1 tsp dried lemon balm
- 1 tsp dried peppermint
- 1 cup boiling water
- Honey to taste

Steps:

1   Put dried lemon balm and peppermint in your teapot.
2   Pour boiling water into the teapot.
3   Allow it to steep for 8-9 minutes.
4   Strain the liquid into a cup.
5   Sweeten with honey, if you like.

Usage Tips: Start your day with this refreshing tea to promote a mindful and serene mindset.

57. MEDITATION SUPPORT INCENSE BLEND

Ingredients:

- Dried lavender flowers (1 part)
- Dried chamomile flowers (1 part)
- Dried rosemary (1 part)
- Dried sage (1 part)

Steps:

1   Combine all dried herbs in a bowl.
2   Mix thoroughly to ensure an even blend.

3 Store the mixture in an airtight container.
4 To use, place a small amount on a charcoal disc or in an incense burner.

Usage Tips: Burn this incense blend during meditation to support focus and relaxation.

---

58. GROUNDING GOTU KOLA BREW

Ingredients:

- 1 tsp dried gotu kola
- 1 cup hot water
- Honey to taste

Steps:

1 Put dried gotu kola in a cup.
2 Pour hot water into the cup.
3 Steep for 12-14 minutes.
4 Strain into a cup.
5 Sweeten with honey, if desired.

Usage Tips: Drink this brew to promote grounding and mental clarity.

---

59. ZEN MATCHA FOCUS DRINK

Ingredients:

- 1 tsp matcha powder
- 1 cup almond milk
- 1 tsp honey
- 1/4 tsp vanilla extract

Steps:

1 Warm the almond milk in a saucepan over low heat.
2 Stir in matcha powder, honey, and vanilla extract.
3 Whisk until well combined and smooth.
4 Pour into a cup and serve warm.

Usage Tips: Enjoy this matcha drink in the morning to enhance focus and promote a Zen-like calm.

---

60. THIRD EYE CHAI

Ingredients:

- 1 cup almond milk
- 1 tsp chai tea blend
- 1/2 tsp gotu kola powder
- 1/2 tsp honey

Steps:

1 Heat the almond milk in a small pot over low heat.
2 Add the chai tea mix and gotu kola powder.
3 Let it simmer for 6-8 minutes, stirring occasionally.
4 Strain into a cup and mix in honey.

Usage Tips: Drink this chai to enhance intuition and promote mental clarity.

---

61. CLARITY ENHANCING SAGE SMUDGE

Ingredients:

- Fresh sage leaves
- Cotton string

Steps:

1 Gather a bundle of fresh sage leaves.
2 Tightly wrap the cotton string around the bundle, starting at the base and working your way up.
3 Allow the smudge stick to dry in a cool, dry place for about 1-2 weeks.

Usage Tips: Light the end of the smudge stick and blow out the flame, allowing the smoke to enhance mental clarity and focus.

---

62. DAILY CALM LEMON BALM CAPSULES

Ingredients:

- 1/3 cup dried lemon balm
- Empty gelatin or vegetarian capsules

Steps:

1 Grind the dried lemon balm into a fine powder using a coffee grinder.
2 Fill the empty capsules with the powdered lemon balm using a capsule machine or by hand.
3 Store the filled capsules in an airtight container.

Usage Tips: Take one capsule daily to promote calm and reduce anxiety.

63.   SOOTHING CINNAMON SPICE INHALER

Ingredients:

- 4 drops cinnamon essential oil
- 4 drops clove essential oil
- 4 drops orange essential oil
- Cotton wick
- Inhaler tube

Steps:

1. Place the cotton wick in a small dish.
2. Add the essential oils to the wick.
3. Insert the wick into the inhaler tube and secure it.

Usage Tips: Inhale deeply to promote relaxation and a sense of well-being.

64.   HOLY BASIL TEMPLE TONIC

Ingredients:

- 1 tsp dried holy basil
- 1 cup boiling water
- Honey to taste

Steps:

1. Put dried holy basil in your teapot.
2. Pour hot water into the teapot.
3. Allow it to steep for 8-9 minutes.
4. Strain the tea into a cup.
5. Sweeten with honey, if preferred.

Usage Tips: Drink this tonic to enhance spiritual clarity and promote a sense of peace.

65.   TRANQUIL TULSI AND LICORICE ELIXIR

Ingredients:

- 1 tsp dried tulsi
- 1 tsp dried licorice root
- 1 cup boiling water
- Honey to taste

Steps:

1. Add dried tulsi and licorice root to a teapot.
2. Pour boiling water into the teapot.
3. Let it steep for 12-14 minutes.
4. Strain the infusion into a cup.
5. Sweeten with honey, if you like.

Usage Tips: Enjoy this elixir in the evening to promote tranquility and relaxation.

66.   HERBAL MINDFULNESS PILLOW MIST

Ingredients:

- 1 cup distilled water
- 12 drops lavender essential oil
- 5 drops chamomile essential oil
- 5 drops sandalwood essential oil
- 1 tbsp witch hazel

Steps:

1. Mix all ingredients in a spray bottle.
2. Mix well.

Usage Tips: Spray this mist on your pillow before bedtime to enhance mindfulness and promote restful sleep.

1.7 Managing Change and Personal Challenges with Herbs

67.   COURAGE BOOSTING COCOA ELIXIR

Ingredients:

- 1 cup almond milk
- 1 tbsp cocoa powder
- 1 tsp maca powder
- 1 tsp honey
- 1/4 tsp cinnamon

Steps:

1. Warm the almond milk in a small saucepan over low heat.
2. Stir in cocoa powder, maca powder, honey, and cinnamon.
3. Whisk until well combined and smooth.
4. Pour into a cup and serve warm.

Usage Tips: Enjoy this elixir in the morning or evening to boost courage and emotional strength.

68.   ELDERFLOWER ENCOURAGEMENT SYRUP

Ingredients:

- 1 cup fresh elderflowers
- 2 cups water
- 2 cups sugar
- 1 lemon, juiced

Steps:

1. Mix elderflowers and water in a saucepan.
2. Bring to a boil, then lower the heat and let it simmer for 20 minutes.
3. Strain the mixture and pour the liquid back into the saucepan.
4. Stir in sugar and lemon juice until fully dissolved.
5. Transfer the syrup to a bottle and refrigerate.

Usage Tips: Take 1-2 tbsp of this syrup daily for encouragement and to uplift your spirits.

69.   ADAPTOGEN BLEND FOR RESILIENCE

Ingredients:

- 1 tsp ashwagandha powder
- 1 tsp reishi mushroom powder
- 1 tsp maca powder
- 1 cup warm almond milk
- Honey to taste

Steps:

1. Combine ashwagandha, reishi, and maca powders in a cup.
2. Pour warm almond milk over the powders and stir well.
3. Add honey to taste, if desired.

Usage Tips: Drink this blend in the morning or evening to help build resilience and manage stress.

70.   NEW BEGINNINGS NETTLE TEA

Ingredients:

- 1 tsp dried nettle leaves
- 1 cup boiling water
- Honey to taste

Steps:

1. Add dried nettle leaves to a teapot.
2. Pour hot water over the leaves.
3. Allow it to steep for 8-9 minutes.
4. Strain the tea into a cup.
5. Sweeten with honey, if preferred.

Usage Tips: Enjoy this tea to support new beginnings and enhance your energy and vitality.

71. CHANGE EMBRACE HERBAL INFUSION

Ingredients:

- 1 tsp dried lemon balm
- 1 tsp dried peppermint
- 1 tsp dried chamomile
- 1 cup boiling water
- Honey to taste

Steps:

1. Add dried lemon balm, peppermint, and chamomile to a teapot.
2. Pour boiling water into the teapot.
3. Steep for 8-9 minutes.
4. Strain the liqui
5. d into a cup.
6. Sweeten with honey, if you like.

Usage Tips: Drink this herbal infusion to help embrace change with a calm and open mind.

72.   RHODIOLA ROSEA ROOT REVIVER

Ingredients:

- 1 tsp dried Rhodiola Rosea root
- 1 cup hot water
- Honey to taste

Steps:

1. Put dried Rhodiola root in a cup.
2. Pour hot water over the root.
3. Allow it to steep for 12-14 minutes.
4. Strain into another cup.
5. Sweeten with honey, if desired.

Usage Tips: Enjoy this invigorating tea in the morning or early afternoon to support energy and mental clarity.

73. PERSONAL GROWTH GREEN JUICE

Ingredients:

- 1 cucumber
- 1 green apple
- 1 cup spinach
- 1/2 lemon, juiced
- 1 tsp spirulina powder
- 1 cup water

Steps:

1. Put all ingredients in a blender.
2. Blend until smooth.
3. Strain if desired and serve right away.

Usage Tips: Enjoy this green juice in the morning to support personal growth and overall wellness.

74. SCHISANDRA STRESS RELIEF SNACK

Ingredients:

- 1 cup dried Schisandra berries
- 1/2 cup almonds
- 1/3 cup dark chocolate chips
- 1 tbsp honey

Steps:

1. Mix all ingredients in a bowl.
2. Stir well until everything is evenly coated with honey.
3. Preserve in an airtight container.

Usage Tips: Enjoy a handful of this snack mix during the day to help manage stress and boost energy.

75. TRANSFORMATIVE TURMERIC TONIC

Ingredients:

- 1/2 tsp turmeric powder
- 1/4 tsp black pepper
- 1 tbsp lemon juice
- 1 cup warm water
- Honey to taste

Steps:

1. Combine turmeric powder, black pepper, and lemon juice in a cup.

2. Add warm water and stir well.
3. Add honey to taste, if desired.

Usage Tips: Take this tonic daily to support transformation and reduce inflammation.

76. LEMON ADAPTOGEN ADE

Ingredients:

- 1 tsp ashwagandha powder
- 1 tsp maca powder
- 1 lemon, juiced
- 2 cups cold water
- Honey to taste
- Ice

Steps:

1. Combine ashwagandha powder, maca powder, and lemon juice in a pitcher.
2. Add cold water and stir well.
3. Add honey to taste, if desired.
4. Serve over ice.

Usage Tips: Drink this refreshing ade to help manage stress and support overall wellness.

77. HERBAL ARMOR FOR CHALLENGING TIMES

Ingredients:

- 1 tsp dried holy basil
- 1 tsp dried ashwagandha root
- 1 tsp dried lemon balm
- 1 cup boiling water
- Honey to taste

Steps:

1. Place dried holy basil, ashwagandha, and lemon balm in your teapot.
2. Pour boiling water into the teapot.
3. Let steep for 12-14 minutes.
4. Strain the tea into a cup.
5. Add honey for sweetness, if desired.

Usage Tips: Drink this herbal tea during challenging times to provide emotional support and resilience.

Chapter 2: Holistic Practices and Wellness Culture

2.1 Caffeine-Free Herbal Energy Support

78.   SIBERIAN GINSENG AND LICORICE ROOT TONIC

Ingredients:

- 1 tsp dried Siberian ginseng root
- 1 tsp dried licorice root
- 1 cup boiling water

Steps:

1 Combine dried Siberian ginseng root and licorice root in your teapot.
2 Pour boiling water into the teapot.
3 Let steep for 12-14 min.
4 Strain into a cup and serve.

Usage Tips: Drink this tonic in the morning for a natural energy boost. Siberian ginseng is important for its adaptogenic properties, that aid to combat fatigue and stress.

79.   ENERGIZING ELEUTHERO AND ORANGE JUICE

Ingredients:

- 1 tsp dried eleuthero root
- 1 cup boiling water
- 1 cup fresh orange juice
- 1 tbsp honey

Steps:

1 Combine dried eleuthero root and boiling water in your teapot.
2 Let steep for 8-9 min.
3 Strain the tea into a cup and let cool.
4 Mix the cooled tea with fresh orange juice and honey.
5 Stir well and serve.

Usage Tips: Start your day with this energizing drink. Eleuthero, also known as Siberian ginseng, is an adaptogen that enhances endurance and reduces fatigue, while orange juice adds a vitamin C boost.

80.   ENERGY BOOSTING SCHISANDRA BERRY SYRUP

Ingredients:

- 1 cup dried schisandra berries
- 4 cups water
- 1 cup honey

Steps:

1 Combine dried schisandra berries and water in a pot.
2 Bring to a boil, then simmer for 45 min.
3 Strain the mixture and return the liquid to the pot.
4 Stir in honey and simmer until thickened.
5 Pour into a jar and preserve in the refrigerator.

Usage Tips: Take 1 tbsp of this syrup daily to boost your energy levels. Schisandra berries support adrenal health and improve stamina and endurance.

81. CORDYCEPS MUSHROOM SPORTS DRINK

Ingredients:

- 1 tsp cordyceps mushroom powder
- 1 cup coconut water
- 1 tbsp honey
- 1/2 tsp sea salt

Steps:

1 Transfer all ingredients in a shaker bottle.
2 Stir well to mix.
3 Pour into a glass and serve.

Usage Tips: Use this drink before or after workouts to enhance athletic performance. Cordyceps mushrooms are known to boost energy and improve oxygen utilization.

82. RHODIOLA ROSEA MORNING ELIXIR

Ingredients:

- 1 tsp dried Rhodiola rosea root
- 1 cup boiling water
- 1 tbsp honey
- 1 tsp lemon juice

Steps:

1 Combine dried Rhodiola rosea root and boiling water in a cup.
2 Let steep for 8-9 min.
3 Strain the tea into another cup.
4 Stir in honey and lemon juice, then serve.

Usage Tips: Start your day with this elixir to enhance mental clarity and energy. Rhodiola rosea is an adaptogen that helps the body resist physical and mental stress.

83. INVIGORATING PEPPERMINT AND LEMON BALM TEA

Ingredients:

- 1 tsp dried peppermint leaves
- 1 tsp dried lemon balm leaves
- 1 cup boiling water

Steps:

1 Transfer dried peppermint and lemon balm leaves in your teapot.
2 Pour boiling water into the teapot.
3 Let steep for 8-9 min.
4 Strain into a cup and serve.

Usage Tips: Enjoy this refreshing tea in the afternoon to combat fatigue. Peppermint and lemon balm both have uplifting and invigorating properties.

84. ASHWAGANDHA AND DATE SMOOTHIE

Ingredients:

- 1 banana
- 1 cup almond milk
- 1 tbsp ashwagandha powder
- 2 dates, pitted
- 1 tbsp almond butter

Steps:

1 Transfer all ingredients in a blender.
2 Mix until smooth.
3 Pour into a glass and serve immediately.

Usage Tips: Drink this smoothie in the morning for sustained energy. Ashwagandha helps to reduce stress and increase vitality, while dates provide natural sweetness and nutrients.

85. REVITALIZING GUARANA SEED BREW

Ingredients:

- 1 tsp ground guarana seeds
- 1 cup hot water
- 1 tbsp honey

Steps:

1 Combine ground guarana seeds and hot water in a cup.
2 Let steep for 5 minutes.
3 Strain into another cup.
4 Stir in honey and serve.

Usage Tips: Drink this brew in the morning for a natural energy boost. Guarana seeds contain natural caffeine that provides a steady release of energy without jitters.

86. HERBAL MATE ENERGY DRINK

Ingredients:

- 1 tbsp dried yerba mate leaves
- 1 cup boiling water
- 1 tsp honey
- 1 slice lemon

Steps:

1 Transfer dried yerba mate leaves and boiling water in your teapot.
2 Let steep for 7-8 min.

3 Strain into a cup.

4 Stir in honey and add a slice of lemon before serving.

Usage Tips: Enjoy this drink in the morning or early afternoon for a smooth energy lift. Yerba mate is rich in antioxidants and provides a balanced energy boost without causing anxiety.

87. CAROB AND DANDELION ROOT COFFEE SUBSTITUTE

Ingredients:

- 1 tsp roasted dandelion root
- 1 tsp roasted carob powder
- 1 cup boiling water
- 1 tbsp coconut milk

Steps:

1 Combine roasted dandelion root and roasted carob powder in a cup.

2 Pour boiling water over the mixture.

3 Let steep for 7-8 min.

4 Strain into another cup.

5 Stir in coconut milk and serve.

Usage Tips: Use this blend as a caffeine-free coffee substitute. Dandelion root supports liver health, and carob provides a rich, chocolaty flavor that satisfies coffee cravings.

88. RED RASPBERRY LEAF AND NETTLE ICED TEA

Ingredients:

- 1 tbsp dried red raspberry leaf
- 1 tbsp dried nettle leaf
- 4 cups boiling water
- 1 tbsp honey
- Ice cubes

Steps:

1 Transfer dried red raspberry leaf and dried nettle leaf in your teapot.

2 Pour boiling water into the teapot.

3 Let steep for 8-9 min.

4 Strain the tea into a pitcher.

5 Stir in honey and let cool.

6 Serve over ice.

Usage Tips: Drink this iced tea on hot days for a refreshing and nourishing boost. Red raspberry leaf and nettle are packed with vitamins and minerals to support overall health.

2.2 Natural Tonics for Seasonal Transition

89. ALLERGY RELIEF NETTLE AND HONEY ELIXIR

Ingredients:

- 1 tsp dried nettle leaf
- 1 cup boiling water
- 1 tbsp honey
- 1 tsp lemon juice

Steps:

1 Transfer dried nettle leaf and boiling water in a cup.

2 Let steep for 8-9 min.

3 Strain the tea into another cup.

4 Stir in honey and lemon juice, then serve.

Usage Tips: Drink this elixir during allergy season to reduce symptoms. Nettle has natural antihistamine properties that help to alleviate allergy symptoms, and honey soothes the throat.

90. REVITALIZING GREEN TEA AND JASMINE BLEND

Ingredients:

- 1 tsp green tea leaves
- 1 tsp dried jasmine flowers
- 1 cup boiling water

Steps:

1 Combine green tea leaves and dried jasmine flowers in your teapot.

2 Pour boiling water into the teapot.

3 Let steep for about 4 min.

4 Strain into a cup and serve.

Usage Tips: Enjoy this tea blend for a revitalizing and fragrant experience. Green tea provides a gentle caffeine boost, while jasmine flowers add a calming aroma.

91. SPRING RENEWAL DANDELION AND BURDOCK TONIC

Ingredients:

- 1 tsp dried dandelion root
- 1 tsp dried burdock root
- 1 cup boiling water
- 1 tbsp honey

Steps:

1. Transfer dried dandelion root and dried burdock root in your teapot.
2. Pour boiling water into the teapot.
3. Let steep for 8-9 min.
4. Strain into a cup.
5. Stir in honey and serve.

Usage Tips: Drink this tonic during the spring to support detoxification and renewal. Dandelion and burdock roots help to cleanse the liver and improve digestion.

92. SUMMER COOLING CUCUMBER AND ALOE VERA DRINK

Ingredients:

- 1 cucumber, peeled and sliced
- 1 tbsp aloe vera gel
- 1 cup water
- 1 tbsp lemon juice
- Ice cubes

Steps:

1. Combine cucumber, aloe vera gel, water, and lemon juice in a blender.
2. Mix until smooth.
3. Pour into a glass over ice cubes and serve.

Usage Tips: Enjoy this drink on hot summer days to stay hydrated and cool. Cucumber and aloe vera are both incredibly hydrating and soothing, perfect for beating the heat.

93. AUTUMN IMMUNE BOOSTER ELDERBERRY AND ECHINACEA SYRUP

Ingredients:

- 1 cup dried elderberries
- 1 tbsp dried echinacea root
- 4 cups water
- 1 cup honey

Steps:

1. Combine dried elderberries, dried echinacea root, and water in a pot.
2. Bring to a boil, then simmer for 45 min.
3. Strain the mixture and return the liquid to the pot.
4. Stir in honey and simmer until thickened.
5. Pour into a jar and preserve in the refrigerator.

Usage Tips: Take 1 tbsp of this syrup daily during autumn to boost your immune system. Elderberries and echinacea are powerful immune boosters that help to prevent colds and flu.

94. WINTER WARMING GINGER AND CINNAMON HOT TONIC

Ingredients:

- 1 tsp grated fresh ginger
- 1 cinnamon stick
- 1 cup boiling water
- 1 tbsp honey

Steps:

1. Combine grated fresh ginger and cinnamon stick in a cup.
2. Pour boiling water over the ingredients.
3. Let steep for 8-9 min.
4. Strain into another cup.
5. Stir in honey and serve.

Usage Tips: Enjoy this warming tonic during winter to stay warm and healthy. Ginger and cinnamon have warming properties that help to improve circulation and boost immunity.

95. MOISTURIZING ROSEHIP AND HIBISCUS TEA FOR DRY WEATHER

Ingredients:

- 1 tsp dried rosehips
- 1 tsp dried hibiscus flowers
- 1 cup boiling water
- 1 tbsp honey

Steps:

1. Transfer dried rosehips and dried hibiscus flowers in your teapot.
2. Pour boiling water into the teapot.
3. Let steep for 8-9 min.
4. Strain into a cup.
5. Stir in honey and serve.

Usage Tips: Drink this tea during dry weather to keep your skin and body hydrated. Rosehips and hibiscus are rich in antioxidants and vitamin C, which help to moisturize and protect the skin.

96. DETOXIFYING MILK THISTLE AND LEMON CLEANSE

Ingredients:

- 1 tsp dried milk thistle seeds
- 1 cup boiling water
- 1 tbsp lemon juice
- 1 tsp honey

Steps:

1. Transfer dried milk thistle seeds and boiling water in your teapot.
2. Let steep for 8-9 min.
3. Strain the tea into another cup.
4. Stir in lemon juice and honey, then serve.

Usage Tips: Use this cleanse periodically to detoxify your liver. Milk thistle is known for its liver-protective properties, and lemon helps to enhance detoxification.

97. SOOTHING LICORICE AND MARSHMALLOW ROOT TEA

Ingredients:

- 1 tsp dried licorice root
- 1 tsp dried marshmallow root
- 1 cup boiling water
- 1 tbsp honey

Steps:

1. Transfer dried licorice root and dried marshmallow root in your teapot.
2. Pour boiling water into the teapot.
3. Let steep for 8-9 min.
4. Strain into a cup.
5. Stir in honey and serve.

Usage Tips: Drink this tea to soothe a sore throat and digestive discomfort. Licorice and marshmallow roots have soothing properties that aid to diminish inflammation and irritation.

98. ANTIOXIDANT RICH BILBERRY AND HAWTHORN DRINK

Ingredients:

- 1 tsp dried bilberries
- 1 tsp dried hawthorn berries
- 1 cup boiling water
- 1 tbsp honey

Steps:

1. Transfer dried bilberries and dried hawthorn berries in your teapot.
2. Pour boiling water into the teapot.
3. Let steep for 8-9 min.
4. Strain into a cup.
5. Stir in honey and serve.

Usage Tips: Enjoy this drink to boost your antioxidant intake. Bilberries and hawthorn berries are rich in antioxidants that support cardiovascular health and overall well-being.

99. CALMING CHAMOMILE AND LAVENDER SLEEP TONIC

Ingredients:

- 1 tsp dried chamomile flowers
- 1 tsp dried lavender flowers
- 1 cup boiling water
- 1 tbsp honey

Steps:

1. Transfer dried chamomile flowers and dried lavender flowers in your teapot.
2. Pour boiling water into the teapot.

3 Let steep for 8-9 min.
4 Strain into a cup.
5 Stir in honey and serve.

Usage Tips: Drink this tonic before bedtime to promote restful sleep. Chamomile and lavender have natural calming properties that help to relax the mind and body, ensuring a good night's rest.

2.3 Ancient Practices for Modern Wellness

100. JAPANESE MATCHA CEREMONY FOR MENTAL CLARITY

Ingredients:

- 1 tsp matcha powder
- 1/2 cup hot water

Steps:

1 Sift matcha powder into a bowl.
2 Add hot water and whisk until frothy.
3 Pour into a cup and enjoy.

Usage Tips: Perform this matcha ceremony in the morning to enhance mental clarity and focus. Matcha provides a gentle caffeine boost and is rich in antioxidants that support brain health.

101. AYURVEDIC TRIPHALA MORNING RINSE

Ingredients:

- 1 tsp triphala powder
- 1 cup warm water

Steps:

1 Combine triphala powder and warm water in a cup.
2 Stir well to dissolve the powder.
3 Drink the mixture first thing in the morning on an empty stomach.

Usage Tips: Use this rinse daily to support digestion and detoxification. Triphala is a traditional Ayurvedic blend of three fruits known for their cleansing and rejuvenating properties.

102. MEDITERRANEAN OLIVE LEAF EXTRACT FOR HEART HEALTH

Ingredients:

- 1 cup dried olive leaves
- 2 cups water

Steps:

1 Combine dried olive leaves and water in a pot.
2 Bring to a boil, then simmer for about 25-28 min.
3 Strain the mixture and let the liquid cool.
4 Preserve in a glass bottle in the refrigerator.

Usage Tips: Take 1 tbsp of this extract daily to support heart health. Olive leaves contain compounds that help to lower blood pressure and improve cardiovascular function.

103. NATIVE AMERICAN WHITE SAGE SMUDGING FOR CLEARING ENERGY

Ingredients:

- 1 bundle of dried white sage
- A fireproof bowl or shell

Steps:

1 Light the end of the white sage bundle until it begins to smolder.
2 Blow out the flame, allowing the sage to produce smoke.
3 Use your hand or a feather to direct the smoke around your space.

Usage Tips: Use white sage smudging to clear negative energy and purify your environment. This Native American practice helps to create a calm and balanced atmosphere.

104. MIDDLE EASTERN ZA'ATAR FOR DIGESTIVE HEALTH

Ingredients:

- 2 tbsp dried thyme
- 2 tbsp dried oregano
- 1 tbsp sumac
- 1 tbsp toasted sesame seeds
- 1/2 tsp salt

Steps:

1 Transfer all ingredients in a bowl.
2 Stir well to combine.
3 Preserve in an airtight container.

Usage Tips: Sprinkle za'atar on salads, bread, or yogurt for added flavor and digestive benefits. Thyme and oregano support digestion, while sumac adds a tangy, antioxidant-rich boost.

105. NORDIC BIRCH SAP TONIC FOR SPRING VITALITY

Ingredients:

- 1 cup fresh birch sap
- 1 tsp honey
- 1 tsp lemon juice

Steps:

1 Combine fresh birch sap, honey, and lemon juice in a glass.
2 Stir well to combine.
3 Serve chilled.

Usage Tips: Drink this tonic in the spring to rejuvenate and refresh your body. Birch sap is a traditional Nordic beverage that supports vitality and overall health.

106. SOUTH AMERICAN YERBA MATE RITUAL FOR COMMUNITY AND STAMINA

Ingredients:

- 1 tbsp dried yerba mate leaves
- 1 cup hot water
- Lemon or mint (optional)

Steps:

1 Place dried yerba mate leaves in a gourd or cup.
2 Pour hot water over the leaves.

3 Let steep for a few minutes.
4 Add lemon or mint if desired.
5 Drink through a bombilla or metal straw.

Usage Tips: Use this yerba mate ritual to boost stamina and foster a sense of community. Yerba mate is a traditional South American drink that provides sustained energy and is often shared among friends.

107. AFRICAN BAOBAB FRUIT SMOOTHIE FOR ANTIOXIDANTS

Ingredients:

- 1 tbsp baobab powder
- 1 banana
- 1 cup almond milk
- 1 tbsp honey

Steps:

1 Transfer all ingredients in a blender.
2 Mix until smooth.
3 Pour into a glass and serve.

Usage Tips: Enjoy this smoothie for a powerful antioxidant boost. Baobab fruit is rich in vitamin C and other antioxidants that help to protect cells from damage and support overall health.

108. TRADITIONAL CHINESE MEDICINE JUJUBE AND GOJI BERRY TEA

Ingredients:

- 1 tbsp dried jujube dates
- 1 tbsp dried goji berries
- 2 cups boiling water

Steps:

1 Transfer dried jujube dates and dried goji berries in your teapot.
2 Pour boiling water into the teapot.
3 Let steep for 15-20 min.
4 Strain into cups and serve.

Usage Tips: Drink this tea to boost your energy and immune system. Jujube dates and goji berries are staples in Traditional Chinese Medicine for their nourishing and tonic effects.

109. EUROPEAN HERBAL POULTICE FOR MUSCLE AND JOINT PAIN

Ingredients:

- 1 tbsp dried comfrey leaves
- 1 tbsp dried arnica flowers
- 1 cup hot water
- Cheesecloth or muslin

Steps:

1 Transfer dried comfrey leaves and dried arnica flowers in a bowl.
2 Pour hot water into the bowl and let steep for 8-9 min.
3 Strain the mixture and place the herbs in cheesecloth or muslin.
4 Apply the poultice to the affected area for 15-20 minutes.

Usage Tips: Use this herbal poultice to relieve muscle and joint pain. Comfrey and arnica have anti-inflammatory properties that aid to diminish swelling and promote healing.

110. INDIAN GOLDEN TURMERIC PASTE FOR INFLAMMATION

Ingredients:

- 1/3 cup ground turmeric
- 1/2 cup water
- 1/4 tsp black pepper
- 1 tbsp coconut oil

Steps:

1 Combine ground turmeric and water in a saucepan.
2 Simmer over low heat for 7-8-9 min until a thick paste forms.
3 Remove from heat and stir in black pepper and coconut oil.
4 Preserve in a glass jar in the refrigerator.

Usage Tips: Use this turmeric paste in smoothies, teas, or as a cooking ingredient to reduce inflammation. The combination of turmeric and black pepper enhances the absorption of curcumin.

2.4 Holistic Approaches to Longevity and Vitality

111. LONGEVITY ELIXIR WITH REISHI AND CHAGA MUSHROOMS

Ingredients:

- 1 tsp reishi mushroom powder
- 1 tsp chaga mushroom powder
- 1 cup hot water
- 1 tbsp honey

Steps:

1 Combine reishi mushroom powder and chaga mushroom powder in a cup.
2 Pour hot water over the powders.
3 Stir well and let steep for 7-8 min.
4 Stir in honey and serve.

Usage Tips: Drink this elixir daily to support longevity and overall health. Reishi and chaga mushrooms have adaptogenic and immune-boosting properties that promote vitality and resilience.

112. ANTI-AGING GINKGO BILOBA AND GOTU KOLA TEA

Ingredients:

- 1 tsp dried ginkgo biloba leaves
- 1 tsp dried gotu kola leaves
- 1 cup boiling water

Steps:

1 Transfer dried ginkgo biloba leaves and dried gotu kola leaves in your teapot.
2 Pour boiling water into the teapot.
3 Let steep for 8-9 min.
4 Strain into a cup and serve.

Usage Tips: Drink this tea to support brain health and cognitive function. Ginkgo biloba and gotu kola are known for their neuroprotective and anti-aging effects.

113. VITALITY-BOOSTING MACA AND COCOA SMOOTHIE

Ingredients:

- 1 banana
- 1 cup almond milk
- 1 tbsp maca powder
- 1 tbsp cocoa powder
- 1 tbsp honey

Steps:

1 Transfer all ingredients in a blender.
2 Mix until smooth.
3 Pour into a glass and serve.

Usage Tips: Enjoy this smoothie in the morning for a vitality boost. Maca and cocoa provide energy and stamina, while the banana and almond milk add creaminess and nutrients.

114. HERBAL ADAPTOGEN BLEND FOR STRESS RESISTANCE

Ingredients:

- 1 tsp ashwagandha powder
- 1 tsp rhodiola rosea powder
- 1 cup hot water
- 1 tbsp honey

Steps:

1 Combine ashwagandha powder and rhodiola rosea powder in a cup.
2 Pour hot water over the powders.
3 Stir well and let steep for 7-8 min.
4 Stir in honey and serve.

Usage Tips: Use this blend to enhance stress resistance and resilience. Ashwagandha and rhodiola are powerful adaptogens that help the body adapt to physical and mental stress.

115. SEA BUCKTHORN AND ROSEHIP ANTIOXIDANT JUICE

Ingredients:

- 1 tbsp sea buckthorn juice
- 1 tbsp rosehip syrup
- 1 cup water
- 1 tbsp honey

Steps:

1 Combine sea buckthorn juice, rosehip syrup, water, and honey in a glass.
2 Stir well to combine.
3 Serve immediately.

Usage Tips: Drink this juice daily for a potent dose of antioxidants. Sea buckthorn and rosehip are both rich in vitamins and antioxidants that protect against aging and support overall health.

116. HEART HEALTH HAWTHORN BERRY SYRUP

Ingredients:

- 1 cup dried hawthorn berries
- 4 cups water
- 1 cup honey

Steps:

1 Combine dried hawthorn berries and water in a pot.
2 Bring to a boil, then simmer for 45 min.
3 Strain the mixture and return the liquid to the pot.
4 Stir in honey and simmer until thickened.
5 Pour into a jar and preserve in the refrigerator.

Usage Tips: Take 1 tbsp of this syrup daily to support heart health. Hawthorn berries are known for their ability to strengthen the heart and improve circulation.

117. BRAIN-BOOSTING BACOPA AND SAGE TONIC

Ingredients:

- 1 tsp dried bacopa leaves
- 1 tsp dried sage leaves
- 1 cup boiling water
- 1 tbsp honey

Steps:

1 Transfer dried bacopa leaves and dried sage leaves in your teapot.
2 Pour boiling water into the teapot.
3 Let steep for 8-9 min.
4 Strain into a cup.
5 Stir in honey and serve.

Usage Tips: Drink this tonic to enhance cognitive function and memory. Bacopa and sage have been used traditionally to support brain health and improve mental clarity.

118. LIVER CLEANSING MILK THISTLE AND DANDELION DRINK

Ingredients:

- 1 tsp dried milk thistle seeds
- 1 tsp dried dandelion root
- 1 cup boiling water
- 1 tbsp lemon juice

Steps:

1 Combine dried milk thistle seeds and dried dandelion root in your teapot.
2 Pour boiling water into the teapot.
3 Let steep for 8-9 min.
4 Strain the tea into another cup.
5 Stir in lemon juice and serve.

Usage Tips: Use this drink periodically to cleanse and support your liver. Milk thistle and dandelion are known for their detoxifying and liver-protective properties.

119. BONE STRENGTHENING HORSETAIL AND NETTLE DECOCTION

Ingredients:

- 1 tsp dried horsetail
- 1 tsp dried nettle
- 2 cups water

Steps:

1 Combine dried horsetail and dried nettle in a pot.
2 Add water and bring to a boil.
3 Simmer for about 18 min.
4 Strain into cups and serve.

Usage Tips: Drink this decoction to support bone health. Horsetail and nettle are rich in minerals like silica and calcium, which are essential for strong bones.

120. ANTI-INFLAMMATORY TURMERIC AND CHERRY JUICE

Ingredients:

- 1 tsp ground turmeric
- 1 cup tart cherry juice
- 1 tbsp honey

Steps:

1 Combine ground turmeric and tart cherry juice in a glass.
2 Stir well to combine.
3 Stir in honey and serve.

Usage Tips: Enjoy this juice to reduce inflammation and support joint health. Turmeric and tart cherries are both powerful anti-inflammatory agents that help to relieve pain and swelling.

121. SKIN REJUVENATING ALOE VERA AND CUCUMBER GEL

Ingredients:

- 1/3 cup fresh aloe vera gel
- 1/3 cup grated cucumber
- 1 tsp lemon juice

Steps:

1 Combine fresh aloe vera gel, grated cucumber, and lemon juice in a bowl.
2 Mix well to combine.
3 Apply the gel to your skin and let sit for 18-20 minutes.
4 Rinse off with cool water.

Usage Tips: Use this gel to rejuvenate and hydrate your skin. Aloe vera and cucumber provide soothing and moisturizing properties, while lemon juice helps to brighten the complexion.

122. IMMUNE-BOOSTING GARLIC AND HONEY TINCTURE

Ingredients:

- 1/2 cup peeled garlic cloves
- 1 cup honey
- 1 cup apple cider vinegar

Steps:

1. Combine peeled garlic cloves, honey, and apple cider vinegar in a jar.
2. Seal the jar and let sit for 10 days, shaking daily.
3. Strain the mixture and store the liquid in a glass bottle.

Usage Tips: Take 1 tsp of this tincture daily to boost your immune system. Garlic and honey have potent antimicrobial properties that help to prevent infections.

123. DAILY DETOXIFYING HERBAL TEA BLEND

Ingredients:

- 1 tsp dried dandelion root
- 1 tsp dried burdock root
- 1 tsp dried milk thistle seeds
- 1 cup boiling water

Steps:

1. Combine dried dandelion root, dried burdock root, and dried milk thistle seeds in your teapot.
2. Pour boiling water into the teapot.
3. Let steep for 8-9 min.
4. Strain into a cup and serve.

Usage Tips: Drink this tea daily to support detoxification and liver health. Dandelion, burdock, and milk thistle are powerful detoxifying herbs that help to cleanse the body.

124. DIGESTIVE AID FENNEL AND PEPPERMINT LOZENGES

Ingredients:

- 1/2 cup honey
- 1/3 cup fennel seed tea
- 1 tbsp dried peppermint leaves

Steps:

1. Combine honey, fennel seed tea, and dried peppermint leaves in a saucepan.
2. Heat over low heat until the mixture reaches 300°F (150°C) on a candy thermometer.
3. Pour the mixture into a candy mold and let cool completely.
4. Remove the lozenges from the mold and store in an airtight container.

Usage Tips: Suck on these lozenges after meals to aid digestion. Fennel and peppermint help to reduce bloating and gas, making them effective digestive aids.

125. RELAXATION SUPPORT LAVENDER INFUSED BATH SALTS

Ingredients:

- 1 cup Epsom salts
- 1/2 cup sea salt
- 1/3 cup dried lavender flowers
- 12 drops lavender essential oil

Steps:

1. Combine Epsom salts, sea salt, and dried lavender flowers in a bowl.
2. Add lavender essential oil and mix well.
3. Store in an airtight container.

Usage Tips: Add 1/2 cup of these bath salts to your bathwater to promote relaxation. Lavender has soothing properties that help to calm the mind and relax the muscles.

126. SLEEP INDUCING VALERIAN ROOT NIGHTCAP

Ingredients:

- 1 tsp dried valerian root
- 1 cup boiling water
- 1 tbsp honey

Steps:

1 Transfer dried valerian root and boiling water in a cup.
2 Let steep for 8-9 min.
3 Strain the tea into another cup.
4 Stir in honey and serve.

Usage Tips: Drink this nightcap before bed to promote restful sleep. Valerian root is a natural sedative that helps to calm the mind and body, ensuring a good night's rest.

127. ENERGIZING MORNING HERBAL TONIC

Ingredients:

- 1 tsp dried ginseng root
- 1 tsp dried licorice root
- 1 cup boiling water
- 1 tbsp honey

Steps:

1 Transfer dried ginseng root and dried licorice root in your teapot.
2 Pour boiling water into the teapot.
3 Let steep for 8-9 min.
4 Strain into a cup.
5 Stir in honey and serve.

Usage Tips: Drink this tonic in the morning to boost your energy levels. Ginseng and licorice root are adaptogens that help to increase stamina and reduce fatigue.

128. HERBAL COLD AND FLU PREVENTION INHALER

Ingredients:

- 12 drops eucalyptus essential oil
- 12 drops peppermint essential oil
- 12 drops tea tree essential oil
- 1 inhaler tube

Steps:

1 Combine eucalyptus, peppermint, and tea tree essential oils in a small bowl.
2 Soak the inhaler wick in the oil blend.
3 Insert the wick into the inhaler tube and seal.

Usage Tips: Use this inhaler at the first sign of a cold or flu to prevent symptoms. The essential oils have antimicrobial properties that help to clear nasal passages and boost immunity.

129. NATURAL HERBAL MOUTHWASH WITH THYME AND MINT

Ingredients:

- 1 tsp dried thyme
- 1 tsp dried mint leaves
- 1 cup boiling water
- 1 tsp baking soda

Steps:

1 Transfer dried thyme and dried mint leaves in your teapot.
2 Pour boiling water into the teapot.
3 Let steep for 8-9 min.
4 Strain into a cup.
5 Stir in baking soda and let cool.
6 Store in a glass bottle.

Usage Tips: Use this mouthwash daily to maintain oral health. Thyme and mint have antibacterial properties that help to freshen breath and reduce plaque.

130. HERBAL FIRST AID SPRAY FOR CUTS AND SCRAPES

Ingredients:

- 1 cup witch hazel
- 1 tsp dried calendula flowers
- 1 tsp dried chamomile flowers
- 12 drops tea tree essential oil

Steps:

1 Combine witch hazel, dried calendula flowers, and dried chamomile flowers in a jar.
2 Seal the jar and let sit for about 10 days, shaking daily.

3 Strain the mixture and add tea tree essential oil.
4 Pour into a spray bottle.

Usage Tips: Spray this mixture on cuts and scrapes to promote healing. Calendula, chamomile, and tea tree oil have antiseptic and anti-inflammatory properties that aid to prevent infection and diminish inflammation.

---

131.   NATURAL ANXIETY RELIEF LEMON BALM TEA

Ingredients:

- 1 tsp dried lemon balm leaves
- 1 cup boiling water
- 1 tbsp honey

Steps:

1 Transfer dried lemon balm leaves and boiling water in a cup.
2 Let steep for 8-9 min.
3 Strain the tea into another cup.
4 Stir in honey and serve.

Usage Tips: Drink this tea to reduce anxiety and promote relaxation. Lemon balm has calming properties that help to soothe the mind and body, making it effective for anxiety relief.

---

132.   HOMEGROWN HERBAL SALAD MIX

Ingredients:

- 1 cup mixed greens (lettuce, spinach, arugula)
- 1/3 cup fresh herbs (basil, parsley, cilantro)
- 1/3 cup edible flowers (nasturtiums, violets)
- 1 tbsp olive oil
- 1 tbsp lemon juice
- Salt and pepper to taste

Steps:

1 Combine mixed greens, fresh herbs, and edible flowers in a bowl.
2 Drizzle with olive oil and lemon juice.
3 Mix well.
4 Season with salt and pepper.

Usage Tips: Enjoy this salad for a fresh and nutritious meal. Growing your own herbs and edible flowers ensures a constant supply of fresh, nutrient-rich ingredients for your salads.

2.6 Ancient Remedies for Modern Anxiety

133.   ASHWAGANDHA ROOT STRESS REDUCTION TINCTURE

Ingredients:

- 1/2 cup dried ashwagandha root
- 1 cup vodka or brandy

Steps:

1 Combine dried ashwagandha root and vodka or brandy in a jar.
2 Seal the jar and let sit for about 1 month, shaking daily.
3 Strain the mixture and store the liquid in a glass bottle.

Usage Tips: Take 1 tsp of this tincture daily to reduce stress. Ashwagandha is an adaptogen that helps to balance cortisol levels and promote relaxation.

---

134.   CALMING PASSIONFLOWER AND HOPS SLEEP AID

Ingredients:

- 1 tsp dried passionflower
- 1 tsp dried hops
- 1 cup boiling water
- 1 tbsp honey

Steps:

1 Transfer dried passionflower and dried hops in your teapot.
2 Pour boiling water into the teapot.
3 Let steep for 8-9 min.

4 Strain into a cup.
5 Stir in honey and serve.

Usage Tips: Drink this sleep aid before bedtime to promote restful sleep. Passionflower and hops have natural sedative properties that help to calm the mind and induce sleep.

135. ADAPTOGENIC HOLY BASIL AND LICORICE TEA

Ingredients:

- 1 tsp dried holy basil leaves
- 1 tsp dried licorice root
- 1 cup boiling water

Steps:

1 Transfer dried holy basil leaves and dried licorice root in your teapot.
2 Pour boiling water into the teapot.
3 Let steep for 8-9 min.
4 Strain into a cup and serve.

Usage Tips: Enjoy this tea to reduce stress and support adrenal health. Holy basil and licorice root are adaptogens that help to balance stress hormones and improve resilience.

136. ANXIETY-SOOTHING VALERIAN AND CHAMOMILE CAPSULES

Ingredients:

- 1/2 cup dried valerian root
- 1/2 cup dried chamomile flowers
- Empty gelatin capsules

Steps:

1 Grind dried valerian root and dried chamomile flowers into a fine powder.
2 Fill empty gelatin capsules with the powder.
3 Store the capsules in an airtight container.

Usage Tips: Take 1-2 capsules before bedtime to reduce anxiety and promote sleep. Valerian and chamomile have calming properties that help to relax the mind and body.

137. GROUNDING CEDARWOOD AROMATHERAPY OIL

Ingredients:

- 12 drops cedarwood essential oil
- 1 tbsp carrier oil (such as jojoba or almond oil)

Steps:

1 Transfer cedarwood essential oil and jojoba or almond oil in a small bottle.
2 Stir well to mix.

Usage Tips: Apply some drops of this oil to your wrists or neck to promote grounding and relaxation. Cedarwood has a calming and centering effect that helps to reduce anxiety.

138. PROTECTIVE AMETHYST AND SAGE ENERGY CLEARING MIST

Ingredients:

- 1 small amethyst crystal
- 12 drops sage essential oil
- 1/2 cup distilled water
- 1 tbsp witch hazel

Steps:

1 Place the amethyst crystal in a spray bottle.
2 Add sage essential oil, distilled water, and witch hazel.
3 Stir well to mix.

Usage Tips: Spray this mist around your space to clear negative energy and promote protection. Amethyst and sage work together to create a balanced and positive environment.

139. LEMON BALM AND LAVENDER ANTI-ANXIETY SPRAY

Ingredients:

- 12 drops lemon balm essential oil
- 12 drops lavender essential oil
- 1/2 cup distilled water
- 1 tbsp witch hazel

Steps:

1. Combine lemon balm essential oil, lavender essential oil, distilled water, and witch hazel in a spray bottle.
2. Stir well to mix.

Usage Tips: Spray this blend around your home or on your pillow to reduce anxiety. Lemon balm and lavender have calming effects that help to create a relaxing environment.

140. EMOTIONAL BALANCE FLOWER ESSENCE FORMULA

Ingredients:

- 2 drops Bach Rescue Remedy
- 2 drops Bach Olive
- 2 drops Bach White Chestnut
- 1/2 cup spring water
- 1 tbsp brandy

Steps:

1. Combine Bach flower essences, spring water, and brandy in a dropper bottle.
2. Stir well to mix.

Usage Tips: Take 4 drops of this formula under the tongue as needed to balance emotions. Bach flower remedies are known for their gentle, supportive effects on emotional well-being.

141. SOOTHING SKULLCAP AND CATNIP TEA BLEND

Ingredients:

- 1 tsp dried skullcap
- 1 tsp dried catnip
- 1 cup boiling water
- 1 tbsp honey

Steps:

1. Combine dried skullcap and dried catnip in your teapot.
2. Pour boiling water into the teapot.
3. Let steep for 8-9 min.
4. Strain into a cup.
5. Stir in honey and serve.

Usage Tips: Drink this tea blend to reduce anxiety and promote relaxation. Skullcap and catnip have calming properties that help to soothe the nervous system.

142. ST. JOHN'S WORT MOOD STABILIZER TEA

Ingredients:

- 1 tsp dried St. John's wort
- 1 cup boiling water
- 1 tbsp honey

Steps:

1. Combine dried St. John's wort and boiling water in a cup.
2. Let steep for 8-9 min.
3. Strain the tea into another cup.
4. Stir in honey and serve.

Usage Tips: Drink this tea to support mood stability and reduce symptoms of depression. St. John's wort is known for its natural antidepressant properties.

143. STRESS RELIEF RHODIOLA AND SCHISANDRA BERRY ELIXIR

Ingredients:

- 1 tsp dried rhodiola root
- 1 tsp dried schisandra berries
- 1 cup boiling water
- 1 tbsp honey

Steps:

1. Transfer dried rhodiola root and dried schisandra berries in your teapot.
2. Pour boiling water into the teapot.
3. Let steep for 8-9 min.
4. Strain into a cup.
5. Stir in honey and serve.

Usage Tips: Enjoy this elixir to reduce stress and enhance resilience. Rhodiola and schisandra are adaptogens that help to balance stress hormones and support overall well-being.

Chapter 3: Holistic Practices and Wellness Culture

3.1 Caffeine-Free Herbal Energy Support

144. SIBERIAN GINSENG AND LICORICE ROOT TONIC

Ingredients:

- 1 tsp dried Siberian ginseng root
- 1 tsp dried licorice root
- 1 cup boiling water

Steps:

1. Combine dried Siberian ginseng root and licorice root in your teapot.
2. Pour boiling water into the teapot.
3. Let steep for 12-14 min.
4. Strain into a cup and serve.

Usage Tips: Drink this tonic in the morning for a natural energy boost. Siberian ginseng is important for its adaptogenic properties, that aid to combat fatigue and stress.

145. ASHWAGANDHA AND DATE SMOOTHIE

Ingredients:

- 1 banana
- 1 cup almond milk
- 1 tbsp ashwagandha powder
- 2 dates, pitted
- 1 tbsp almond butter

Steps:

1. Transfer all ingredients in a blender.
2. Mix until smooth.
3. Pour into a glass and serve immediately.

Usage Tips: Drink this smoothie in the morning for sustained energy. Ashwagandha helps to reduce stress and increase vitality, while dates provide natural sweetness and nutrients.

146. REVITALIZING GUARANA SEED BREW

Ingredients:

- 1 tsp ground guarana seeds
- 1 cup hot water
- 1 tbsp honey

Steps:

1. Combine ground guarana seeds and hot water in a cup.
2. Let steep for 5 minutes.
3. Strain into another cup.
4. Stir in honey and serve.

Usage Tips: Drink this brew in the morning for a natural energy boost. Guarana seeds contain natural caffeine that provides a steady release of energy without jitters.

147. CORDYCEPS MUSHROOM SPORTS DRINK

Ingredients:

- 1 tsp cordyceps mushroom powder
- 1 cup coconut water
- 1 tbsp honey
- 1/2 tsp sea salt

Steps:

1. Transfer all ingredients in a shaker bottle.
2. Stir well to mix.
3. Pour into a glass and serve.

Usage Tips: Use this drink before or after workouts to enhance athletic performance. Cordyceps mushrooms are known to boost energy and improve oxygen utilization.

148. ENERGY BOOSTING SCHISANDRA BERRY SYRUP

Ingredients:

- 1 cup dried schisandra berries
- 4 cups water
- 1 cup honey

Steps:

1 Combine dried schisandra berries and water in a pot.
2 Bring to a boil, then simmer for 45 min.
3 Strain the mixture and return the liquid to the pot.
4 Stir in honey and simmer until thickened.
5 Pour into a jar and preserve in the refrigerator.

Usage Tips: Take 1 tbsp of this syrup daily to boost your energy levels. Schisandra berries support adrenal health and improve stamina and endurance.

149. INVIGORATING PEPPERMINT AND LEMON BALM TEA

Ingredients:

- 1 tsp dried peppermint leaves
- 1 tsp dried lemon balm leaves
- 1 cup boiling water

Steps:

1 Transfer dried peppermint and lemon balm leaves in your teapot.
2 Pour boiling water into the teapot.
3 Let steep for 8-9 min.
4 Strain into a cup and serve.

Usage Tips: Enjoy this refreshing tea in the afternoon to combat fatigue. Peppermint and lemon balm both have uplifting and invigorating properties.

150. RHODIOLA ROSEA MORNING ELIXIR

Ingredients:

- 1 tsp dried Rhodiola rosea root
- 1 cup boiling water
- 1 tbsp honey
- 1 tsp lemon juice

Steps:

1 Combine dried Rhodiola rosea root and boiling water in a cup.
2 Let steep for 8-9 min.
3 Strain the tea into another cup.
4 Stir in honey and lemon juice, then serve.

Usage Tips: Start your day with this elixir to enhance mental clarity and energy. Rhodiola rosea is an adaptogen that helps the body resist physical and mental stress.

151. HERBAL MATE ENERGY DRINK

Ingredients:

- 1 tbsp dried yerba mate leaves
- 1 cup boiling water
- 1 tsp honey
- 1 slice lemon

Steps:

1 Transfer dried yerba mate leaves and boiling water in your teapot.
2 Let steep for 7-8 min.
3 Strain into a cup.
4 Stir in honey and add a slice of lemon before serving.

Usage Tips: Enjoy this drink in the morning or early afternoon for a smooth energy lift. Yerba mate is rich in antioxidants and provides a balanced energy boost without causing anxiety.

152. CAROB AND DANDELION ROOT COFFEE SUBSTITUTE

Ingredients:

- 1 tsp roasted dandelion root
- 1 tsp roasted carob powder
- 1 cup boiling water
- 1 tbsp coconut milk

Steps:

1 Combine roasted dandelion root and roasted carob powder in a cup.
2 Pour boiling water over the mixture.
3 Let steep for 7-8 min.
4 Strain into another cup.
5 Stir in coconut milk and serve.

Usage Tips: Use this blend as a caffeine-free coffee substitute. Dandelion root supports liver health, and carob provides a rich, chocolaty flavor that satisfies coffee cravings.

153. RED RASPBERRY LEAF AND NETTLE ICED TEA

Ingredients:

- 1 tbsp dried red raspberry leaf
- 1 tbsp dried nettle leaf
- 4 cups boiling water
- 1 tbsp honey
- Ice cubes

Steps:

1. Transfer dried red raspberry leaf and dried nettle leaf in your teapot.
2. Pour boiling water into the teapot.
3. Let steep for 8-9 min.
4. Strain the tea into a pitcher.
5. Stir in honey and let cool.
6. Serve over ice.

Usage Tips: Drink this iced tea on hot days for a refreshing and nourishing boost. Red raspberry leaf and nettle are packed with vitamins and minerals to support overall health.

154. ENERGIZING ELEUTHERO AND ORANGE JUICE

Ingredients:

- 1 tsp dried eleuthero root
- 1 cup boiling water
- 1 cup fresh orange juice
- 1 tbsp honey

Steps:

1. Combine dried eleuthero root and boiling water in your teapot.
2. Let steep for 8-9 min.
3. Strain the tea into a cup and let cool.
4. Mix the cooled tea with fresh orange juice and honey.
5. Stir well and serve.

Usage Tips: Start your day with this energizing drink. Eleuthero, also known as Siberian ginseng, is an adaptogen that enhances endurance and reduces fatigue, while orange juice adds a vitamin C boost.

3.2 Natural Tonics for Seasonal Transition

155. SPRING RENEWAL DANDELION AND BURDOCK TONIC

Ingredients:

- 1 tsp dried dandelion root
- 1 tsp dried burdock root
- 1 cup boiling water
- 1 tbsp honey

Steps:

1. Transfer dried dandelion root and dried burdock root in your teapot.
2. Pour boiling water into the teapot.
3. Let steep for 8-9 min.
4. Strain into a cup.
5. Stir in honey and serve.

Usage Tips: Drink this tonic during the spring to support detoxification and renewal. Dandelion and burdock roots help to cleanse the liver and improve digestion.

156. SUMMER COOLING CUCUMBER AND ALOE VERA DRINK

Ingredients:

- 1 cucumber, peeled and sliced
- 1 tbsp aloe vera gel
- 1 cup water
- 1 tbsp lemon juice
- Ice cubes

Steps:

1. Combine cucumber, aloe vera gel, water, and lemon juice in a blender.
2. Mix until smooth.
3. Pour into a glass over ice cubes and serve.

Usage Tips: Enjoy this drink on hot summer days to stay hydrated and cool. Cucumber and aloe vera are both incredibly hydrating and soothing, perfect for beating the heat.

157. WINTER WARMING GINGER AND CINNAMON HOT TONIC

Ingredients:

- 1 tsp grated fresh ginger
- 1 cinnamon stick
- 1 cup boiling water
- 1 tbsp honey

Steps:

1 Combine grated fresh ginger and cinnamon stick in a cup.
2 Pour boiling water over the ingredients.
3 Let steep for 8-9 min.
4 Strain into another cup.
5 Stir in honey and serve.

Usage Tips: Enjoy this warming tonic during winter to stay warm and healthy. Ginger and cinnamon have warming properties that help to improve circulation and boost immunity.

158. ALLERGY RELIEF NETTLE AND HONEY ELIXIR

Ingredients:

- 1 tsp dried nettle leaf
- 1 cup boiling water
- 1 tbsp honey
- 1 tsp lemon juice

Steps:

1 Transfer dried nettle leaf and boiling water in a cup.
2 Let steep for 8-9 min.
3 Strain the tea into another cup.
4 Stir in honey and lemon juice, then serve.

Usage Tips: Drink this elixir during allergy season to reduce symptoms. Nettle has natural antihistamine properties that help to alleviate allergy symptoms, and honey soothes the throat.

159. MOISTURIZING ROSEHIP AND HIBISCUS TEA FOR DRY WEATHER

Ingredients:

- 1 tsp dried rosehips
- 1 tsp dried hibiscus flowers
- 1 cup boiling water
- 1 tbsp honey

Steps:

1 Transfer dried rosehips and dried hibiscus flowers in your teapot.
2 Pour boiling water into the teapot.
3 Let steep for 8-9 min.
4 Strain into a cup.
5 Stir in honey and serve.

Usage Tips: Drink this tea during dry weather to keep your skin and body hydrated. Rosehips and hibiscus are rich in antioxidants and vitamin C, which help to moisturize and protect the skin.

160. REVITALIZING GREEN TEA AND JASMINE BLEND

Ingredients:

- 1 tsp green tea leaves
- 1 tsp dried jasmine flowers
- 1 cup boiling water

Steps:

1 Combine green tea leaves and dried jasmine flowers in your teapot.
2 Pour boiling water into the teapot.
3 Let steep for about 4 min.
4 Strain into a cup and serve.

Usage Tips: Enjoy this tea blend for a revitalizing and fragrant experience. Green tea provides a gentle caffeine boost, while jasmine flowers add a calming aroma.

161. AUTUMN IMMUNE BOOSTER ELDERBERRY AND ECHINACEA SYRUP

Ingredients:

- 1 cup dried elderberries
- 1 tbsp dried echinacea root
- 4 cups water
- 1 cup honey

Steps:

1 Combine dried elderberries, dried echinacea root, and water in a pot.
2 Bring to a boil, then simmer for 45 min.
3 Strain the mixture and return the liquid to the pot.
4 Stir in honey and simmer until thickened.
5 Pour into a jar and preserve in the refrigerator.

Usage Tips: Take 1 tbsp of this syrup daily during autumn to boost your immune system. Elderberries and echinacea are powerful immune boosters that help to prevent colds and flu.

162. SOOTHING LICORICE AND MARSHMALLOW ROOT TEA

Ingredients:

- 1 tsp dried licorice root
- 1 tsp dried marshmallow root
- 1 cup boiling water
- 1 tbsp honey

Steps:

1 Transfer dried licorice root and dried marshmallow root in your teapot.
2 Pour boiling water into the teapot.
3 Let steep for 8-9 min.
4 Strain into a cup.
5 Stir in honey and serve.

Usage Tips: Drink this tea to soothe a sore throat and digestive discomfort. Licorice and marshmallow roots have soothing properties that aid to diminish inflammation and irritation.

163. DETOXIFYING MILK THISTLE AND LEMON CLEANSE

Ingredients:

- 1 tsp dried milk thistle seeds
- 1 cup boiling water
- 1 tbsp lemon juice
- 1 tsp honey

Steps:

1 Transfer dried milk thistle seeds and boiling water in your teapot.
2 Let steep for 8-9 min.

3 Strain the tea into another cup.
4 Stir in lemon juice and honey, then serve.

Usage Tips: Use this cleanse periodically to detoxify your liver. Milk thistle is known for its liver-protective properties, and lemon helps to enhance detoxification.

164. CALMING CHAMOMILE AND LAVENDER SLEEP TONIC

Ingredients:

- 1 tsp dried chamomile flowers
- 1 tsp dried lavender flowers
- 1 cup boiling water
- 1 tbsp honey

Steps:

1 Transfer dried chamomile flowers and dried lavender flowers in your teapot.
2 Pour boiling water into the teapot.
3 Let steep for 8-9 min.
4 Strain into a cup.
5 Stir in honey and serve.

Usage Tips: Drink this tonic before bedtime to promote restful sleep. Chamomile and lavender have natural calming properties that help to relax the mind and body, ensuring a good night's rest.

165. ANTIOXIDANT RICH BILBERRY AND HAWTHORN DRINK

Ingredients:

- 1 tsp dried bilberries
- 1 tsp dried hawthorn berries
- 1 cup boiling water
- 1 tbsp honey

Steps:

1 Transfer dried bilberries and dried hawthorn berries in your teapot.
2 Pour boiling water into the teapot.
3 Let steep for 8-9 min.
4 Strain into a cup.
5 Stir in honey and serve.

Usage Tips: Enjoy this drink to boost your antioxidant intake. Bilberries and hawthorn berries are rich in antioxidants that support cardiovascular health and overall well-being.

166. JAPANESE MATCHA CEREMONY FOR MENTAL CLARITY

Ingredients:

- 1 tsp matcha powder
- 1/2 cup hot water

Steps:

1. Sift matcha powder into a bowl.
2. Add hot water and whisk until frothy.
3. Pour into a cup and enjoy.

Usage Tips: Perform this matcha ceremony in the morning to enhance mental clarity and focus. Matcha provides a gentle caffeine boost and is rich in antioxidants that support brain health.

167. AYURVEDIC TRIPHALA MORNING RINSE

Ingredients:

- 1 tsp triphala powder
- 1 cup warm water

Steps:

1. Combine triphala powder and warm water in a cup.
2. Stir well to dissolve the powder.
3. Drink the mixture first thing in the morning on an empty stomach.

Usage Tips: Use this rinse daily to support digestion and detoxification. Triphala is a traditional Ayurvedic blend of three fruits known for their cleansing and rejuvenating properties.

168. SOUTH AMERICAN YERBA MATE RITUAL FOR COMMUNITY AND STAMINA

Ingredients:

- 1 tbsp dried yerba mate leaves
- 1 cup hot water
- Lemon or mint (optional)

Steps:

1. Place dried yerba mate leaves in a gourd or cup.
2. Pour hot water over the leaves.
3. Let steep for a few minutes.
4. Add lemon or mint if desired.
5. Drink through a bombilla or metal straw.

Usage Tips: Use this yerba mate ritual to boost stamina and foster a sense of community. Yerba mate is a traditional South American drink that provides sustained energy and is often shared among friends.

169. NATIVE AMERICAN WHITE SAGE SMUDGING FOR CLEARING ENERGY

Ingredients:

- 1 bundle of dried white sage
- A fireproof bowl or shell

Steps:

1. Light the end of the white sage bundle until it begins to smolder.
2. Blow out the flame, allowing the sage to produce smoke.
3. Use your hand or a feather to direct the smoke around your space.

Usage Tips: Use white sage smudging to clear negative energy and purify your environment. This Native American practice helps to create a calm and balanced atmosphere.

170. MIDDLE EASTERN ZA'ATAR FOR DIGESTIVE HEALTH

Ingredients:

- 2 tbsp dried thyme
- 2 tbsp dried oregano
- 1 tbsp sumac
- 1 tbsp toasted sesame seeds
- 1/2 tsp salt

Steps:

1. Transfer all ingredients in a bowl.
2. Stir well to combine.
3. Preserve in an airtight container.

Usage Tips: Sprinkle za'atar on salads, bread, or yogurt for added flavor and digestive benefits. Thyme and oregano support digestion, while sumac adds a tangy, antioxidant-rich boost.

171. TRADITIONAL CHINESE MEDICINE JUJUBE AND GOJI BERRY TEA

Ingredients:

- 1 tbsp dried jujube dates
- 1 tbsp dried goji berries
- 2 cups boiling water

Steps:

1 Transfer dried jujube dates and dried goji berries in your teapot.
2 Pour boiling water into the teapot.
3 Let steep for 15-20 min.
4 Strain into cups and serve.

Usage Tips: Drink this tea to boost your energy and immune system. Jujube dates and goji berries are staples in Traditional Chinese Medicine for their nourishing and tonic effects.

172. AFRICAN BAOBAB FRUIT SMOOTHIE FOR ANTIOXIDANTS

Ingredients:

- 1 tbsp baobab powder
- 1 banana
- 1 cup almond milk
- 1 tbsp honey

Steps:

1 Transfer all ingredients in a blender.
2 Mix until smooth.
3 Pour into a glass and serve.

Usage Tips: Enjoy this smoothie for a powerful antioxidant boost. Baobab fruit is rich in vitamin C and other antioxidants that help to protect cells from damage and support overall health.

173. NORDIC BIRCH SAP TONIC FOR SPRING VITALITY

Ingredients:

- 1 cup fresh birch sap
- 1 tsp honey
- 1 tsp lemon juice

Steps:

1 Combine fresh birch sap, honey, and lemon juice in a glass.
2 Stir well to combine.
3 Serve chilled.

Usage Tips: Drink this tonic in the spring to rejuvenate and refresh your body. Birch sap is a traditional Nordic beverage that supports vitality and overall health.

174. MEDITERRANEAN OLIVE LEAF EXTRACT FOR HEART HEALTH

Ingredients:

- 1 cup dried olive leaves
- 2 cups water

Steps:

1 Combine dried olive leaves and water in a pot.
2 Bring to a boil, then simmer for about 25-28 min.
3 Strain the mixture and let the liquid cool.
4 Preserve in a glass bottle in the refrigerator.

Usage Tips: Take 1 tbsp of this extract daily to support heart health. Olive leaves contain compounds that help to lower blood pressure and improve cardiovascular function.

175. EUROPEAN HERBAL POULTICE FOR MUSCLE AND JOINT PAIN

Ingredients:

- 1 tbsp dried comfrey leaves
- 1 tbsp dried arnica flowers
- 1 cup hot water
- Cheesecloth or muslin

Steps:

1 Transfer dried comfrey leaves and dried arnica flowers in a bowl.
2 Pour hot water into the bowl and let steep for 8-9 min.
3 Strain the mixture and place the herbs in cheesecloth or muslin.
4 Apply the poultice to the affected area for 15-20 minutes.

Usage Tips: Use this herbal poultice to relieve muscle and joint pain. Comfrey and arnica have anti-inflammatory properties that aid to diminish swelling and promote healing.

176. INDIAN GOLDEN TURMERIC PASTE FOR INFLAMMATION

Ingredients:

- 1/3 cup ground turmeric
- 1/2 cup water
- 1/4 tsp black pepper
- 1 tbsp coconut oil

Steps:

1 Combine ground turmeric and water in a saucepan.
2 Simmer over low heat for 7-8-9 min until a thick paste forms.
3 Remove from heat and stir in black pepper and coconut oil.

4 Preserve in a glass jar in the refrigerator.

Usage Tips: Use this turmeric paste in smoothies, teas, or as a cooking ingredient to reduce inflammation. The combination of turmeric and black pepper enhances the absorption of curcumin.

3.4 Holistic Approaches to Longevity and Vitality

177. LONGEVITY ELIXIR WITH REISHI AND CHAGA MUSHROOMS

Ingredients:

- 1 tsp reishi mushroom powder
- 1 tsp chaga mushroom powder
- 1 cup hot water
- 1 tbsp honey

Steps:

1 Combine reishi mushroom powder and chaga mushroom powder in a cup.
2 Pour hot water over the powders.
3 Stir well and let steep for 7-8 min.
4 Stir in honey and serve.

Usage Tips: Drink this elixir daily to support longevity and overall health. Reishi and chaga mushrooms have adaptogenic and immune-boosting properties that promote vitality and resilience.

178. ANTI-AGING GINKGO BILOBA AND GOTU KOLA TEA

Ingredients:

- 1 tsp dried ginkgo biloba leaves
- 1 tsp dried gotu kola leaves
- 1 cup boiling water

Steps:

1 Transfer dried ginkgo biloba leaves and dried gotu kola leaves in your teapot.
2 Pour boiling water into the teapot.
3 Let steep for 8-9 min.
4 Strain into a cup and serve.

Usage Tips: Drink this tea to support brain health and cognitive function. Ginkgo biloba and gotu kola are known for their neuroprotective and anti-aging effects.

179. VITALITY-BOOSTING MACA AND COCOA SMOOTHIE

Ingredients:

- 1 banana
- 1 cup almond milk
- 1 tbsp maca powder
- 1 tbsp cocoa powder
- 1 tbsp honey

Steps:

1 Transfer all ingredients in a blender.
2 Mix until smooth.
3 Pour into a glass and serve.

Usage Tips: Enjoy this smoothie in the morning for a vitality boost. Maca and cocoa provide energy and stamina, while the banana and almond milk add creaminess and nutrients.

180. HERBAL ADAPTOGEN BLEND FOR STRESS RESISTANCE

Ingredients:

- 1 tsp ashwagandha powder
- 1 tsp rhodiola rosea powder
- 1 cup hot water
- 1 tbsp honey

Steps:

1 Combine ashwagandha powder and rhodiola rosea powder in a cup.
2 Pour hot water over the powders.
3 Stir well and let steep for 7-8 min.
4 Stir in honey and serve.

Usage Tips: Use this blend to enhance stress resistance and resilience. Ashwagandha and rhodiola are powerful adaptogens that help the body adapt to physical and mental stress.

181. SKIN REJUVENATING ALOE VERA AND CUCUMBER GEL

Ingredients:

- 1/3 cup fresh aloe vera gel
- 1/3 cup grated cucumber
- 1 tsp lemon juice

Steps:

1 Combine fresh aloe vera gel, grated cucumber, and lemon juice in a bowl.
2 Mix well to combine.
3 Apply the gel to your skin and let sit for 18-20 minutes.
4 Rinse off with cool water.

Usage Tips: Use this gel to rejuvenate and hydrate your skin. Aloe vera and cucumber provide soothing and moisturizing properties, while lemon juice helps to brighten the complexion.

182. SEA BUCKTHORN AND ROSEHIP ANTIOXIDANT JUICE

Ingredients:

- 1 tbsp sea buckthorn juice
- 1 tbsp rosehip syrup
- 1 cup water
- 1 tbsp honey

Steps:

1 Combine sea buckthorn juice, rosehip syrup, water, and honey in a glass.
2 Stir well to combine.
3 Serve immediately.

Usage Tips: Drink this juice daily for a potent dose of antioxidants. Sea buckthorn and rosehip are both rich in vitamins and antioxidants that protect against aging and support overall health.

183. HEART HEALTH HAWTHORN BERRY SYRUP

Ingredients:

- 1 cup dried hawthorn berries
- 4 cups water
- 1 cup honey

Steps:

1 Combine dried hawthorn berries and water in a pot.
2 Bring to a boil, then simmer for 45 min.
3 Strain the mixture and return the liquid to the pot.
4 Stir in honey and simmer until thickened.
5 Pour into a jar and preserve in the refrigerator.

Usage Tips: Take 1 tbsp of this syrup daily to support heart health. Hawthorn berries are known for their ability to strengthen the heart and improve circulation.

184. BRAIN-BOOSTING BACOPA AND SAGE TONIC

Ingredients:

- 1 tsp dried bacopa leaves
- 1 tsp dried sage leaves
- 1 cup boiling water
- 1 tbsp honey

Steps:

1 Transfer dried bacopa leaves and dried sage leaves in your teapot.
2 Pour boiling water into the teapot.
3 Let steep for 8-9 min.
4 Strain into a cup.
5 Stir in honey and serve.

Usage Tips: Drink this tonic to enhance cognitive function and memory. Bacopa and sage have been used traditionally to support brain health and improve mental clarity.

185. LIVER CLEANSING MILK THISTLE AND DANDELION DRINK

Ingredients:

- 1 tsp dried milk thistle seeds
- 1 tsp dried dandelion root
- 1 cup boiling water
- 1 tbsp lemon juice

Steps:

1 Combine dried milk thistle seeds and dried dandelion root in your teapot.
2 Pour boiling water into the teapot.
3 Let steep for 8-9 min.
4 Strain the tea into another cup.
5 Stir in lemon juice and serve.

Usage Tips: Use this drink periodically to cleanse and support your liver. Milk thistle and dandelion are known for their detoxifying and liver-protective properties.

186. BONE STRENGTHENING HORSETAIL AND NETTLE DECOCTION

Ingredients:

- 1 tsp dried horsetail
- 1 tsp dried nettle
- 2 cups water

Steps:

1 Combine dried horsetail and dried nettle in a pot.
2 Add water and bring to a boil.
3 Simmer for about 18 min.
4 Strain into cups and serve.

Usage Tips: Drink this decoction to support bone health. Horsetail and nettle are rich in minerals like silica and calcium, which are essential for strong bones.

187. ANTI-INFLAMMATORY TURMERIC AND CHERRY JUICE

Ingredients:

- 1 tsp ground turmeric
- 1 cup tart cherry juice
- 1 tbsp honey

Steps:

1 Combine ground turmeric and tart cherry juice in a glass.
2 Stir well to combine.
3 Stir in honey and serve.

Usage Tips: Enjoy this juice to reduce inflammation and support joint health. Turmeric and tart cherries are both powerful anti-inflammatory agents that help to relieve pain and swelling.

188. IMMUNE-BOOSTING GARLIC AND HONEY TINCTURE

Ingredients:

- 1/2 cup peeled garlic cloves
- 1 cup honey
- 1 cup apple cider vinegar

Steps:

1 Combine peeled garlic cloves, honey, and apple cider vinegar in a jar.
2 Seal the jar and let sit for 10 days, shaking daily.
3 Strain the mixture and store the liquid in a glass bottle.

Usage Tips: Take 1 tsp of this tincture daily to boost your immune system. Garlic and honey have potent antimicrobial properties that help to prevent infections.

189. NATURAL HERBAL MOUTHWASH WITH THYME AND MINT

Ingredients:

- 1 tsp dried thyme
- 1 tsp dried mint leaves
- 1 cup boiling water
- 1 tsp baking soda

Steps:

1 Transfer dried thyme and dried mint leaves in your teapot.
2 Pour boiling water into the teapot.
3 Let steep for 8-9 min.
4 Strain into a cup.
5 Stir in baking soda and let cool.
6 Store in a glass bottle.

Usage Tips: Use this mouthwash daily to maintain oral health. Thyme and mint have antibacterial properties that help to freshen breath and reduce plaque.

190. DIGESTIVE AID FENNEL AND PEPPERMINT LOZENGES

Ingredients:

- 1/2 cup honey
- 1/3 cup fennel seed tea
- 1 tbsp dried peppermint leaves

Steps:

1 Combine honey, fennel seed tea, and dried peppermint leaves in a saucepan.
2 Heat over low heat until the mixture reaches 300°F (150°C) on a candy thermometer.
3 Pour the mixture into a candy mold and let cool completely.
4 Remove the lozenges from the mold and store in an airtight container.

Usage Tips: Suck on these lozenges after meals to aid digestion. Fennel and peppermint help to reduce bloating and gas, making them effective digestive aids.

191. DAILY DETOXIFYING HERBAL TEA BLEND

Ingredients:

- 1 tsp dried dandelion root
- 1 tsp dried burdock root
- 1 tsp dried milk thistle seeds
- 1 cup boiling water

Steps:

1 Combine dried dandelion root, dried burdock root, and dried milk thistle seeds in your teapot.
2 Pour boiling water into the teapot.
3 Let steep for 8-9 min.
4 Strain into a cup and serve.

Usage Tips: Drink this tea daily to support detoxification and liver health. Dandelion, burdock, and milk thistle are powerful detoxifying herbs that help to cleanse the body.

192. RELAXATION SUPPORT LAVENDER INFUSED BATH SALTS

Ingredients:

- 1 cup Epsom salts
- 1/2 cup sea salt
- 1/3 cup dried lavender flowers
- 12 drops lavender essential oil

Steps:

1 Combine Epsom salts, sea salt, and dried lavender flowers in a bowl.
2 Add lavender essential oil and mix well.
3 Store in an airtight container.

Usage Tips: Add 1/2 cup of these bath salts to your bathwater to promote relaxation. Lavender has soothing properties that help to calm the mind and relax the muscles.

193. ENERGIZING MORNING HERBAL TONIC

Ingredients:

- 1 tsp dried ginseng root
- 1 tsp dried licorice root
- 1 cup boiling water
- 1 tbsp honey

Steps:

1 Transfer dried ginseng root and dried licorice root in your teapot.
2 Pour boiling water into the teapot.
3 Let steep for 8-9 min.
4 Strain into a cup.
5 Stir in honey and serve.

Usage Tips: Drink this tonic in the morning to boost your energy levels. Ginseng and licorice root are adaptogens that help to increase stamina and reduce fatigue.

194. SLEEP INDUCING VALERIAN ROOT NIGHTCAP

Ingredients:

- 1 tsp dried valerian root
- 1 cup boiling water
- 1 tbsp honey

Steps:

1 Transfer dried valerian root and boiling water in a cup.
2 Let steep for 8-9 min.
3 Strain the tea into another cup.
4 Stir in honey and serve.

Usage Tips: Drink this nightcap before bed to promote restful sleep. Valerian root is a natural sedative that helps to calm the mind and body, ensuring a good night's rest.

195. HERBAL COLD AND FLU PREVENTION INHALER

Ingredients:

- 12 drops eucalyptus essential oil
- 12 drops peppermint essential oil
- 12 drops tea tree essential oil
- 1 inhaler tube

Steps:

1 Combine eucalyptus, peppermint, and tea tree essential oils in a small bowl.
2 Soak the inhaler wick in the oil blend.
3 Insert the wick into the inhaler tube and seal.

Usage Tips: Use this inhaler at the first sign of a cold or flu to prevent symptoms. The essential oils have antimicrobial properties that help to clear nasal passages and boost immunity.

196. HERBAL FIRST AID SPRAY FOR CUTS AND SCRAPES

Ingredients:

- 1 cup witch hazel
- 1 tsp dried calendula flowers
- 1 tsp dried chamomile flowers
- 12 drops tea tree essential oil

Steps:

1 Combine witch hazel, dried calendula flowers, and dried chamomile flowers in a jar.
2 Seal the jar and let sit for about 10 days, shaking daily.
3 Strain the mixture and add tea tree essential oil.
4 Pour into a spray bottle.

Usage Tips: Spray this mixture on cuts and scrapes to promote healing. Calendula, chamomile, and tea tree oil have antiseptic and anti-inflammatory properties that aid to prevent infection and diminish inflammation.

197. NATURAL ANXIETY RELIEF LEMON BALM TEA

Ingredients:

- 1 tsp dried lemon balm leaves
- 1 cup boiling water
- 1 tbsp honey

Steps:

1 Transfer dried lemon balm leaves and boiling water in a cup.
2 Let steep for 8-9 min.
3 Strain the tea into another cup.
4 Stir in honey and serve.

Usage Tips: Drink this tea to reduce anxiety and promote relaxation. Lemon balm has calming properties that help to soothe the mind and body, making it effective for anxiety relief.

198. HOMEGROWN HERBAL SALAD MIX

Ingredients:

- 1 cup mixed greens (lettuce, spinach, arugula)
- 1/3 cup fresh herbs (basil, parsley, cilantro)
- 1/3 cup edible flowers (nasturtiums, violets)
- 1 tbsp olive oil
- 1 tbsp lemon juice
- Salt and pepper to taste

Steps:

1 Combine mixed greens, fresh herbs, and edible flowers in a bowl.
2 Drizzle with olive oil and lemon juice.
3 Mix well.
4 Season with salt and pepper.

Usage Tips: Enjoy this salad for a fresh and nutritious meal. Growing your own herbs and edible flowers ensures a constant supply of fresh, nutrient-rich ingredients for your salads.

3.6 Ancient Remedies for Modern Anxiety

199. ASHWAGANDHA ROOT STRESS REDUCTION TINCTURE

Ingredients:

- 1/2 cup dried ashwagandha root
- 1 cup vodka or brandy

Steps:

1 Combine dried ashwagandha root and vodka or brandy in a jar.
2 Seal the jar and let sit for about 1 month, shaking daily.
3 Strain the mixture and store the liquid in a glass bottle.

Usage Tips: Take 1 tsp of this tincture daily to reduce stress. Ashwagandha is an adaptogen that helps to balance cortisol levels and promote relaxation.

200. ANXIETY-SOOTHING VALERIAN AND CHAMOMILE CAPSULES

Ingredients:

- 1/2 cup dried valerian root
- 1/2 cup dried chamomile flowers
- Empty gelatin capsules

Steps:

1 Grind dried valerian root and dried chamomile flowers into a fine powder.
2 Fill empty gelatin capsules with the powder.
3 Store the capsules in an airtight container.

Usage Tips: Take 1-2 capsules before bedtime to reduce anxiety and promote sleep. Valerian and chamomile have calming properties that help to relax the mind and body.

201. ADAPTOGENIC HOLY BASIL AND LICORICE TEA

Ingredients:

- 1 tsp dried holy basil leaves
- 1 tsp dried licorice root
- 1 cup boiling water

Steps:

1 Transfer dried holy basil leaves and dried licorice root in your teapot.
2 Pour boiling water into the teapot.
3 Let steep for 8-9 min.
4 Strain into a cup and serve.

Usage Tips: Enjoy this tea to reduce stress and support adrenal health. Holy basil and licorice root are adaptogens that help to balance stress hormones and improve resilience.

202. GROUNDING CEDARWOOD AROMATHERAPY OIL

Ingredients:

- 12 drops cedarwood essential oil
- 1 tbsp carrier oil (such as jojoba or almond oil)

Steps:

1 Transfer cedarwood essential oil and jojoba or almond oil in a small bottle.
2 Stir well to mix.

Usage Tips: Apply some drops of this oil to your wrists or neck to promote grounding and relaxation. Cedarwood has a calming and centering effect that helps to reduce anxiety.

203. ST. JOHN'S WORT MOOD STABILIZER TEA

Ingredients:

- 1 tsp dried St. John's wort
- 1 cup boiling water
- 1 tbsp honey

Steps:

1 Combine dried St. John's wort and boiling water in a cup.
2 Let steep for 8-9 min.

3 Strain the tea into another cup.
4 Stir in honey and serve.

Usage Tips: Drink this tea to support mood stability and reduce symptoms of depression. St. John's wort is known for its natural antidepressant properties.

204. LEMON BALM AND LAVENDER ANTI-ANXIETY SPRAY

Ingredients:

- 12 drops lemon balm essential oil
- 12 drops lavender essential oil
- 1/2 cup distilled water
- 1 tbsp witch hazel

Steps:

1 Combine lemon balm essential oil, lavender essential oil, distilled water, and witch hazel in a spray bottle.
2 Stir well to mix.

Usage Tips: Spray this blend around your home or on your pillow to reduce anxiety. Lemon balm and lavender have calming effects that help to create a relaxing environment.

205. CALMING PASSIONFLOWER AND HOPS SLEEP AID

Ingredients:

- 1 tsp dried passionflower
- 1 tsp dried hops
- 1 cup boiling water
- 1 tbsp honey

Steps:

1 Transfer dried passionflower and dried hops in your teapot.
2 Pour boiling water into the teapot.
3 Let steep for 8-9 min.
4 Strain into a cup.
5 Stir in honey and serve.

Usage Tips: Drink this sleep aid before bedtime to promote restful sleep. Passionflower and hops have natural sedative properties that help to calm the mind and induce sleep.

206. SOOTHING SKULLCAP AND CATNIP TEA BLEND

Ingredients:

- 1 tsp dried skullcap
- 1 tsp dried catnip
- 1 cup boiling water
- 1 tbsp honey

Steps:

1. Combine dried skullcap and dried catnip in your teapot.
2. Pour boiling water into the teapot.
3. Let steep for 8-9 min.
4. Strain into a cup.
5. Stir in honey and serve.

Usage Tips: Drink this tea blend to reduce anxiety and promote relaxation. Skullcap and catnip have calming properties that help to soothe the nervous system.

207. STRESS RELIEF RHODIOLA AND SCHISANDRA BERRY ELIXIR

Ingredients:

- 1 tsp dried rhodiola root
- 1 tsp dried schisandra berries
- 1 cup boiling water
- 1 tbsp honey

Steps:

1. Transfer dried rhodiola root and dried schisandra berries in your teapot.
2. Pour boiling water into the teapot.
3. Let steep for 8-9 min.
4. Strain into a cup.
5. Stir in honey and serve.

Usage Tips: Enjoy this elixir to reduce stress and enhance resilience. Rhodiola and schisandra are adaptogens that help to balance stress hormones and support overall well-being.

208. EMOTIONAL BALANCE FLOWER ESSENCE FORMULA

Ingredients:

- 2 drops Bach Rescue Remedy
- 2 drops Bach Olive
- 2 drops Bach White Chestnut
- 1/2 cup spring water
- 1 tbsp brandy

Steps:

1. Combine Bach flower essences, spring water, and brandy in a dropper bottle.
2. Stir well to mix.

Usage Tips: Take 4 drops of this formula under the tongue as needed to balance emotions. Bach flower remedies are known for their gentle, supportive effects on emotional well-being.

209. PROTECTIVE AMETHYST AND SAGE ENERGY CLEARING MIST

Ingredients:

- 1 small amethyst crystal
- 12 drops sage essential oil
- 1/2 cup distilled water
- 1 tbsp witch hazel

Steps:

1. Place the amethyst crystal in a spray bottle.
2. Add sage essential oil, distilled water, and witch hazel.
3. Stir well to mix.

Usage Tips: Spray this mist around your space to clear negative energy and promote protection. Amethyst and sage work together to create a balanced and positive environment.

Chapter 3: Integrating Herbal Practices into Daily Life

3.1 The Holistic Approach to Wellness

Viewing wellness through a holistic lens is essential for achieving a balanced and harmonious life. This approach emphasizes the integration of mind, body, and spirit, recognizing that these aspects are interconnected and influence each other. Herbs play a vital role in this integrative perspective, offering a natural and effective means to support overall well-being. By addressing physical health, mental clarity, and emotional stability, herbs can help create a foundation for lasting wellness.

The mind-body connection is pivotal in holistic health. When the mind is stressed or anxious, the body often manifests these feelings through physical symptoms such as tension, headaches, or digestive issues. Conversely, physical ailments can impact mental and emotional health. Herbs like chamomile, lavender, and ashwagandha are renowned for their ability to soothe both the mind and body. Chamomile, for instance, is known for its calming effects on the nervous system, making it an excellent choice for reducing anxiety and promoting restful sleep. Lavender, with its soothing aroma, can alleviate stress and tension, while ashwagandha helps balance the body's stress response, supporting both mental clarity and physical resilience.

Incorporating herbs into daily rituals can further enhance this mind-body connection and foster overall well-being. Simple practices such as starting the day with a cup of herbal tea can set a positive tone. Teas made from herbs like lemon balm, peppermint, or holy basil can provide a gentle energy boost while calming the mind. Evening rituals, such as taking a warm herbal bath infused with rose petals or eucalyptus, can promote relaxation and prepare the body for restful sleep. Creating a calming bedtime routine with herbal sachets under the pillow or using lavender essential oil in a diffuser can also improve sleep quality.

Moreover, using herbs in mindfulness practices can deepen the sense of inner peace and clarity. For example, drinking a cup of green tea before meditation can enhance focus, while burning sage or palo santo can cleanse the space and set a tranquil atmosphere. Incorporating these simple herbal practices into daily life helps cultivate a consistent state of balance and well-being.

Embracing a holistic approach to wellness by integrating herbs into daily routines supports the interconnectedness of mind, body, and spirit. This holistic perspective not only addresses individual health issues but also fosters a sense of overall harmony and resilience, paving the way for a healthier, more balanced life.

3.2 Embracing Spiritual Herbal Practices

Herbal practices can significantly enhance spiritual growth and self-awareness by connecting us to the natural world and our inner selves. Embracing the spiritual dimensions of herbalism involves recognizing the subtle energies of plants and how they can support our spiritual journey. Herbs have long been used in various cultures to deepen spiritual practices, promote inner peace, and foster a sense of connection to the divine.

Incorporating herbs into mindfulness and meditation practices can greatly aid in achieving focus and clarity. Certain herbs, such as holy basil, frankincense, and gotu kola, are known for their ability to calm the mind and enhance concentration. Holy basil, revered in Ayurvedic tradition, helps balance the mind and reduce stress, making it an excellent companion for meditation. Frankincense, often used in religious ceremonies, has a grounding and centering effect, helping to create a serene environment for meditation. Gotu kola is another herb that supports mental clarity and enhances cognitive function, making it ideal for deepening mindfulness practices.

Creating sacred spaces at home using herbs can further enrich spiritual practices. A sacred space is a dedicated area where one can meditate, relax, and reflect, free from the distractions of daily life. Herbs can play a crucial role in establishing these spaces. Smudging with sage or palo santo, for example, is a traditional practice that involves burning these herbs to cleanse and purify the environment, removing negative energies and fostering a sense of peace. Adding potted herbs like rosemary or lavender can also enhance the atmosphere, as their presence and aroma promote tranquility and spiritual awareness.

Additionally, making use of herbal incense, candles, and essential oils can transform a regular space into a sacred sanctuary. Incense made from herbs such as sandalwood, myrrh, and cedar can elevate the spiritual ambiance, while herbal candles infused with essential oils can create a soothing light and scent. Essential oils like lavender, jasmine, and patchouli can be diffused to enhance the meditative experience, promoting relaxation and deeper introspection.

Incorporating these spiritual herbal practices into daily life fosters a deeper connection with the self and the natural world. By integrating herbs into mindfulness, meditation, and the creation of sacred spaces, we can cultivate an environment that supports spiritual growth, self-awareness, and inner peace. This holistic approach to spirituality not only enhances our daily practices but also helps us navigate life's challenges with greater clarity and resilience. Embracing the spiritual dimensions of herbalism can lead to profound personal transformation and a more harmonious existence.

3.3 Long-Term Benefits and Lifestyle Integration

Embracing herbal practices is not just about achieving immediate benefits but also about fostering sustainable habits that contribute to long-term health and environmental stewardship. Sustainable herbal practices ensure that we use resources wisely and protect the natural environments that provide us with these valuable plants. By cultivating our own herbs, practicing wildcrafting with respect, and supporting organic and sustainable agriculture, we can make a positive impact on the planet while enhancing our own well-being. This approach not only preserves the environment for future generations but also ensures the purity and potency of the herbs we use.

Lifelong learning is a crucial aspect of integrating herbal practices into our lives. The world of herbalism is vast and continually evolving, offering endless opportunities for exploration and discovery. Encouraging readers to continue their education in herbal medicine can lead to a deeper understanding and appreciation of the diverse properties and applications of herbs. This can be achieved through various means such as attending workshops, reading books, participating in online courses, and engaging with herbal communities. Expanding one's herbal knowledge not only empowers individuals to make informed choices for their health but also fosters a sense of connection to the rich traditions and wisdom of herbal medicine.

Personal transformation is a profound benefit of consistent herbal practice. Over time, integrating herbs into daily routines can foster resilience, balance, and harmony in one's life. The gentle, supportive nature of herbs helps to nurture the body, mind, and spirit, promoting overall well-being. For example, regularly using adaptogenic herbs like ashwagandha and rhodiola can enhance the body's ability to cope with stress, leading to greater emotional and physical resilience. Similarly, incorporating calming herbs such as lavender and chamomile into daily rituals can help maintain emotional balance and inner peace.

Furthermore, the mindful practice of using herbs encourages a deeper connection to oneself and the natural world. This connection can lead to a greater sense of harmony and fulfillment, as individuals become more attuned to their body's needs and the rhythms of nature. The transformative power of herbal practices lies in their ability to support holistic health, fostering a state of equilibrium that permeates all aspects of life. By committing to these practices, individuals can experience profound shifts in their health and well-being, leading to a more balanced and harmonious existence.

In conclusion, the long-term benefits of integrating herbal practices into daily life are vast and multifaceted. Sustainable herbal practices promote environmental stewardship, lifelong learning enriches knowledge and appreciation of herbal medicine, and consistent use of herbs fosters personal transformation. By embracing these practices, individuals can achieve lasting health and well-being, cultivating resilience, balance, and harmony in their lives.

Your Voice Matters!

Dear reader,

*You have completed **"The Ultimate Collection of Barbara O'Neill: 550+ Revolutionary Herbal and Natural Remedies for Everyday Ailments, Life-Changing Holistic Health and Wellness"**.*

I hope you found inspiration and useful advice.

I want to be honest: your reviews are crucial. Believe it or not, a positive review can help me expand my audience and enable more and more people to discover the benefits of these practices.

Leaving feedback is simple, and I treasure each piece of insight. Just go to the ORDERS section of your Amazon account and click on the "Write a product review" button, or SCAN THIS QR CODE to go directly to the review section.

If you enjoyed this book, I ask you to take a moment to leave a review on Amazon. It doesn't have to be long, just sincere.

Your opinion can help to improve the lives of other readers.

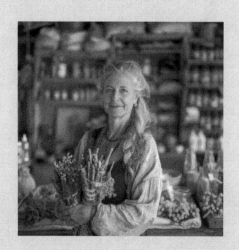

Thank you so much for your time and sincerity.

__Serena Moss__

Conclusion

Incorporating herbal remedies into daily routines can significantly enhance mental wellness and manage stress. Herbs such as lavender, chamomile, and ashwagandha are excellent for promoting relaxation and reducing anxiety. Regular use of these herbs can help manage daily stress and support a serene mind. Herbal infusions and teas can be integrated into your daily routine to help manage stress naturally. Techniques such as mindfulness meditation, supported by calming herbs, can provide a balanced approach to handling life's challenges.

Herbs like calendula, aloe vera, and rosemary play a vital role in maintaining radiant skin and healthy hair. These natural remedies are beneficial for all ages, offering solutions for hydration, anti-aging, and overall skin health. Gentle and safe herbs such as chamomile, fennel, and lemon balm are excellent choices for children. These herbs can help with common issues like digestion, sleep, and calming effects, ensuring holistic wellness for the younger members of the family.

Herbal infusions for vitality, natural baths, and essential oil massages are wonderful ways to incorporate the benefits of herbs into body care routines. These practices not only enhance physical well-being but also provide emotional and mental relaxation. Creating a natural first aid kit, making salves and balms, and practicing therapeutic gardening are excellent ways to incorporate herbs into your home. These practices promote a healthy living environment and support overall well-being.

The integration of herbs into your diet can provide numerous health benefits. From using spices for wellness to creating healing gardens, the nutritional use of herbs is essential for holistic health. Herbs support various holistic practices that contribute to long-term health and vitality. Integrating naturopathy into everyday life and using ancient remedies for modern issues can lead to a more balanced and harmonious lifestyle.

Herbal remedies for seasonal wellness, relaxing moments with herbal teas, and the benefits of herbal poultices are simple yet effective ways to maintain health and well-being. Embracing these natural methods ensures a holistic approach to personal care. Sustainable practices in herbalism, including eco-friendly preparations and herbal cultivation, are crucial for long-term health and environmental stewardship. Innovations in herbal preparation and sustainable use of resources highlight the importance of integrating these practices into daily life.

Final Thoughts

Embracing the holistic approach to wellness through herbal practices can lead to significant personal transformation. By continuing to learn about and integrate herbs into daily routines, individuals can achieve greater resilience, balance, and harmony in their lives. The journey of herbalism is ongoing, offering endless opportunities for growth and well-being.